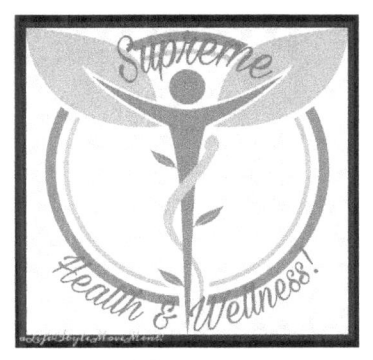

I0481896

Understanding Our Immune System!

*How To Create Health, Wellness & Abundant Life!

Supreme Health
Staff & Scientist

Kareem Tyree
Khalil Malik

Gabriella Monique
Sean Ali

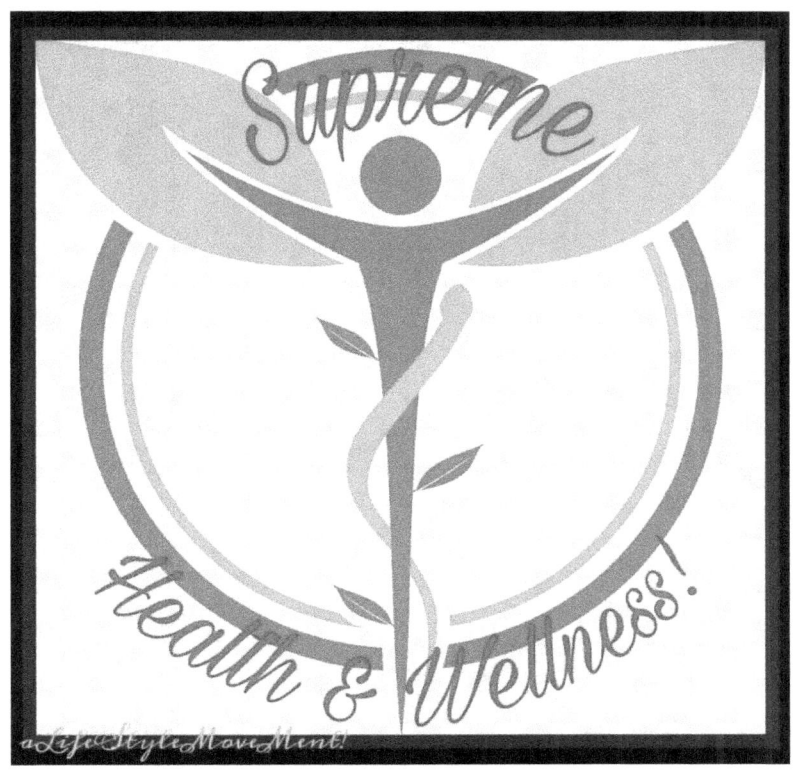

Supreme Health & Fitness by Sean Ali!

Achieving and Maintaining Supreme Health and Fitness by increasing the level of

Knowledge and Science of Life!

PAGE 2

Supreme Health & Fitness!   Health & Wellness Series Vol. 1

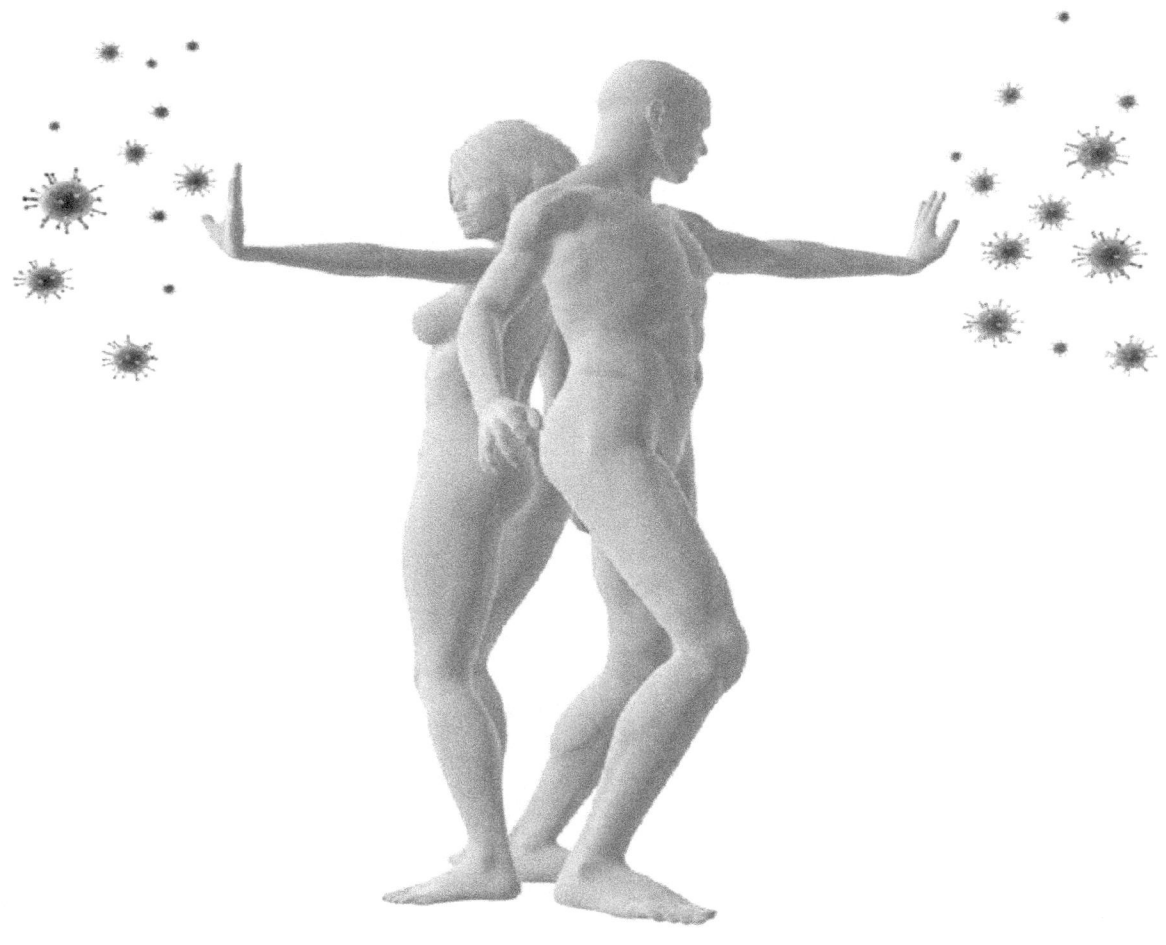

Table of Contents

*****

Supreme Health & Fitness!   Health & Wellness Series Vol. 1

PAGE 6

IMMUNE SYSTEM

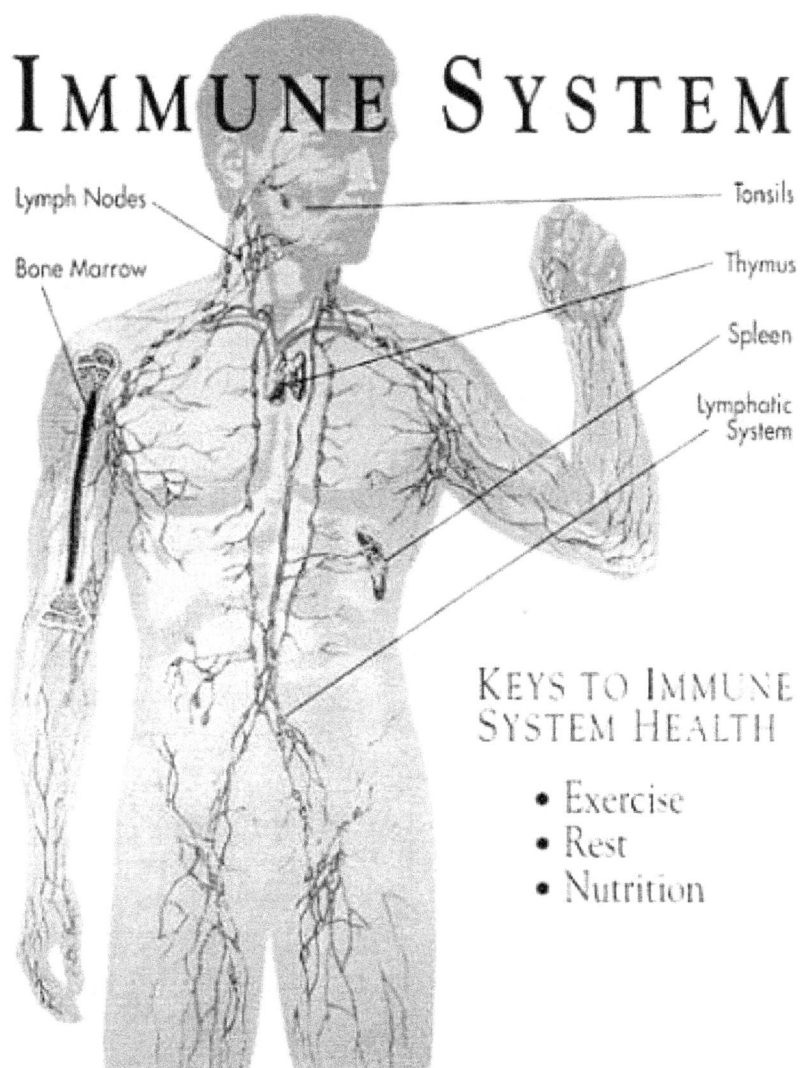

Lymph Nodes

Bone Marrow

Tonsils

Thymus

Spleen

Lymphatic System

KEYS TO IMMUNE SYSTEM HEALTH

- Exercise
- Rest
- Nutrition

*****

Introduction

*****

Peace and Blessings of Life!

In the Creator's Name I Greet You with Peace and Pray that this Humble Offering can Help Us to BE that which HE Created Us to BE and fulfill the Divine Promise of Life Abundant!

This small work represents Volume One of my Health and Wellness Series. In this Volume we focus on our Gift from The CREATOR = Our Immune System. We have an Awesome Immune System that is designed to eliminate Any and All pathogens, dis-eases, bacteria and viruses that can interfere with our bodies ability to achieve and maintain Balance or Homeostasis.

Most of us don't really think about our immune systems, except just before when winter begins to sets-in and a lot of health practitioners in the news, on the radio, in social media and on television are talking about the upcoming flu season and what we should do, e.g. get a flu shot or not.

Unfortunately, most of us will also run out and pick up a bunch of herbs, vitamins, teas and other concoctions, hoping to avoid catching a cold or the flu this year.

PAGE 10

Supreme Health & Fitness!   Health & Wellness Series Volume 1

Our immune system is one of the 10 major systems in the human body. It protects us from ALL invading microbes and pathogens such as bacteria, fungi, viruses, parasites, etc. In addition, the immune system plays another major role that most people (including most doctors) don't really know that much about -- have any idea what it is?

We know that our immune system is important regardless of our current specific health problem, it also plays an even bigger role in protecting you by helping to heal damaged cells and tissues.

Your immune system plays a major role in helping to protect you from cancer and helping to repair and heal your body if you happen to have cancer. This is especially important since the conventional medical treatment for cancer patients is to poison them with chemotherapy and/or radiation, which severely weakens the immune system and the patient – which ultimately causes their death.

Your immune system protects your body against disease by identifying and killing pathogens and tumor cells. It is created to detect any and all agents, from viruses to parasitic worms, and needs to distinguish them from your own healthy cells and tissues in order to function properly. Detection is complicated as pathogens can evolve rapidly and adapt to avoid the immune system but we cause the most damage by compromising our own immunity through Poor dietary habits and detrimental thoughts and lifestyle activities.

Our physical bodies are Perfectly Crafted Vehicles, designed to keep Us right Here and in Motion through Time. There is no set time limit or table for the expiration of our physical body. It is all dependent on our commitment to Eat 2 Live!

Supreme Health & Fitness! Health & Wellness Series Volume 1

PAGE 11

Our Bodies are Created to work to achieve and Maintain Homeostasis – Balance – LIFE. When our bodies cannot achieve Homeostasis this is what is scientifically referred to as a state of Dis-ease or Sickness.

Our bodies number 1 function is to achieve and maintain Homeostasis or Balance so that we can LIVE A LONG YOUTHFUL LIFE!!

Everything from a Fever to Sweating to Inflammation or Swelling is our bodies Natural attempts to Resolve an Imbalance issue (dis-ease/sickness) and to once again Be BALANCED!

Death is a permanent State of Imbalance … meaning the Body can longer Achieve and Maintain Homeostasis!

Everything in our physical body is food Based and Dependent … Meaning that You Are What You Eat … And that what you Eat will have a transforming effect on our bodies. This Transforming Effect takes place whether it's in a Positive or Negative direction … Or towards Life or Death.

Our Immune System is the part of our Physical that is designed to AUTOMATICALLY produce the necessary Agent to combat ANY and ALL invaders that can enter us. There are several levels/layers tour Immune System that can be utilized to eradicate everything from the Common Cold to the deadlier invaders of HIV and Cancer.

*Then WHY are we still getting Sick?

*And WHY are We Still Dying from all these different dis-eases and sicknesses?

PAGE 12

Supreme Health & Fitness!   Health & Wellness Series Volume 1

These 2 questions represent the constant theme as we examine the function and role of each Immunity level. As we see the Awesome Power of the Immune System, from the individual elements to the entire system, it will be Very CLEAR that our Immune System is Truly a GIFT ... and that it's all based on What We Do With It ... and NOT Anyone else.

In this Volume, we will look at our many levels or layers of Immunity and their respective anatomical structure and functions.

As we learn of their specific roles in keeping us Healthy, Well and Alive, a common theme of Proper Nutrition will continuously display that is vital to their success of Immune protection.

Our Immune System is intricately related to our Digestive System. Everything we consume is either Decreasing our Increasing our Natural Immune Defense. From our Skin, to Mucus and from Phagocytes to White Blood Cells, all of our Natural defenses and their ability to function, as well as our bodies ability to produce them are Food Related!

Blotchy, itchy and excessively oily or dry skin can easily be resolved with proper Hydration and/or specific dietary changes. Skin is also our 1st Line of Defense. Blotchy, itchy and excessively oily or dry Skin has a significantly Decreased Ability to protect and repel pathogens and bacteria.

Mucous Membrane covers all the openings of our body that our Skin doesn't – Mouth, Eyes, inside Nose, etc. this Mucous Membrane functions in a similar fashion to our Skin and is scientifically recognized as our 2nd Line of defense. Mucus is secreted as a protective fluid to keeps pathogens and bacteria out and simultaneously expelling any that may already be inside.

PAGE 13

Supreme Health & Fitness!   Health & Wellness Series Volume 1

A condition of Dehydration or Nutritional Deficiency severely hampers and decreases the Strength and Condition of the Mucous Membrane as well as the ability to secrete Mucus.

These are our first 2 Lines of Immune Defense and we can see how what we eat can and does effect their respective Protective abilities and get a glimpse at how EASILY pathogens and bacteria can ENTER our bodies and manifest as dis-eases.

Eating 2 LIVE is a vital Life Function!!

Every food choice we make and every food item we place in our mouths will Decrease or Increase that ability to Maintain Balance and this will in-turn be the catalyst of Dis-ease, Sickness and Pre-Mature Death ... OR ... Health, Wellness and Abundant LIFE!!!!!!

Our Immune System is our Gift of Eternal Life from The CREATOR!

Open this book and learn how Awesome your Healing Power is! Understanding Our Immune System gives us the ability to improve our Health and Increase our Life-Span into the Successful Enjoyment of Your Abundant Life!

Achieving and Maintaining Supreme Health and Wellness by increasing the level of Knowledge and Science of LIFE!

Peace and Blessings Of Life!

Your Brother Sean Ali

PAGE 14

Supreme Health & Fitness!　　　　Health & Wellness Series Volume 1

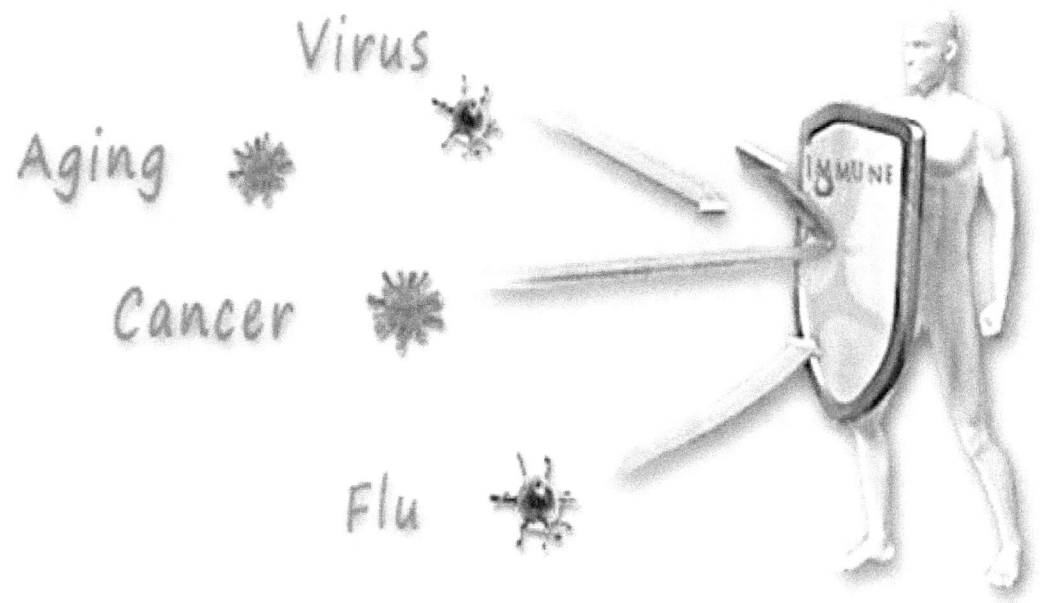

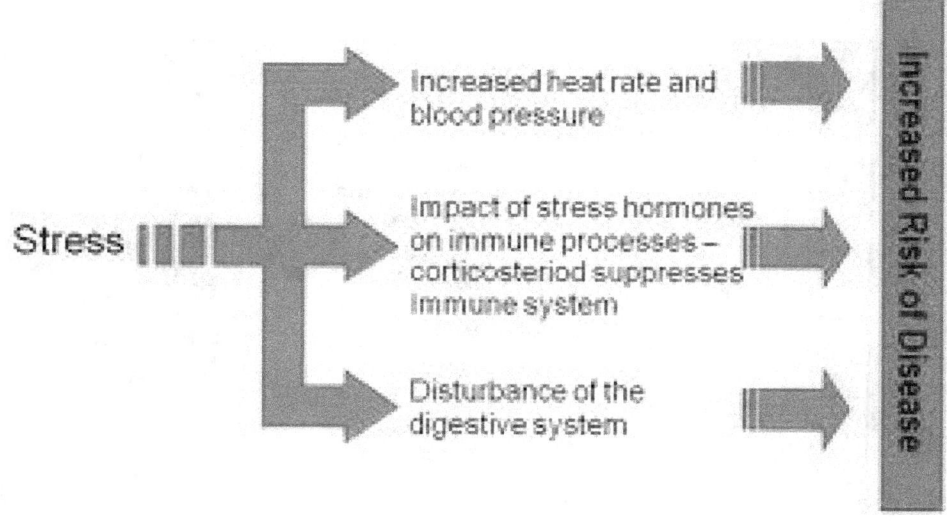

*****

Chapter 1 ... Understanding Dis-Ease, Stress & Stressors

*****

Dis-Ease can be looked at as a dis-connection in the Communication of our Cells known as Intercellular Communication. The dis-connection can manifest from several different sources and present in different from pain to inflammation. If we don't know **HOW** to resolve the disconnect, the dis-ease can cause serious Cellular damage, ranging from mutation to cellular DEATH!

Stress comes in many shapes and sizes, but scientifically, we define stress as **any force that pushes the body out of optimum Homeostatic conditions**. Therefore, **stress** can arise from many situations that we do not normally consider stressful, such as digesting food, exercising, waking after a long sleep, or even walking outdoors after a few hours indoors. Indeed, if you think about it, the events that take place during daily living affect our body's internal chemistry, causing an imbalance, or **stress**, that must be corrected.

Technically, a "**stressor**" is **any factor that causes stress**. Some stressors are obvious. We know that events like having an infectious disease, ingesting a toxic chemical, or being exposed to winter storms also stresses the body.

If the original stress resulted from moving to a cold area, you might generate heat by shivering.

If the stressor is an increase in blood sugar caused by eating an ice cream sundae, the pancreas will secrete insulin to reduce blood sugar levels.

Stress and Disease

- Negative emotions and health-related consequences

Persistent stressors and negative emotions	Release of stress hormones	Heart disease
		Immune suppression
Unhealthy behaviors (smoking, drinking, poor nutrition and sleep)		Autonomic nervous system effects (headaches, hypertension)

Invasions of **fungal**, **bacterial**, or **viral** pathogens are a very important and deadly category of stressors. A pathogen is any agent that can cause disease.

To a **pathogenic bacterium**, we are a walking meal of proteins, sugars, fats, and other good things to eat.

To a **virus**, we are an uncountable number of cells that can be converted into "factories" for making thousands of new viruses.

Despite the huge array of pathogens waiting to infect us, most of us are healthy, most of the time. That is because we have a very sophisticated **defensive** and **counterattacking** system in our bodies – A Gift from The CREATOR – our **Immune System**.

SKIN • NON-SPECIFIC • SPECIFIC

fence   foot soldiers   special forces

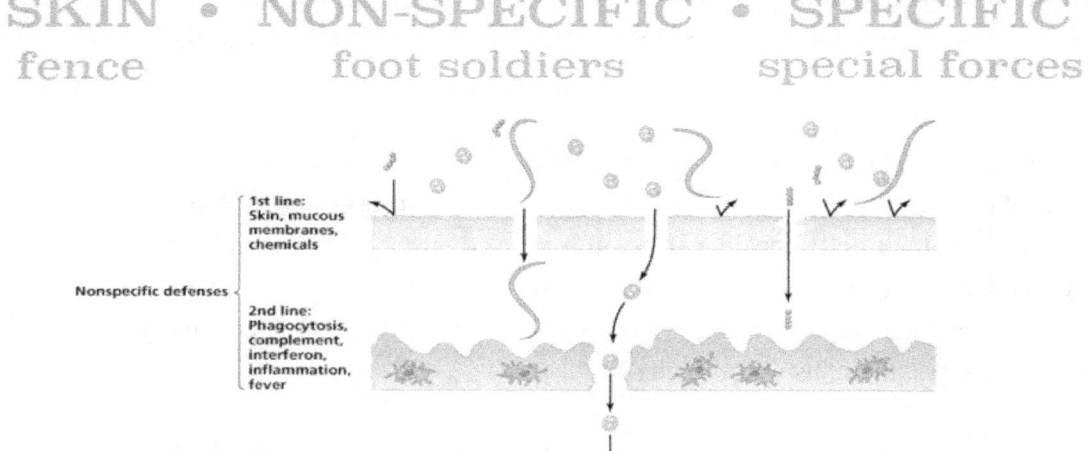

Our immune system is essentially **3 lines of defense**—2 we are **born with** and 1 we **acquire** throughout our lives. Our in-born ability to **defend** against pathogens is called **Innate Immunity**, or **Nonspecific Immunity**.

The most obvious of our innate defenses is our outer layer of **epithelium**— the **Cutaneous membrane** or our **Skin**, which along with **mucous membranes** is often called our 1st line of defense.

Skin disorders, acne, dry or oily skin are all indicators of a comprised immune system and the door is OPEN for us to encounter a dis-ease, pathogen or virus.

Our **2nd line of defense**, also present from birth, is a set of general internal pathogen-fighting measures: antimicrobial proteins like interferon, fever, inflammation, and "eating cells" called phagocytes.

These innate defenses are equally active regardless of whether the threat is a bacterial invasion in the moist environment of your throat or a long wait in line.

Whatever the stress is, these Nonspecific, Innate Defenses will respond the only way they can, repeating the same defense each time. See following Table for a summary of our innate defenses.

Pathogen: An agent that produces disease.

Interferon: A protein produced by virally infected cells that helps other cells respond to viral infection.

Phagocytes: Cells that endocytose (engulf) pathogens

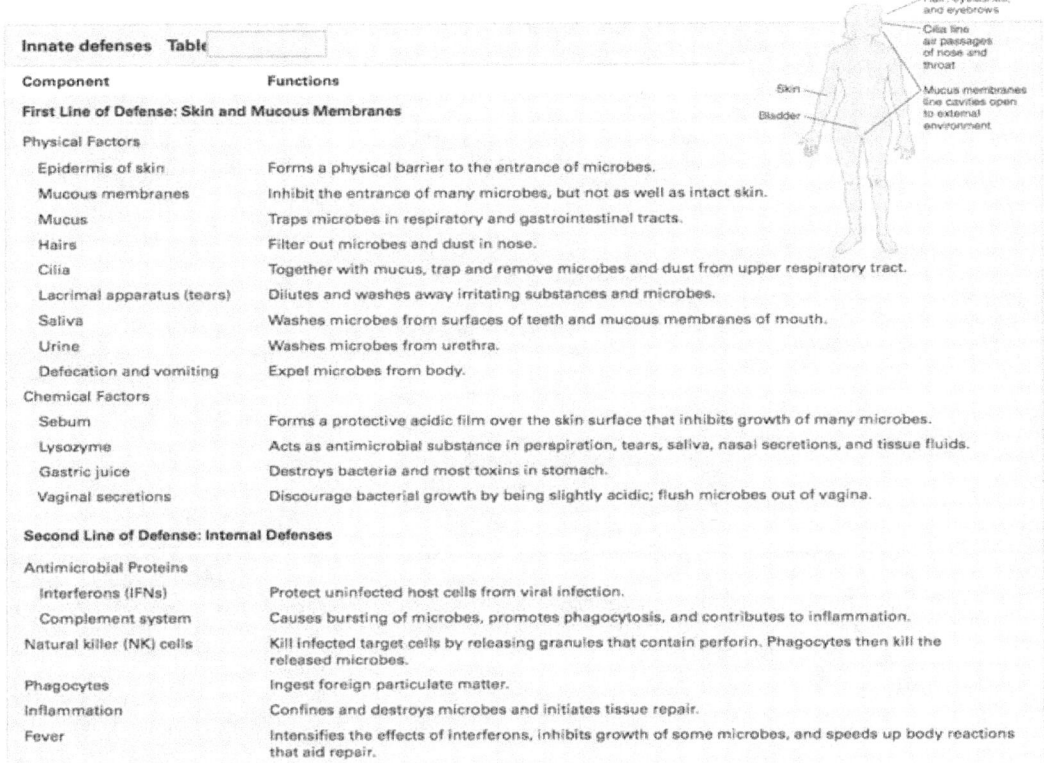

Innate defenses Table

Component	Functions
First Line of Defense: Skin and Mucous Membranes	
Physical Factors	
Epidermis of skin	Forms a physical barrier to the entrance of microbes.
Mucous membranes	Inhibit the entrance of many microbes, but not as well as intact skin.
Mucus	Traps microbes in respiratory and gastrointestinal tracts.
Hairs	Filter out microbes and dust in nose.
Cilia	Together with mucus, trap and remove microbes and dust from upper respiratory tract.
Lacrimal apparatus (tears)	Dilutes and washes away irritating substances and microbes.
Saliva	Washes microbes from surfaces of teeth and mucous membranes of mouth.
Urine	Washes microbes from urethra.
Defecation and vomiting	Expel microbes from body.
Chemical Factors	
Sebum	Forms a protective acidic film over the skin surface that inhibits growth of many microbes.
Lysozyme	Acts as antimicrobial substance in perspiration, tears, saliva, nasal secretions, and tissue fluids.
Gastric juice	Destroys bacteria and most toxins in stomach.
Vaginal secretions	Discourage bacterial growth by being slightly acidic; flush microbes out of vagina.
Second Line of Defense: Internal Defenses	
Antimicrobial Proteins	
Interferons (IFNs)	Protect uninfected host cells from viral infection.
Complement system	Causes bursting of microbes, promotes phagocytosis, and contributes to inflammation.
Natural killer (NK) cells	Kill infected target cells by releasing granules that contain perforin. Phagocytes then kill the released microbes.
Phagocytes	Ingest foreign particulate matter.
Inflammation	Confines and destroys microbes and initiates tissue repair.
Fever	Intensifies the effects of interferons, inhibits growth of some microbes, and speeds up body reactions that aid repair.

If these defenses fail to ward off the threat, our third line of defense and counterattack comes into play. It is called **specific immunity** because it attempts to eradicate that specific invader.

All stressors place physiological demands on the body, which can cause cells to halt routine activities and instead respond to the immediate demands of that stressor and can easily manifest into what we call a dis-ease or sickness. With the Cell focused on Stress it begins to DIE!

The physiological changes associated with stress are known to alter sleep patterns or even personality. These alterations are not for the betterment of Self. Our body doesn't begin to Heal until it is ASLEEP. With a disruption sleep pattern means a LACK of Healing. The Stress and LACK of sleep both create a Negative attitude, often making it hard to be Peaceful and Happy.

Regardless of the stressor, however, the body's response follows a general pattern: opposing the stressor, accommodating to it, and finally succumbing to it. This pattern, called the General Adaptation Syndrome, is a common method our bodies use when handling stress.

PAGE 21

Supreme Health & Fitness!   Health & Wellness Series Volume 1

The General Adaptation Syndrome Helps Overcome Stress

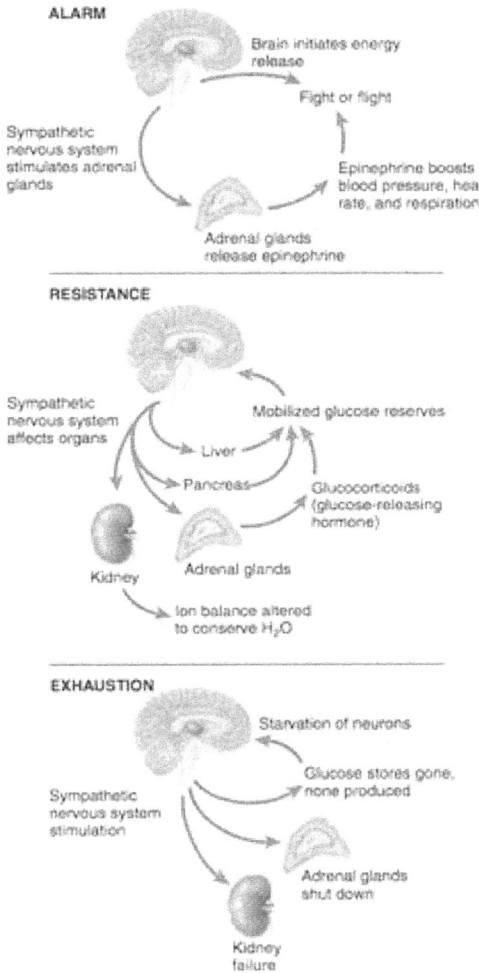

ALARM

Brain initiates energy release

Fight or flight

Sympathetic nervous system stimulates adrenal glands

Epinephrine boosts blood pressure, heart rate, and respirations

Adrenal glands release epinephrine

RESISTANCE

Sympathetic nervous system affects organs

Mobilized glucose reserves

Liver

Pancreas

Glucocorticoids (glucose-releasing hormone)

Kidney

Adrenal glands

Ion balance altered to conserve H₂O

EXHAUSTION

Starvation of neurons

Glucose stores gone, none produced

Sympathetic nervous system stimulation

Adrenal glands shut down

Kidney failure

You may have heard that "fight or flight" is a common response to danger. Fight or flight is one of our innate, automatic physiologic responses to stress, and in fact is the first of the three stages of General Adaptation Syndrome, or GAS. This series of predictable responses to stress is an attempt to adapt and deal with the original stressor. The three stages of this reaction are (1) **Alarm**, (2) **Resistance**, and (3) **Exhaustion**.

During the **alarm stage**, we feel a sudden rush of adrenaline, an immediate jolt of energy that provides the speed, power, and quickness of wit to remove ourselves from danger.

The alarm stage is initiated by the autonomic nervous system.

The alarm phase is controlled by the release of the hormone epinephrine also known as adrenaline. The changes effected during the alarm phase will help the body operate at peak performance while confronting or avoiding a stressor; however, these changes are less appropriate as responses to social stressors. Increased heart rate and blood glucose levels will not speed up a checkout line, but they will boost your frustration level. We call a severe and inappropriate triggering of the alarm phase a "**panic attack**."

If this fight-or-flight response fails to overcome the stress, however, the body continues working through the other two stages of GAS: Resistance and Exhaustion.

The **Resistance phase** is a response to prolonged stress. During the resistance phase, the body concentrates on surviving the stress rather than evading it. The individual is likely to feel tired, irritable, and emotionally fragile.

During the resistance phase, the brain consumes immense amounts of glucose that it obtains from the blood. A series of hormones ensure that lipid and protein reserves are continuously tapped to maintain the high blood sugar level needed by the brain.

The skeletal muscles become more concerned with survival than with rapid movement, and they begin to break down proteins. The break-down of lipids sustains the high fuel supply even during starvation, as the liver begins converting stored carbohydrates into glucose.

In addition, blood volume is conserved by maintaining water and sodium in the body, which unfortunately simultaneously raises blood pressure. Potassium and hydrogen ions are lost at abnormally high rates.

The resistance phase lasts until the stress is removed, lipid reserves are depleted, or complications arise from the altered body chemistry. Poor nutrition, physical damage to the heart, liver, or kidneys, or even emotional trauma can abruptly end the resistance phase.

The **Exhaustion phase** can be terminal. Resistance requires us to maintain extreme physiological conditions, and prolonged resistance can lead to the exhaustion phase, which is a polite way of saying, "death through organ failure and system shutdown."

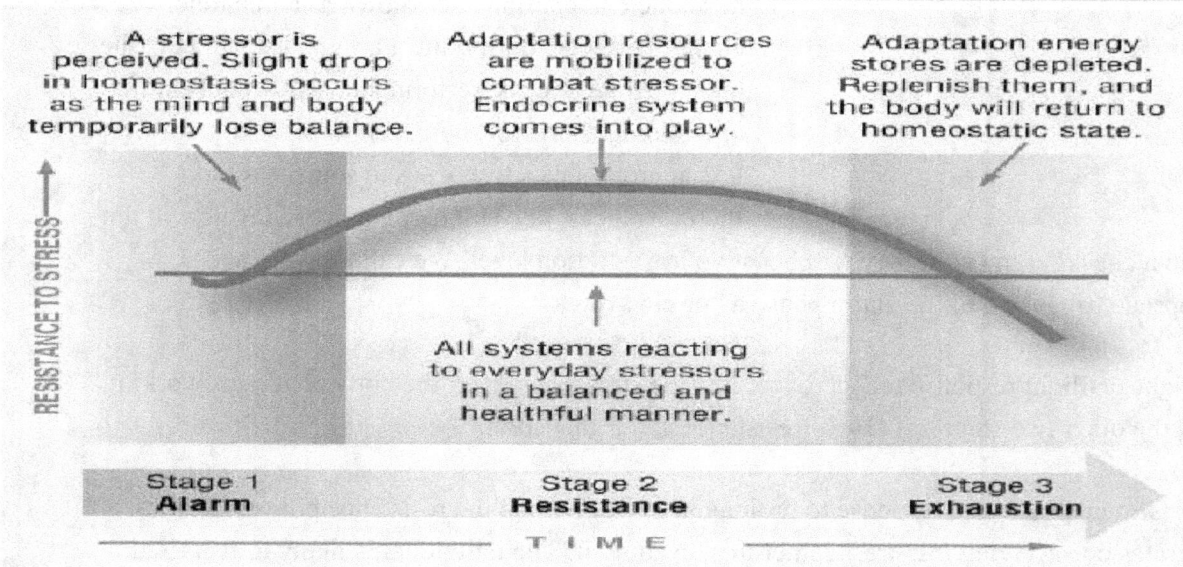

The General Adaptation Syndrome

A stressor is perceived. Slight drop in homeostasis occurs as the mind and body temporarily lose balance.

Adaptation resources are mobilized to combat stressor. Endocrine system comes into play.

Adaptation energy stores are depleted. Replenish them, and the body will return to homeostatic state.

RESISTANCE TO STRESS

All systems reacting to everyday stressors in a balanced and healthful manner.

Stage 1
Alarm

Stage 2
Resistance

Stage 3
Exhaustion

TIME

Understanding Post-Traumatic Stress Disorder

After severe stress, such as witnessing or being victimized by warfare, rape, or violent crime, some people develop post-traumatic stress disorder (PTSD). This disorder is a type of stress reaction that may get worse, not better, with time. Biologically, PTSD looks like a prolonged resistance phase of GAS. In addition, research has shown that victims of PTSD show abnormal brain patterns and changes in the volume of certain areas of the brain.

The amygdala, a center associated with emotion and fear, and the hypothalamus, the homeostasis center, are most often affected. These changes help explain the symptoms of PTSD: fear, heightened vigilance, panic reactions, inability to concentrate, and memory disorders.

Western medical approaches treating PTSD with psychotherapy or psychoactive drugs. But this approach doesn't cure or heal – they just mask and become an unnatural addictive element that changes the body to depend on it to function.

Occasionally, a person may experience episodes of free-floating panic, with a racing heart, profuse sweating, and an inexplicable feeling of dizziness and nausea. These symptoms are characteristic of panic disorder, a chronic state characterized by panic attacks that often occur during times of prolonged stress or life-changing steps, such as during pregnancy or before marriage or graduation.

Unfortunately, these physiological responses are inappropriate for the situation, and often do little more than foster more panic. That is not a welcome response to the festivities surrounding the wedding day and night.

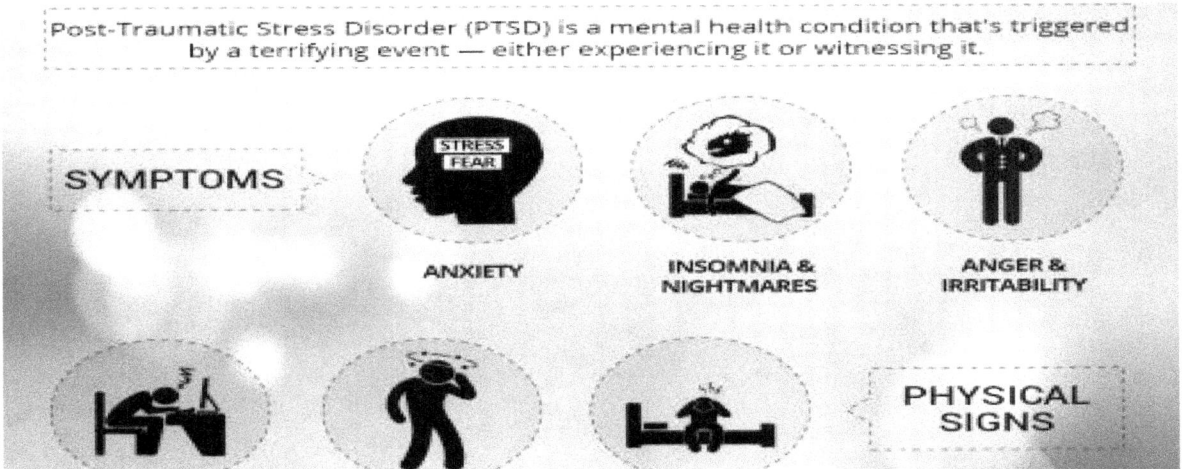

Think Critically

1. What is the main organ of the body responsible for the initial panic feelings associated with life-changing events?

2. What sort of events or situations might trigger a panic attack in an otherwise healthy person?

3. Knowing this, can you prescribe some techniques that might help alleviate this feeling should you ever begin to experience a panic attack?

4. What are the innate defenses?

5. What are the defining characteristics of specific and nonspecific immunity?

6. How do the symptoms of PTSD relate to the changes seen in?

PAGE 25

Supreme Health & Fitness!   Health & Wellness Series Volume 1

Immune system responses to pathogens

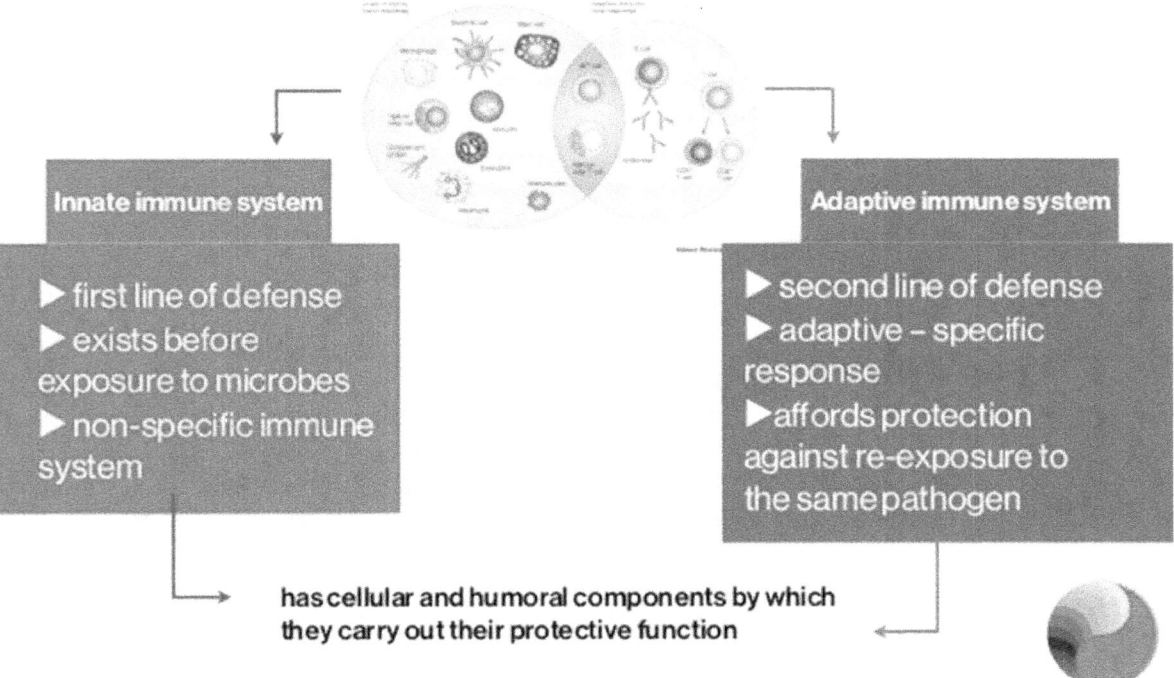

Innate immune system

▶ first line of defense
▶ exists before exposure to microbes
▶ non-specific immune system

Adaptive immune system

▶ second line of defense
▶ adaptive – specific response
▶ affords protection against re-exposure to the same pathogen

has cellular and humoral components by which they carry out their protective function

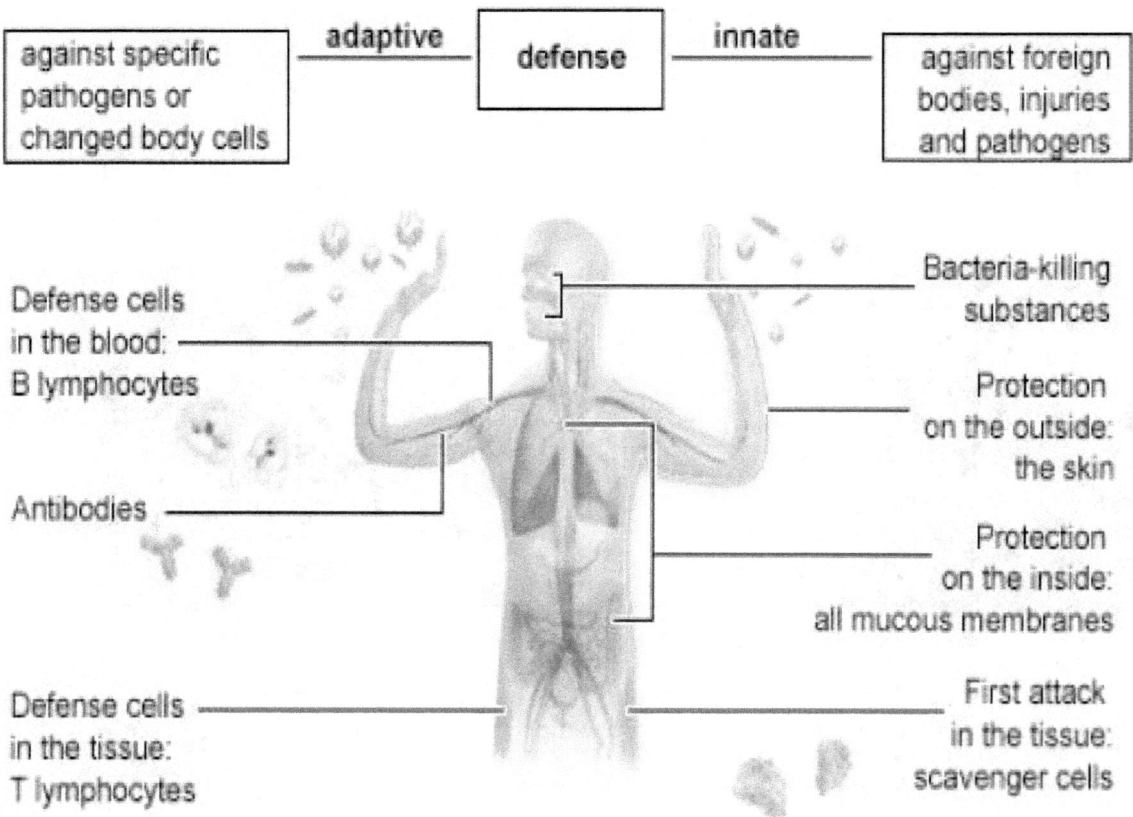

against specific
pathogens or
changed body cells

adaptive — defense — innate

against foreign
bodies, injuries
and pathogens

Defense cells
in the blood:
B lymphocytes

Bacteria-killing
substances

Protection
on the outside:
the skin

Antibodies

Protection
on the inside:
all mucous membranes

Defense cells
in the tissue:
T lymphocytes

First attack
in the tissue:
scavenger cells

THE IMMUNE SYSTEM

Immunity:

"Free from burden". Ability of an organism to recognize and defend itself against *specific* pathogens or antigens.

Immune Response:

"Third line of defense". Involves production of antibodies and generation of specialized lymphocytes against specific antigens.

Antigen:

Molecules from a pathogen or foreign organism that "provoke a specific immune response".

PAGE 28

Supreme Health & Fitness!   Health & Wellness Series Volume 1

*****

Chapter Two ... Understanding Your Immunity

*****

In this chapter I want to give a general over-view of your Immunity and with the subsequent chapters we will explore each layer of immunity from a closer perspective.

When you catch a cold or the flu; or, when you develop a disease such as diabetes or cancer, the primary reason is due to **inflammation** and a **weakened immune system** that is unable to defend your body against the invading pathogens, viruses, fungi, and parasites. In addition, your (weakened) immune system is unable to protect you from other health issues such as high blood pressure, high cholesterol, chronic fatigue and weight gain.

Consequently, two of the most critical steps in being able to successfully prevent or defeat any illness or disease are to **reduce the inflammation** and **strengthen the immune system**. But, first, let's take a look at how your immune system works.

Immune System: 3 Lines of Defense

Innate Immunity (Non-specific Defense Mechanisms)		Adaptive Immunity (Specific Defense Mechanisms)
Timeline: 0 to 12 hours		Timeline: 1 to 7 Days
1st Line of Defense	2nd Line of Defense	3rd Line of Defense
• Skin • Mucous membranes • Secretions of skin • Secretions of mucous membranes	• Macrophages • Other Phagocytes (i.e. neutrophils, NK cells) • Antimicrobial proteins • The Inflammatory response (e.g. redness, fever)	• Lymphocytes (B & T Cells) • Antigen-specific • Antibodies • Memory

The 1st Line of Defense includes the skin; mucous membranes; hair within the nose; cilia in the upper respiratory tract; urine; perspiration; saliva ; stomach gastric juice; and sebum.

The 2nd Line of Defense includes an inflammatory response and white blood cells (called phagocytes) that ingest pathogens.

The 3rd Line of Defense relies on T cells and B cells, some of which produce antibodies and others which kill pathogens.

Immune System: 3 Lines of Defense

The immune system is a collection of special cells, tissues and molecules that protects the body from numerous pathogenic microbes and toxins, utilizing 3 lines of defense:

1. Physical and Chemical Barriers (Innate Immunity)

2. Nonspecific Resistance (Innate Immunity)

3. Specific Resistance (Acquired or Adaptive Immunity)

1st Line of Defense: Physical and Chemical Barriers

Physical Barriers include: the skin; mucous membranes; hair within the nose; cilia which lines the upper respiratory tract; urine which flushes microbes out of the urethra; defecation and vomiting which expel microorganisms.

Chemical Barriers include: lysozyme, an enzyme produced in tears, perspiration, and saliva can break down cell walls and thus acts as an antibiotic (kills bacteria); stomach gastric juice which destroys bacteria and most toxins; sebum (unsaturated fatty acids) provides a protective film on the skin and inhibits growth.

2nd Line of Defense: Nonspecific Resistance (Innate Immunity)

The second line of defense is nonspecific resistance that destroys invaders in a generalized way without targeting specific individuals. White blood cells (called phagocytes) ingest and destroy all microbes that pass into body tissues.

In addition, there is an inflammatory response in the localized tissue where the pathogen invaded the body or where the tissue was damaged due to a cut or wound. Inflammation brings more white blood cells to the site where the microbes have invaded. The inflammatory response produces swelling, redness, heat, pain and fever. Fever inhibits bacterial growth and increases the rate of tissue repair during an infection.

3rd Line of Defense: Specific Resistance (Acquired Immunity)

The third line of defense is specific resistance. This system relies on antibodies, which are produced by specific immune cells (called B cells) in response to the antigens on the surface of the invading pathogens.

PAGE 31

Supreme Health & Fitness!   Health & Wellness Series Volume 1

Once a lymphocyte has recognised antigen a foreign antigen it expands to eliminate the infection

Some cells then become long lasting >20 years 'memory' cells.

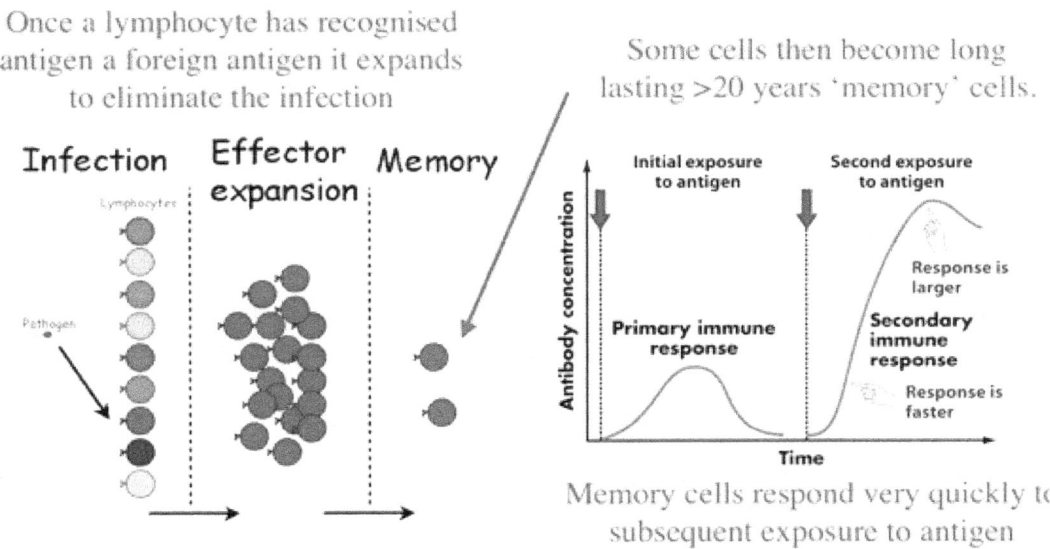

Memory cells respond very quickly to subsequent exposure to antigen

When an antigen is detected by a macrophage, this causes the T cells to become activated. The activation of T cells by a specific antigen is called *cell-mediated immunity*. Your body contains millions of different T cells, each ready and able to respond to one specific antigen.

The T cells secrete the element **interleukin 2**, which causes the proliferation of certain cytotoxic T cells and B cells. Your T cells stimulate the B cells to divide and forming plasma cells that are then able to produce *antibodies* and *memory* B cells.

If the same antigen should happen to enter your body later, your memory B cells divide to make more plasma cells and memory cells that can protect against future attacks by the same antigen.

When the T cells activate (stimulate) the B cells to divide into plasma cells, this is called *antibody-mediated immunity*.

Antibodies (also called *immunoglobulins*) are Y-shaped proteins that circulate through the blood stream and bind to specific antigens, thereby attacking microbes.

The antibodies are then transported through the blood and the lymph to the pathogen invasion site.

Your body contains millions of different B cells, each ready and able to respond to one specific antigen.

Antibodies bind to an antigen, preventing its normal function or making it easier for phagocytic cells to ingest them; or, they activate a complement protein that kills the pathogen or signals other white blood cells; or they bind to the surface of macrophages to further facilitate phagocytosis.

***When you examine and understand this Awesome and Powerful system you have to ask –
HOW CAN ANYONE EVER GET SICK?***

THE IMMUNE SYSTEM
COMPONENTS

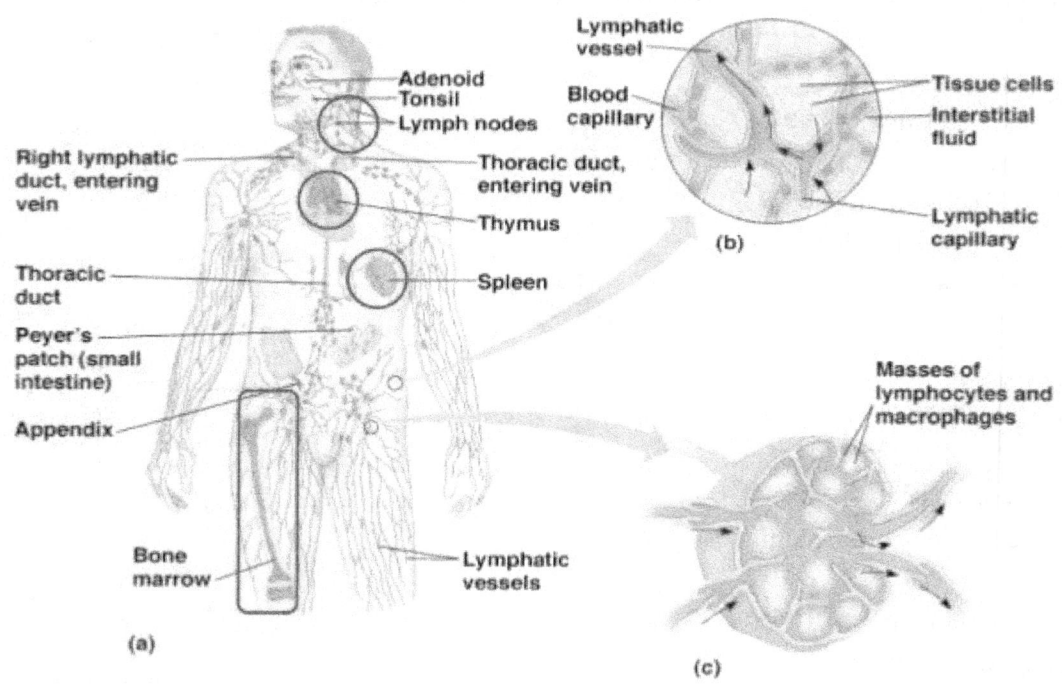

Immune System Components

The major components of Your immune system include the following:

Thymus: is located between your breast bone and your heart and is responsible for producing thymosin, which helps to activate T cells.

As we get older, this organ shrinks over 80% and produces less thymosin and may be one of the factors why our immune system weakens and we become more susceptible to certain diseases.

Thymus:
Is the **_bilobed encapsulated organ_** located behind sternum; above and in front of heart.
Is the major organ for T cell maturation & development.
It remains **highly active during fetal stage** (max) and then atrophies at puberty.

It is comprised of cortical, medullary epithelial cells, stromal cells, interdigitating cells and macrophages.
These accessory cells are important in **the differentiation of immigrating T cell precursors** and their selection prior to their migration to secondary lymphoid tissues.

Spleen: filters the blood looking for foreign cells (the spleen is also looking for old red blood cells in need of replacement). A person missing their spleen gets sick much more often than someone with a spleen.

Lymph system: includes the tissues and organs, including the bone marrow, spleen, thymus, and lymph nodes, that produce and store cells that fight infection and disease. The channels that carry lymph are also part of this system.

Lymph is a clear-like liquid that bathes the cells with water and nutrients. Lymph is blood plasma -- the liquid that makes up blood minus the red and white cells. Each cell has to get food, water, and oxygen to survive and your Blood transfers these materials to the lymph through the capillary walls, and lymph carries it to the cells.

Lymph Nodes:
They are **_small solid structures_** found at varying points along the lymphatic system.
Possess an enveloping capsule beneath which is subcapsular sinus, the cortex, a paracortical region and a medulla.
The cortex contains follicles comprised mainly _of B cells and follicular dendritic cells_.
The paracortical regions contains masses of **T cells**.
Primary function is to produce an immune response against any microbe they trap.

Your cells also produce proteins and waste products and the lymph absorbs these products and carries them away. Any random bacteria that enter the body also find their way into this inter-cell fluid. One job of the lymph system is to drain and filter these fluids to detect and remove the bacteria.

Small lymph vessels collect the liquid and move it toward larger vessels so that the fluid finally arrives at the lymph nodes for processing.

PAGE 34

Supreme Health & Fitness!　　　　　Health & Wellness Series Volume 1

Bone Marrow:
Is the primary source of pluripotent stem cells.
It becomes active only in the last months of fetal development.
Gives rise to all hematopoietic cells including lymphocytes.

Major Organ for B cell maturation.

All lymphoid /precursor cells in turn migrate to thymus for T cell maturation.

they are precursors to different cell types.

Bone marrow: this produces new blood cells, both red and white including B cells. In the case of red blood cells, the cells are fully formed in the marrow and then enter into your bloodstream. In the case of some white blood cells, the cells will mature elsewhere. Your marrow produces all blood cells from stem cells.

They are referred to as "stem cells" because they can branch off and become many different types of cells - Stem cells change into actual, specific types of white blood cells.

White blood cells: also called **leukocytes** and are probably the most important part of your immune system. These cells work together to destroy bacteria and viruses. The different types of white blood cells include: Neutrophils, Eosinophils, Basophils, Monocytes, Lymphocytes, B cells, T cells, Helper T cells, Suppressor T cells, Killer T cells, Granulocytes, Plasma cells, Phagocytes, Dendritic cells, Natural Killer cells, and Macrophages.

Antibodies: (also referred to as **immunoglobulins**) are produced by white blood B cells. They are Y-shaped proteins that each respond to a specific antigen (bacteria, virus or toxin). These Antibodies come in five classes: Immunoglobulin A (IgE), Immunoglobulin D (IgE), Immunoglobulin E (IgE), Immunoglobulin G (IgG), and Immunoglobulin M (IBM).

Antigen: The surface of every cell is covered with molecules that give it a unique set of characteristics and forms its function. These molecules are called antigens. Antigens are generally fragments of protein or carbohydrate molecules. There are millions of different antigens and each one has a unique shape that can be recognized by white blood cells. The white blood cells then produce antibodies to match the shape of the antigens.

Antigens

o Substances that can be recognized by the immunoglobulin receptor of B cells, or by **the T cell receptor when complexed with MHC**, are called *antigens*.

o Although a substance **that induces a specific immune response** is usually called an antigen, it is more appropriately called an *immunogen*.

o *Antigenicity* is the ability to combine specifically with the final products of the above responses (i.e., antibodies and/or cell-surface receptors). *Although all molecules that have the property of immunogenicity also have the property of antigenicity*, the reverse is not true.

o Hapten: Small foreign molecule that is not antigenic. Must be coupled to a carrier molecule to be antigenic. **Once antibodies are formed they will recognize hapten.**

Some antigens (e.g. associated with bacteria, viruses, pollen, etc.) stimulate an immune response by a white blood (B) cell to generate antibodies specific to that antigen that matches the shape of the antigen.

This allows the antibody to be able to bind to that specific antigen to make it easier for other white blood cells to engulf or attack the bacteria or virus who brings the antigen with them.

The antigens on the surface of the invading bacteria, viruses and other pathogenic cells are different from those on the surface of your own cells. This enables your immune system to distinguish pathogens from cells that are part of your body. Antigens are also found in foods like peanuts and on the surface of foreign materials like pollen, pet hairs and house dust where they can be responsible for triggering an allergy, hay-fever or asthma attacks.

Also Note: An antigen can be any substance (not just bacteria or viruses) that causes your immune system to produce antibodies against it, e.g. peanuts, pollen.

Lymphokines: are several hormones generated by components of the immune system. It is also known that certain hormones in the body suppress the immune system. Steroids and corticosteroids (components of adrenaline) suppress the immune system.

Tymosin (thought to be produced by the thymus) is a hormone that encourages lymphocyte production.

Lymphokines

Interleukins are another type of hormone generated by white blood cells. For example, Interleukin-1 is produced by macrophages after they eat a foreign cell. IL-1 has an interesting side-effect - when it reaches the hypothalamus it produces fever and fatigue.

The raised temperature of a fever is a specific reaction designed to kill some bacteria.

▸ Are cytokines secreted by lymphocytes
▸ Usually called interleukin-1, 2, 3 . . . or IL-1, IL-2 . . .

Copyright © The McGraw-Hill Companies, Inc. Permission required for reproduction or display.

Table 15.7   Some Cytokines That Regulate the Immune System

Cytokine	Biological Functions
Interleukin-1 (IL-1)	Induces proliferation and activation of T lymphocytes
Interleukin-2 (IL-2)	Induces proliferation of activated T lymphocytes
Interleukin-3 (IL-3)	Stimulates proliferation of bone marrow stem cells and mast cells
Interleukin-4 (IL-4)	Stimulates proliferation of activated B cells; promotes production of IgE antibodies; increases activity of cytotoxic T cells
Interleukin-5 (IL-5)	Induces activation of cytotoxic T cells; promotes eosinophil differentiation and serves as chemokine for eosinophils
Interleukin-6 (IL-6)	Stimulates proliferation and activation of T and B lymphocytes
Granulocyte/monocyte-macrophage colony-stimulating factor (GM-CSF)	Stimulates proliferation and differentiation of neutrophils, eosinophils, monocytes, and macrophages

Lymphokines are a subset of cytokines that are produced by lymphocytes. They are protein mediators typically produced by T cells to direct the immune system response by signaling between its cells.

Lymphokines have many roles, including the attraction of other immune cells, including macrophages and other lymphocytes, to an infected site and their subsequent activation to prepare them to mount an immune response.

Circulating lymphocytes can detect a very small concentration of lymphokine and then move up the concentration gradient towards where the immune response is required. Lymphokines also aid B cells in the production of antibodies.

Important lymphokines secreted by the T helper cell include: interleukin 2, 3, 4, 5, 6; granulocyte-macrophage colony-stimulating factor; and interferon-gamma.

Cytokines: are small peptides that act as signaling systems within the body. Because they facilitate communication between the innate and adaptive immune systems, cytokines are a key factor in fighting infection and maintaining homeostasis.

Types of CD4⁺ Cells and Cytokines

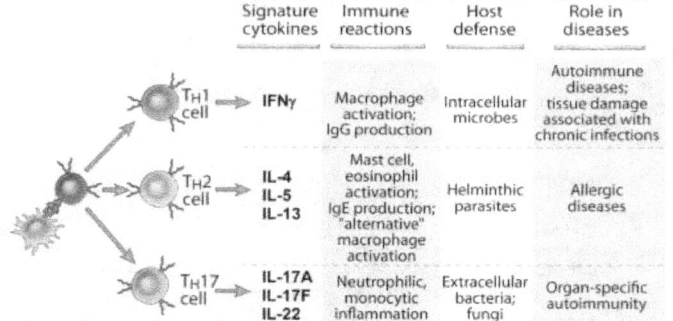

	Signature cytokines	Immune reactions	Host defense	Role in diseases
T$_H$1 cell	IFNγ	Macrophage activation; IgG production	Intracellular microbes	Autoimmune diseases; tissue damage associated with chronic infections
T$_H$2 cell	IL-4 IL-5 IL-13	Mast cell, eosinophil activation; IgE production; "alternative" macrophage activation	Helminthic parasites	Allergic diseases
T$_H$17 cell	IL-17A IL-17F IL-22	Neutrophilic monocytic inflammation	Extracellular bacteria; fungi	Organ-specific autoimmunity

- T$_H$1 and T$_H$2 cells are distinguished by cytokines but also by cytokine receptors and adhesion molecules they express
- Other CD4⁺ cells produce various mixtures of cytokines – not readily classified

Cytokines include chemokines, interferons, interleukins, lymphokines, tumor necrosis factor. Cytokines are produced by a broad range of cells, including immune cells like macrophages, B lymphocytes, T lymphocytes and mast cells, as well as endothelial cells, fibroblasts, and various stromal cells.

Some cytokines are chemical switches that turn certain immune cell types on and off. One cytokine, interleukin 2 (IL-2), triggers the immune system to produce T cells. IL-2's immunity-boosting properties have traditionally made it a promising treatment for several illnesses.

Elevated plasma levels of proinflammatory cytokines are biomarkers of inflammation and/or disease.

An imbalance between the activity of proinflammatory and anti-inflammatory cytokines is believed to affect disease onset, course, and duration.

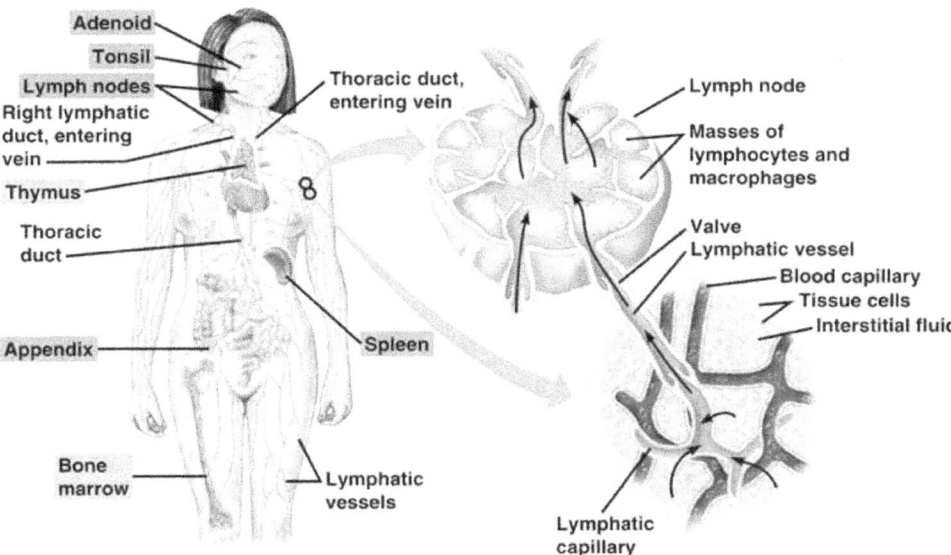

Tonsils: are lymphoepithelial tissues facing into the aerodigestive tract. These tissues are the immune system's first line of defense against ingested or inhaled foreign pathogens. The fundamental immunological roles of tonsils aren't yet understood.

Lymph nodes are distributed widely throughout areas of the body, including the armpit and stomach, and linked by lymphatic vessels. Lymph nodes are garrisons of B, T and other immune cells. These Lymph nodes act as filters or traps for foreign particles and are important in the proper functioning of the immune system. They are packed tightly with the white blood cells, called lymphocytes and macrophages.

Skin: is one of the most important parts of the body because it interfaces with the environment, and is the first line of defense from external factors, acting as an anatomical barrier from pathogens and damage between the internal and external environment in bodily defense. The Langerhans cells in your skin are part of the adaptive immune system.

Liver: has a wide range of functions, including immunological effects—the reticuloendothelial system of the liver contains many immunologically active cells, acting as a "sieve" for antigens carried to it via the portal system.

Bowel: There is lymphatic tissue in the bowel and in other mucous membranes in your body. The bowel plays a central role in defending the body against pathogens.

PAGE 38

Supreme Health & Fitness!   Health & Wellness Series Volume 1

More than half of all cells that produce antibodies are found in the bowel wall, especially in the last part of the small bowel and in the appendix. These cells recognize pathogens and other non-self substances, and mark and destroy them.

They also store information on these non-self substances which enables them to be able to react faster the next time. The large bowel also contains bacteria that belong to the body, called gut flora. These good bacteria in the large bowel make it difficult for other pathogens to settle and to enter the body.

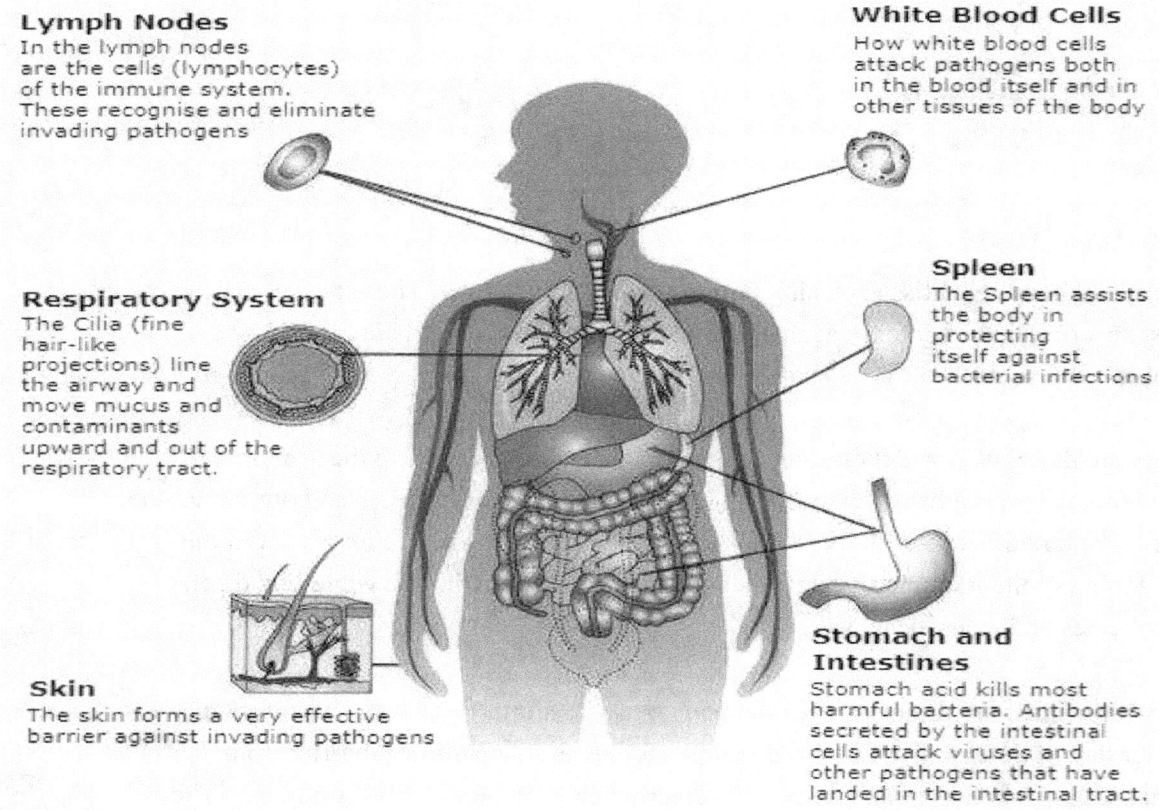

Lymph Nodes
In the lymph nodes are the cells (lymphocytes) of the immune system. These recognise and eliminate invading pathogens

White Blood Cells
How white blood cells attack pathogens both in the blood itself and in other tissues of the body

Respiratory System
The Cilia (fine hair-like projections) line the airway and move mucus and contaminants upward and out of the respiratory tract.

Spleen
The Spleen assists the body in protecting itself against bacterial infections

Skin
The skin forms a very effective barrier against invading pathogens

Stomach and Intestines
Stomach acid kills most harmful bacteria. Antibodies secreted by the intestinal cells attack viruses and other pathogens that have landed in the intestinal tract.

Supreme Health & Fitness!   Health & Wellness Series Volume 1

PAGE 39

Innate and Adaptive Immunity

The protection provided by the immune system is divided into two types of reactions: reactions of innate immunity and reactions of adaptive or acquired immunity.

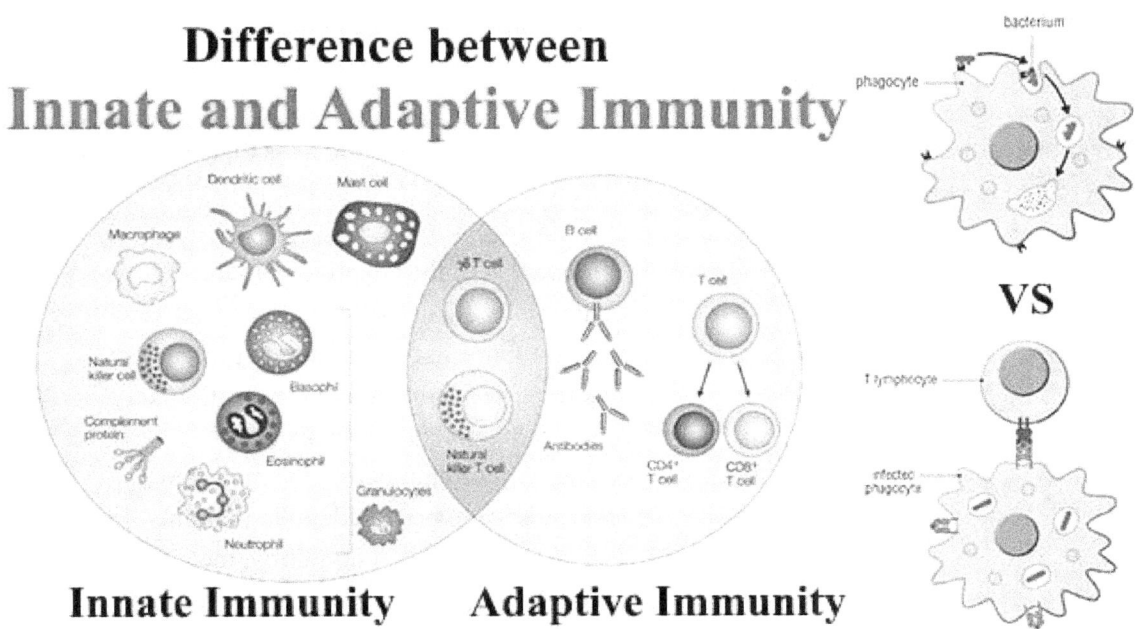

The innate immune system consists of cells and proteins that are always present and ready to mobilize and fight microbes at the site of infection.

The main components of the innate immune system are 1) physical epithelial barriers; 2) phagocytic leukocytes (neutrophils, eosinophils, basophils); 3) monocytes (which develop into macrophages); 4) dendritic cells; 5) a special type of lymphocyte called natural killer (NK) cells; and, 6) circulating plasma proteins. Other participants in innate immunity include the complement system and cytokines such as interleukin 2 (IL-2).

Innate immune cells express genetically encoded receptors, called Toll-like receptors (TLRs), which recognize general danger- or pathogen-associated patterns. Collectively, these receptors can broadly recognize viruses, bacteria, fungi, and even non-infectious problems. However, they cannot distinguish between specific strains of bacteria or viruses.
There are numerous types of innate immune cells with specialized functions.

PAGE 40

Supreme Health & Fitness!　　　　　　　　　　　Health & Wellness Series Volume 1

They include neutrophils, eosinophils, basophils, mast cells, monocytes, dendritic cells, and macrophages.

Their main feature is the ability to respond quickly and broadly when a problem arises, typically leading to inflammation. Innate immune cells also are important for activating adaptive immunity. Innate cells are critical for host defense, and disorders in innate cell function may cause chronic susceptibility to infection.

The adaptive (or acquired) immune system is called into action against pathogens that are able to evade or overcome innate immune defenses.

Adaptive Immunity

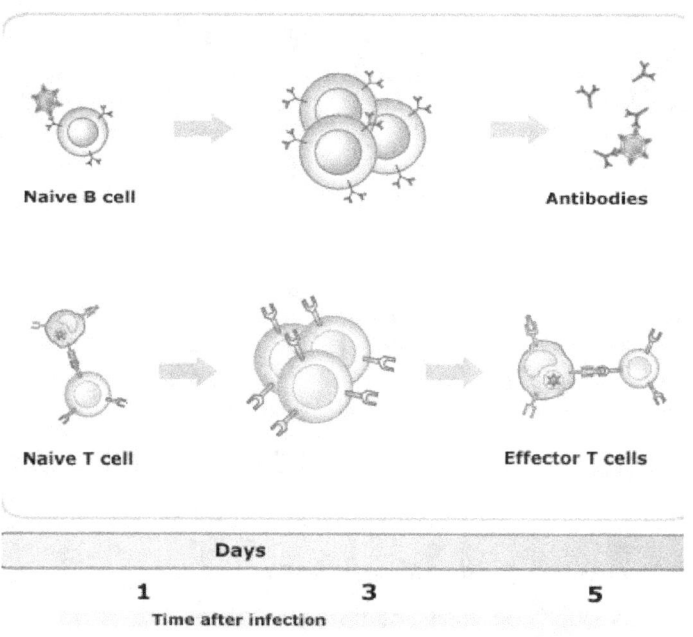

Naive B cell

Antibodies

Naive T cell

Effector T cells

Days

1   3   5

Time after infection

Components of the adaptive immune system are normally silent; however, when activated, these components "adapt" to the presence of infectious agents by activating, proliferating, and creating potent mechanisms for neutralizing or eliminating the microbes. There are two types of adaptive immune responses: 1) humoral immunity, mediated by antibodies produced by B lymphocytes; and, 2) cell-mediated immunity, mediated by T lymphocytes.

The adaptive immune response is more complex than the innate. The antigen first must be processed and recognized. Once an antigen has been recognized, the adaptive immune system creates an army of immune cells specifically designed to attack that antigen.

Adaptive immunity also includes a "memory" that makes future responses against a specific antigen more efficient.

Adaptive immune cells are more specialized, with each adaptive B or T cell bearing unique receptors, B-cell receptors (BCRs) and T-cell receptors (TCRs), that recognize specific signals rather than general patterns.

Each receptor recognizes an antigen, which is simply any molecule that may bind to a BCR or TCR. Antigens are derived from a variety of sources including pathogens, host cells, and allergens. Antigens are typically processed by innate immune cells and presented to adaptive cells in the lymph nodes.

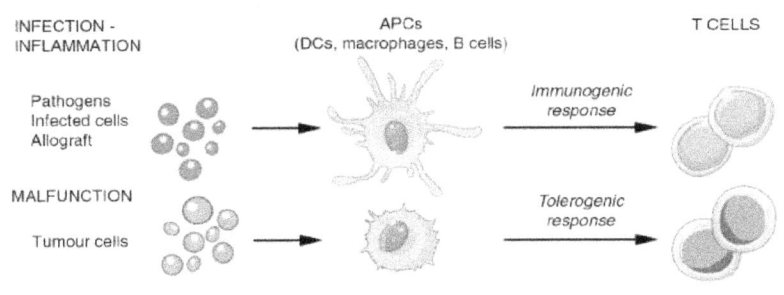

i - Capture of EVs by APCs: modulating the immune response

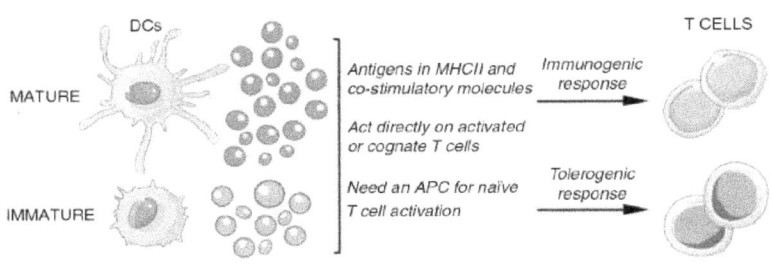

ii - Release of EVs by APCs: another way to present antigens

If a B or T cell has a receptor that recognizes an antigen from a pathogen and also receives cues from innate cells that something is wrong, the B or T cell will activate, divide, and disperse to address the problem.

B cells make antibodies, which neutralize pathogens, rendering them harmless.

T cells carry out multiple functions, including killing infected cells and activating or recruiting other immune cells.

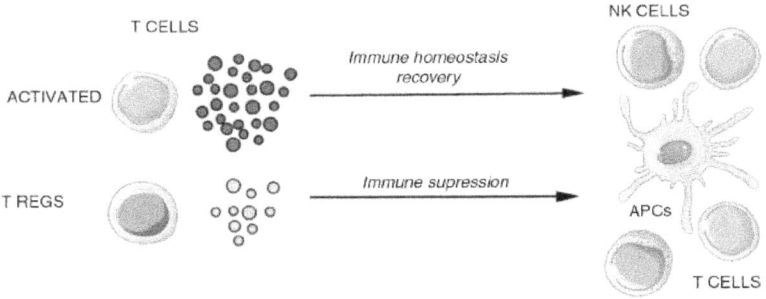

iii - T-cell-derived EVs

Certain T cells (Helper T) help activate B cells to secrete antibodies and macrophages to destroy ingested microbes. They also help activate other T cells called cytotoxic T cells to kill infected target cells.

As dramatically demonstrated in AIDS patients, without Helper T cells we cannot defend ourselves even against many microbes that are normally harmless.

However, Helper T cells themselves can only function when activated to become effector cells. They are activated on the surface of antigen-presenting cells (APC), which mature during the innate immune responses triggered by an infection.

The innate responses also dictate what kind of effector cell a Helper T cell will develop into and thereby determine the nature of the adaptive immune response elicited.

The adaptive immune response has a system of checks and balances to prevent unnecessary activation that could cause damage to the host. If a B or T cell is auto-reactive, meaning its receptor recognizes antigens from the body's own cells, the cell will be deleted. Also, if a B or T cell does not receive signals from innate cells, it will not be optimally activated.

Immune memory is a feature of the adaptive immune response. After B or T cells are activated, they expand rapidly. As the problem resolves, cells stop dividing and are retained in the body as memory cells. The next time this same pathogen enters the body, a memory cell is already poised to react and can clear away the pathogen before it establishes itself.

A further aspect of the adaptive immune system worth mentioning is its role in monitoring body cells to check that they aren't infected by viruses or bacteria, for instance, or in order to make sure that they haven't become cancerous.

Cancer occurs when certain body cells 'go wrong' and start dividing in an uncontrolled way.

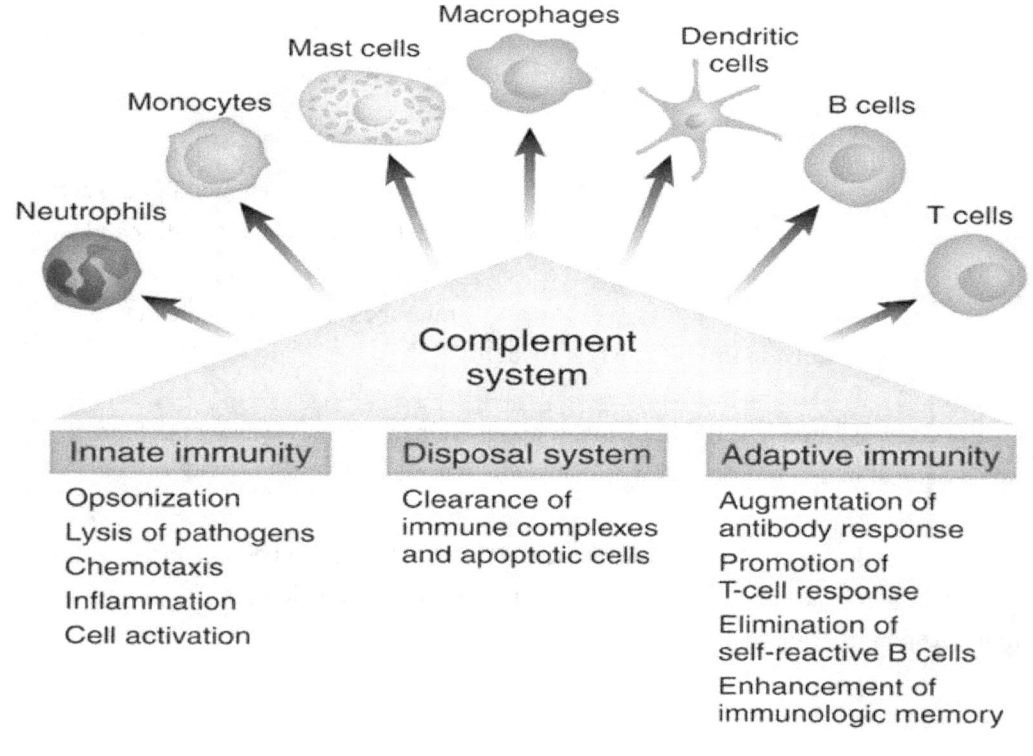

Major Cells of your Immune System

The key tissues and organs involved with the immune system include the lymph nodes, spleen, tonsils, bone marrow, thymus, and lymphatic tissue. The key immune cells are white blood cells (or leukocytes).

The (3) major categories of white blood cells are: granulocytes, lymphocytes and monocytes.

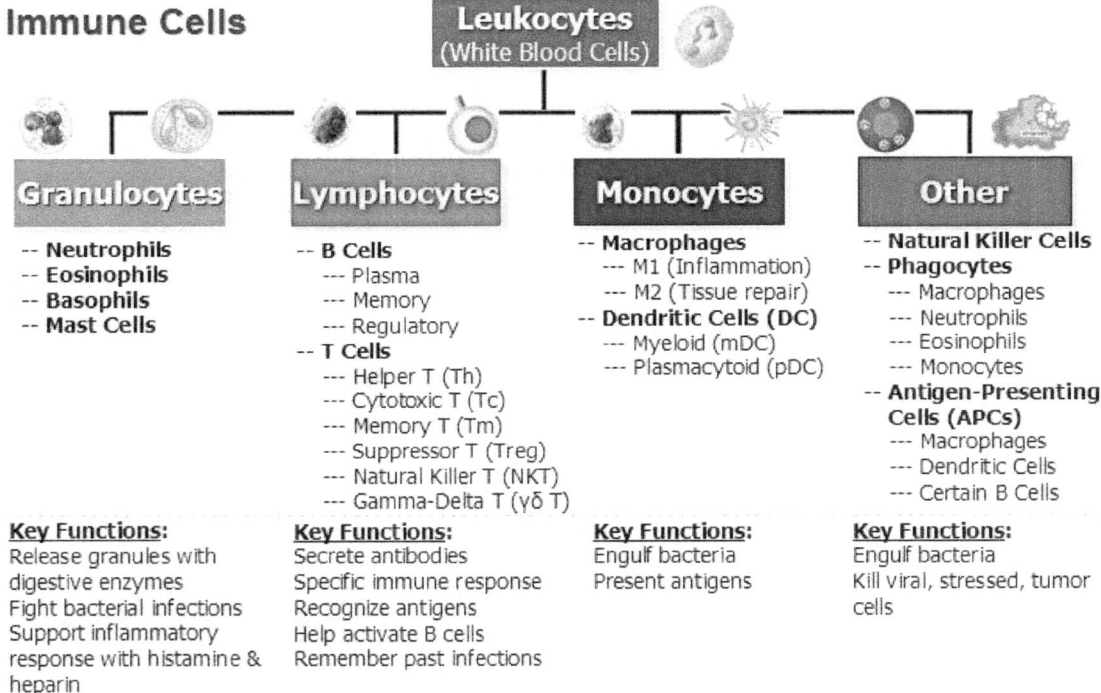

Granulocytes are characterized by the presence of granules in their cytoplasm which contain digestive enzymes that kill various types of bacteria and parasites. Granulocytes are also called polymorphonuclear leukocytes (PMN, PML, or PMNL) because of the varying shapes of the nucleus, which is usually lobed into three segments.

The principal types of granulocytes are neutrophils, eosinophils, basophils, and mast cells.

Lymphocytes come in three major types: B-lymphocytes (or B cells), T-lymphocytes(or T cells) and natural killer (NK) cells.

Supreme Health & Fitness!   Health & Wellness Series Volume 1

PAGE 44

Lymphocytes start out in the bone marrow and either stay there and mature into B cells, or they leave for the thymus gland, where they mature into T cells.

THE CELLS OF THE
IMMUNE SYSTEM

The basic functional units of the immune system are diverse cells derived from lymphoid and reticuloendothelial system.

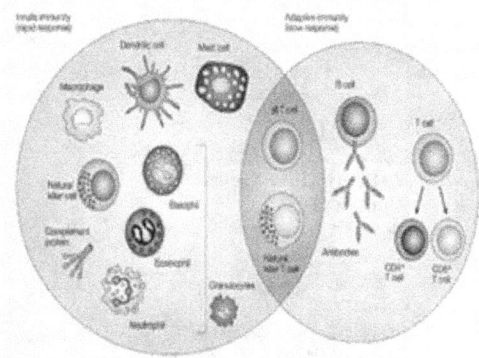

The immunoreactive cells are:
Lymphocytes - T and B cells
Monocytes/macrophages
Natural killer cells
Dendritic cells
Tissue mast cells
Granulocytes - Eosinophils,
basophils and neutrophils.

The disorders of the immune system can result in autoimmune diseases, inflammatory diseases and cancers.

B cells produce antibodies in the humoral immune response and are like the body's military intelligence system, seeking out their targets and sending defenses to lock onto them. With the help of T cells, B cells make special Y-shaped protein antibodies, which stick to antigens on the surface of bacteria, stopping them in their tracks, creating clumps that alert your body to the presence of intruders.

Plasma cells, also called *plasma B cells*, secrete large volumes of antibodies.

Memory B cells are important in generating an accelerated and more robust antibody-mediated immune response in the case of re-infection (also known as a secondary immune response).

PAGE 45

Supreme Health & Fitness!   Health & Wellness Series Volume 1

Regulatory B cells (Bregs) participates in immunomodulations and in suppression of immune responses. via production of anti-inflammatory cytokine interleukin 10 (IL-10).

T cells recognize and kill virus-infected cells directly. Some help B cells to make antibodies, which circulate and bind to antigens. Others send chemical instructions (cytokines) to the rest of the immune system. Types of T cells include Helper T (Th), Memory T (Tm), Cytotoxic T (Tc), Suppressor T (Treg), and Effector T cells.

Helper T Cells (Th) help activate B cells to secrete antibodies and macrophages to destroy ingested microbes, but they also help activate cytotoxic T cells to kill infected target cells. Note: In AIDS patients, without helper T cells we cannot defend ourselves even against many microbes that are normally harmless.

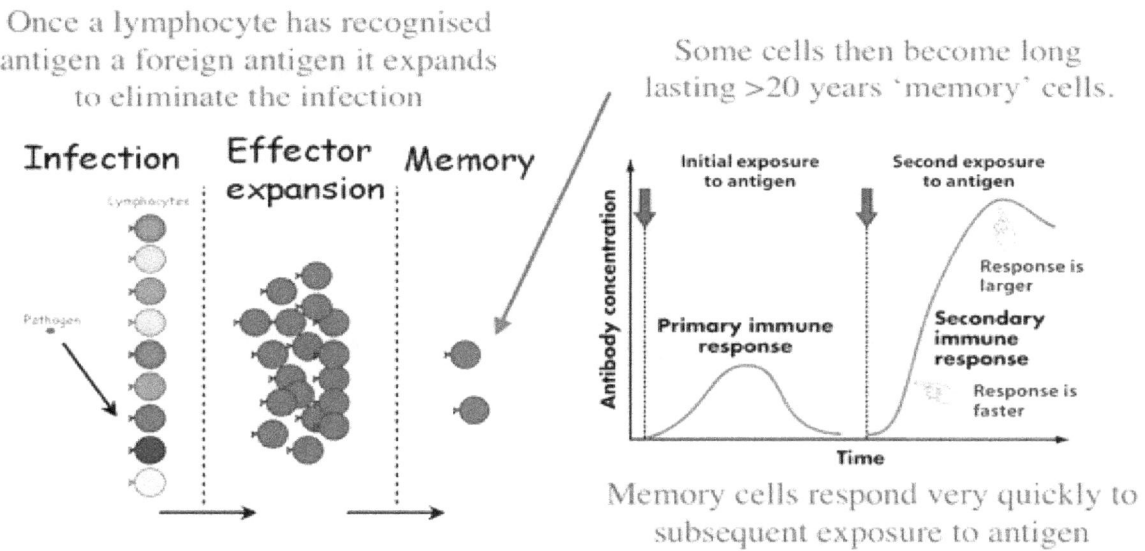

Once a lymphocyte has recognised antigen a foreign antigen it expands to eliminate the infection

Some cells then become long lasting >20 years 'memory' cells.

Memory cells respond very quickly to subsequent exposure to antigen

Memory T Cells (Tm) are derived from normal T cells that have learned how to overcome an invader by 'remembering' the strategy used to defeat previous infections. At a second encounter with the invader, memory T cells can reproduce to mount a faster and stronger immune response than the first time the immune system responded to the invader.

Cytotoxic T Cells (Tc) are lymphocytes that kill invading pathogens including cancer cells, cells that are infected (particularly with viruses), or cells that are damaged in other ways. Tc cells kill their targets by programming them to undergo apoptosis. The successful elimination of infected cells without the destruction of healthy tissue requires the cytotoxic mechanisms of CD8 T cells to be both powerful and accurately targeted.

Suppressor T Cells (Treg) suppress the immune response after invading organisms are destroyed by releasing their own lymphokines to signal all other immune-system participants to cease their attack. This prevents your body from destroying or fighting its own healthy cells.

Effector T cells (also called Helper T (Th) cells), are the functional cells for executing immune functions. Balanced immune responses can only be achieved by proper regulation of the differentiation and function of Th cells.

Natural killer (NK) ***cells*** are cytotoxic cells that participate in the innate immune response and attack in packs by releasing substances that perforate the "skin" of their victims -- this is death by cell lysis.

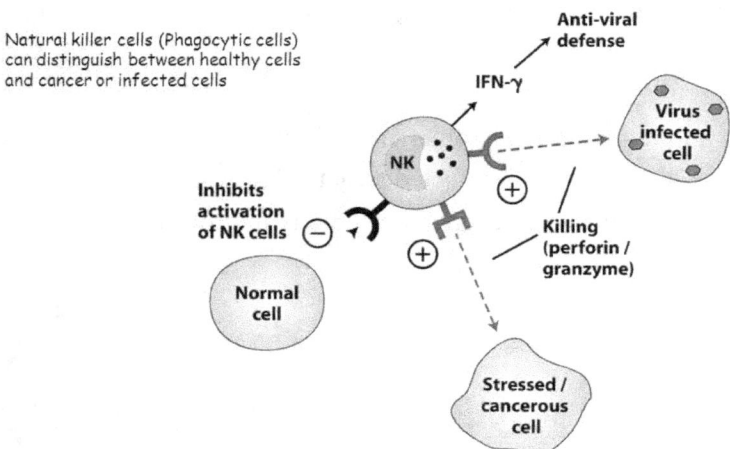

Natural killer cells (Phagocytic cells) can distinguish between healthy cells and cancer or infected cells

Monocytes, which are the largest of all leukocytes, fight off bacteria, viruses and fungi. Originally formed in the bone marrow, they are released into the blood and tissues. When certain germs enter the body, they quickly rush to the site for attack within 8–12 hours.

Monocytes have several functions to help you ward off diseases and infections. To help you remember what they do, note that each function begins with the letter 'M': **Munch**, **Mount** and **Mend**.

<u>**Munch**</u>: Monocytes have the ability to change into another cell form called macrophages before facing the germs. In response to inflammation signals, monocytes move quickly to sites of infection in the tissues and divide/differentiate into macrophages and dendritic cells to elicit an immune response. They change into macrophages when they move from the bloodstream to the tissues. They begin to consume, or munch, on harmful bacteria, fungi and viruses. Then, enzymes in the monocyte kill and break down the germs into pieces.

Monocytes

Structure:
- Largest WBC
- U-shaped nucleus
- Grayish blue cytoplasm

Amount:
- 100-700/mm³

Functions:
- Phagocytosis
- Become macrophages & remove dead cells

Life Span – weeks → months

<u>**Mount**</u>: Monocytes help other white blood cells identify the type of germs that have invaded the body.

After consuming the germs, the monocytes take parts of those germs, called antigens, and mount them outside their body like flags. Other white blood cells see the antigens and make antibodies designed to kill those specific types of germs.

Mend: Monocytes help mend damaged tissue by stopping the inflammation process. They remove dead cells from the sites of infection, which repairs wounds. They have also shown to influence the formation of some organs, like the heart and brain, by helping the components that hold tissues together.

Macrophages are derived from monocytes, granulocyte stem cells, or the cell division of pre-existing macrophages. Macrophages do not have granules but have receptors to detect, capture and ingest pathogens. Macrophages are found throughout the body in almost all tissues and organs, just below the surface of the skin and mucous membranes — any place where a pathogen could get through the first line of defense. Macrophages cause inflammation through the production of interleukin-1, interleukin-6, and TNF-alpha. Macrophages are usually only found in tissue and are rarely seen in blood circulation.

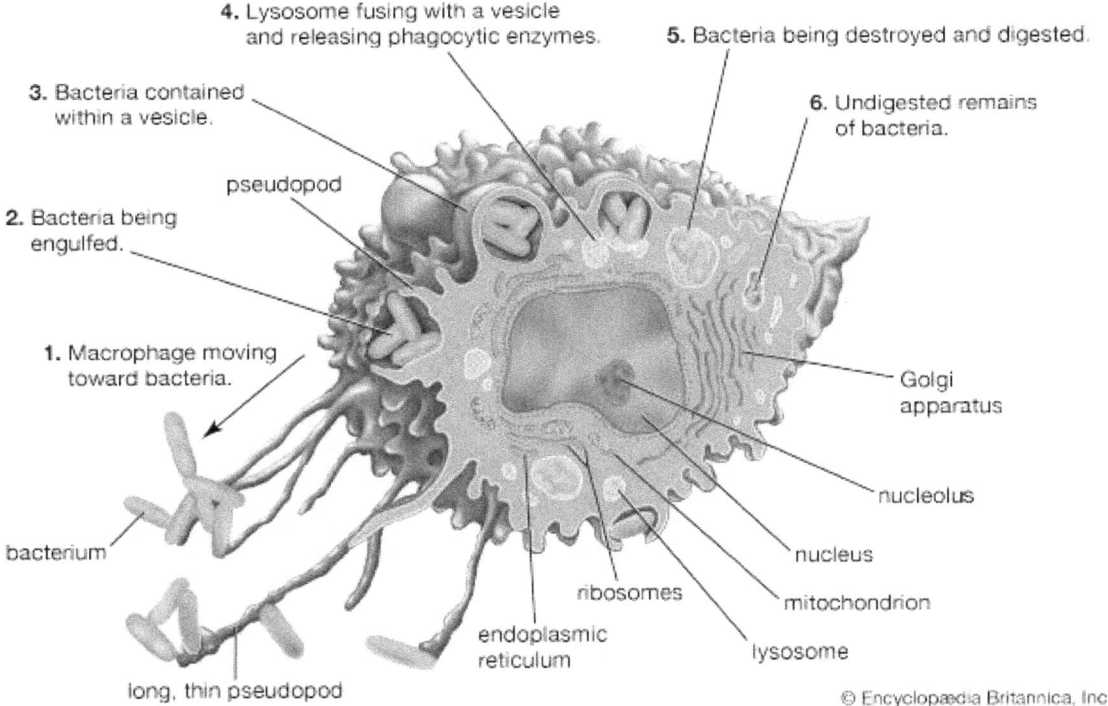

4. Lysosome fusing with a vesicle and releasing phagocytic enzymes.

5. Bacteria being destroyed and digested.

3. Bacteria contained within a vesicle.

6. Undigested remains of bacteria.

pseudopod

2. Bacteria being engulfed.

1. Macrophage moving toward bacteria.

Golgi apparatus

nucleolus

bacterium

nucleus

ribosomes

mitochondrion

endoplasmic reticulum

lysosome

long, thin pseudopod

© Encyclopædia Britannica, Inc.

They take up and destroy necrotic cell debris and foreign material including viruses, bacteria, and tattoo ink. In wound healing, macrophages take on the role of wound protector by fighting infection and overseeing the repair process. Macrophages also produce chemical messengers, called growth factors, which help repair the wound.

When inflammation occurs, monocytes undergo a series of changes to become macrophages and target cells that need eliminating.

Once engulfed, cellular enzymes inside the macrophage destroy the ingested particle. Some macrophages act as scavengers, removing dead cells while others engulf microbes.

Another function of macrophages is to alert the immune system to microbial invasion. After ingesting a microbe, a macrophage presents a protein on its cell surface called an antigen, which signals the presence of the antigen to a corresponding T helper cell.

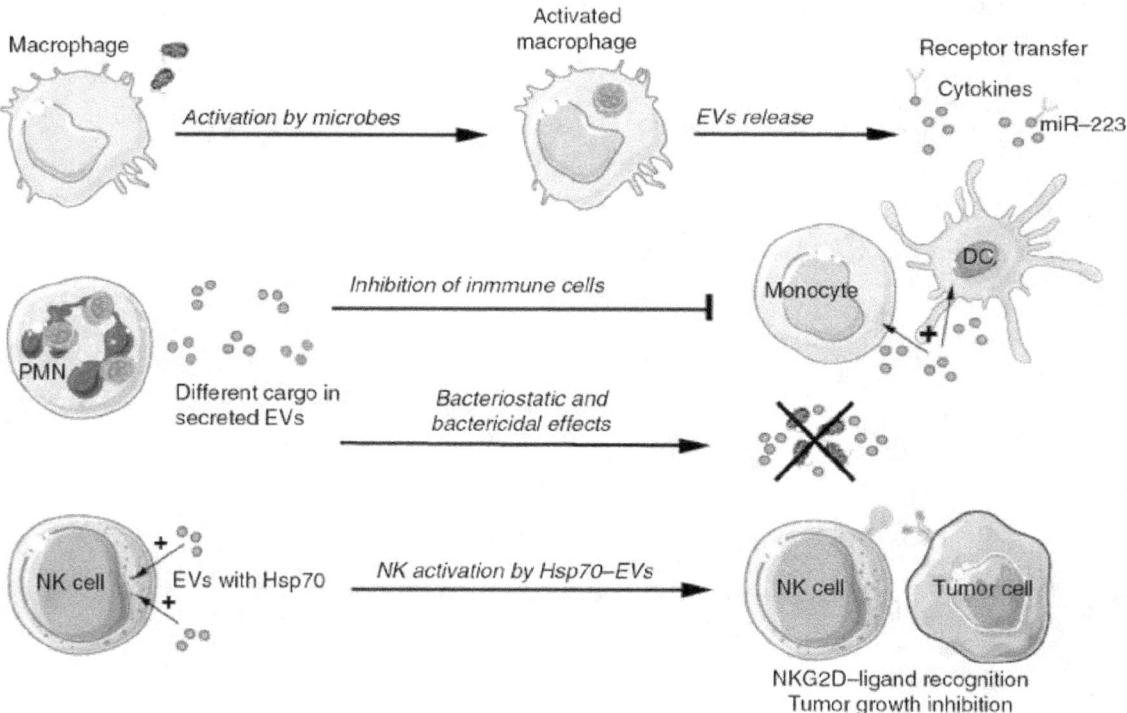

Macrophages also change into foam cells in the blood vessel walls (endothelium), where they try to fight atherosclerosis by engulfing excessive cholesterol engulf large amounts of fatty substances, usually cholesterol. Foam cells are created when the body sends macrophages to the site of a fatty deposit on the blood vessel walls.

The macrophage wraps around the fatty material in an attempt to destroy it and becomes filled with lipids (fats). The lipids engulfed by the macrophage give it a "foamy" appearance.

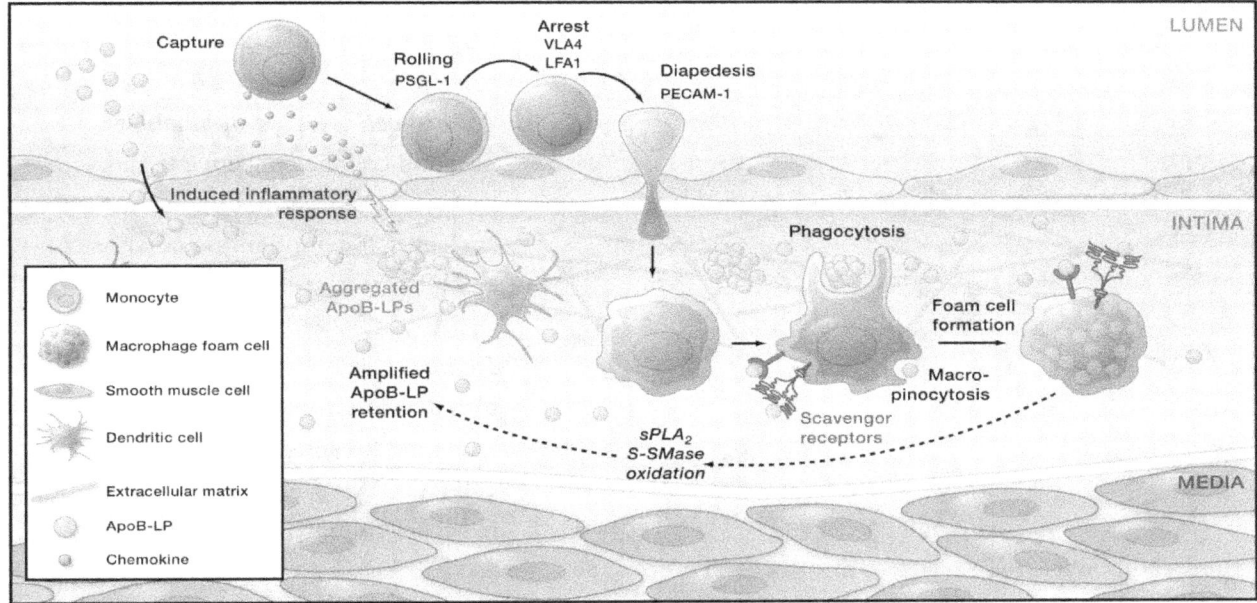

Foam cells are often found in the fatty streaks and plaques inside the blood vessel walls. Foam cells do not give off any specific signs or symptoms, but they are part of the cause of atherosclerosis. Foam cell development can be slowed, however.

Decreasing low density lipoprotein (LDL) cholesterol and increasing high density lipoprotein (HDL) cholesterol will remove the lipids that the macrophages engulf to become foam cells.

In addition to the monocytes and macrophages, the other types of white blood cells include neutrophils, basophils, eosinophils, mast cells and dendritic cells.

Neutrophils defend against bacterial or fungal infection and other very small inflammatory processes. They are usually the first responders to microbial infection; their activity and death in large numbers forms pus.

Basophils are chiefly responsible for allergic reactions and antigen response by releasing the chemical histamine, which helps to trigger inflammation, and heparin, which prevents blood from clotting.

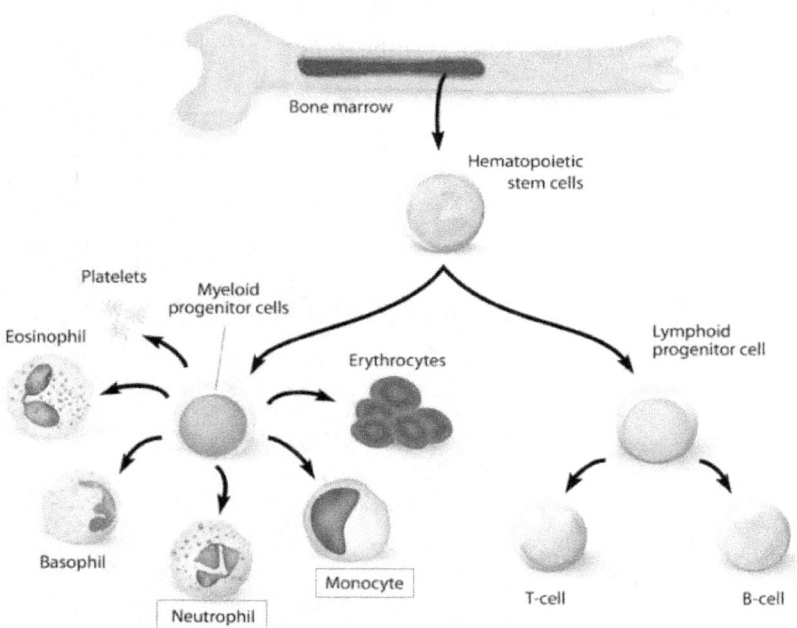

Eosinophils primarily deal with parasitic worm infections. They are also the predominant inflammatory cells in allergic reactions.

A **Mast cell** is a type of granular basophil cell in connective tissue that releases heparin, histamine, and serotonin during inflammation and allergic reactions.

Dendritic cells (DCs), which can also develop from monocytes, are an important antigen-presenting cell (APC) whose main function is to process antigen material and present it on the cell surface to the T cells in order to activate the T cells.

They act as messengers between the innate and the adaptive immune systems. Once activated, dendritic cells migrate to the lymph nodes where they interact with T cells and B cells to initiate and shape the adaptive immune response.

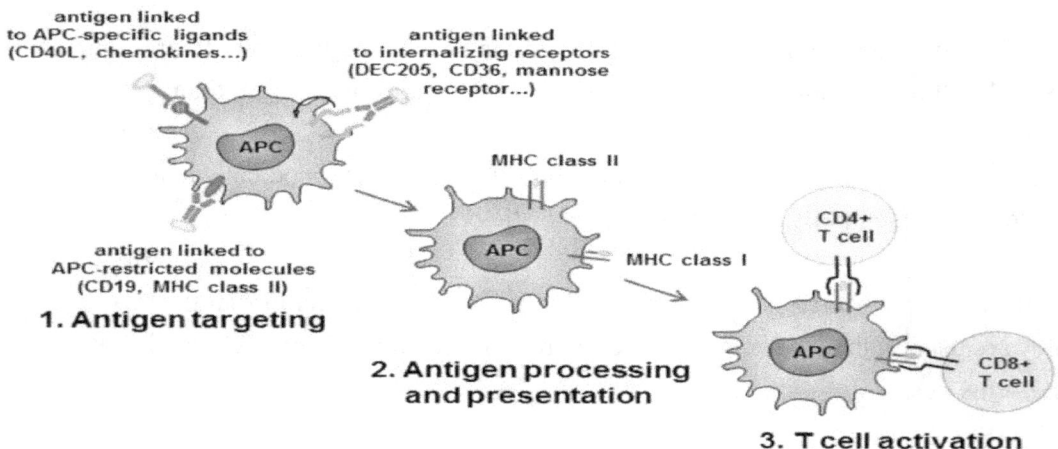

Note: Antigens are molecules from pathogens, host cells, and allergens that may be recognized by adaptive immune cells.

Antigen-presenting cells (APCs) like DCs are responsible for processing large molecules into "readable" fragments (antigens) recognized by adaptive B or T cells in order to activate them. However, antigens alone cannot activate T cells. They must be presented with the appropriate major histocompatibility complex (MHC) molecule "tags" expressed on the APC. MHC provides a checkpoint and helps immune cells distinguish between self and non-self cells.

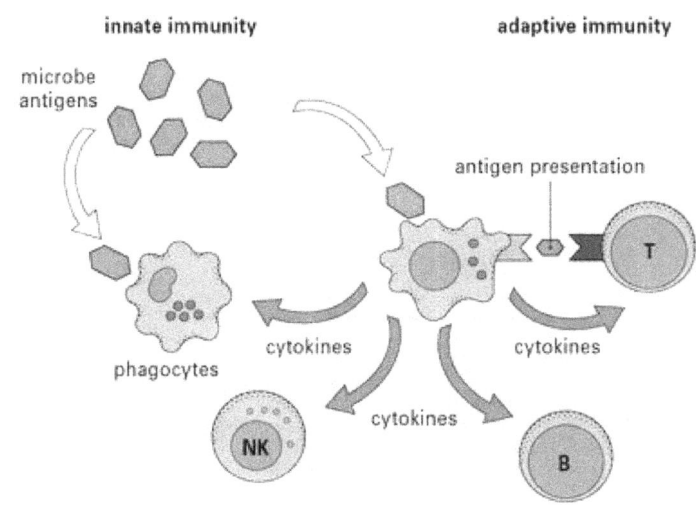

An APC can be any of various cells (as a macrophage or a B cell) that take up and process an antigen into a form that when displayed at the cell surface in combination with an MHC molecule is recognized by and serves to activate a specific helper T cell using their T-cell receptors (TCRs).

We have an Awesome Gift from The Creator – Our Immune System!

Getting an Understanding of our Immune System lets us see how POWERFUL we are or can be. Just be getting this brief introduction into the anatomy and function of our Immune System, we surely have to wonder and ask – HOW DO WE GET SICK WITH THIS POWERFUL SYSTEM???

Through the rest of the book we will take a closer look at key elements of our Immune System and research some of the foods that cause damage to our Immunity and the Foods that INCREASE it!

Cell-Mediated Immune Response

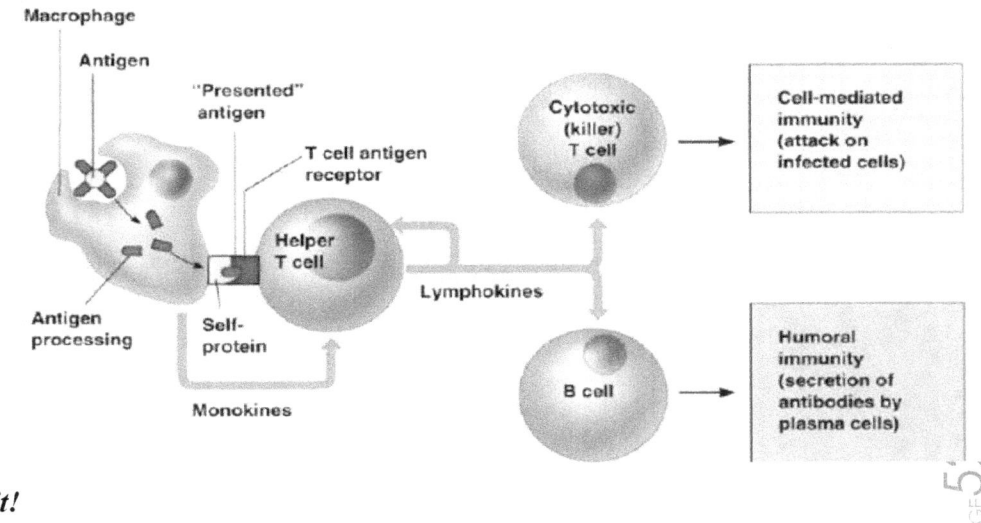

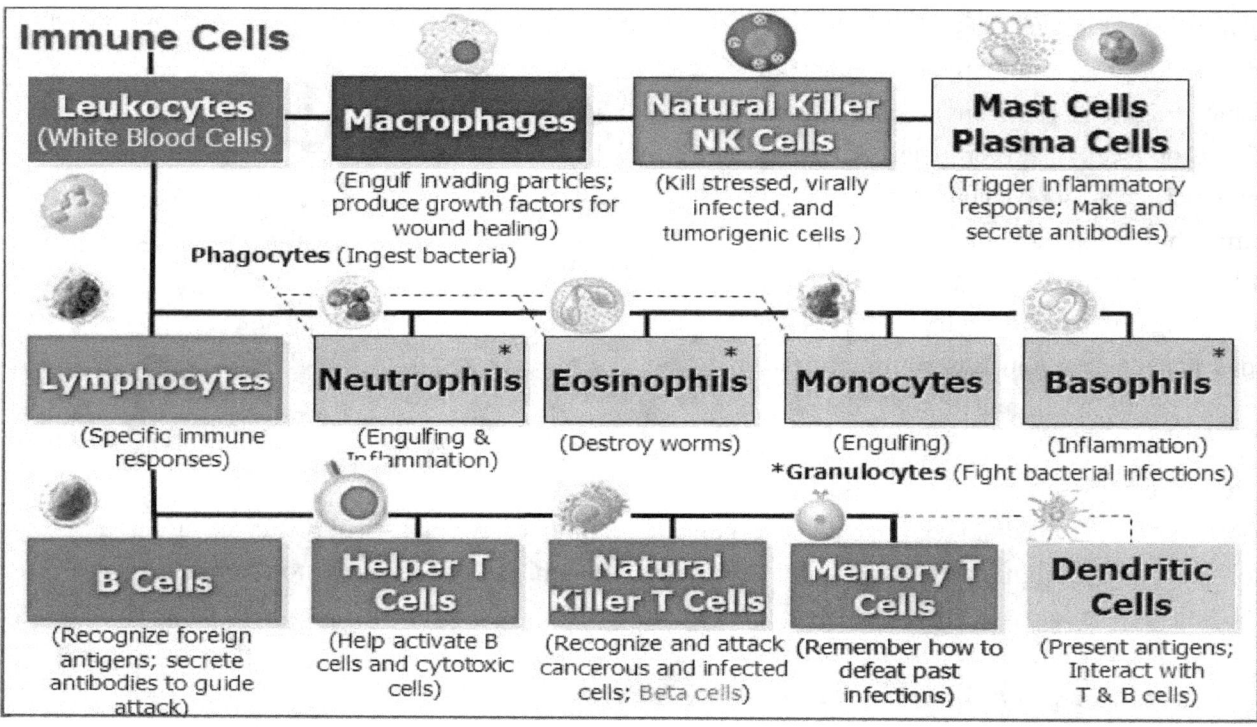

Immune Cells

Leukocytes (White Blood Cells)

Macrophages
(Engulf invading particles; produce growth factors for wound healing)

Natural Killer NK Cells
(Kill stressed, virally infected, and tumorigenic cells)

Mast Cells Plasma Cells
(Trigger inflammatory response; Make and secrete antibodies)

Phagocytes (Ingest bacteria)

Lymphocytes
(Specific immune responses)

Neutrophils *
(Engulfing & Inflammation)

Eosinophils *
(Destroy worms)

Monocytes
(Engulfing)

Basophils *
(Inflammation)

*Granulocytes (Fight bacterial infections)

B Cells
(Recognize foreign antigens; secrete antibodies to guide attack)

Helper T Cells
(Help activate B cells and cytotoxic cells)

Natural Killer T Cells
(Recognize and attack cancerous and infected cells; Beta cells)

Memory T Cells
(Remember how to defeat past infections)

Dendritic Cells
(Present antigens; Interact with T & B cells)

CELL-MEDIATED IMMUNE RESPONSE

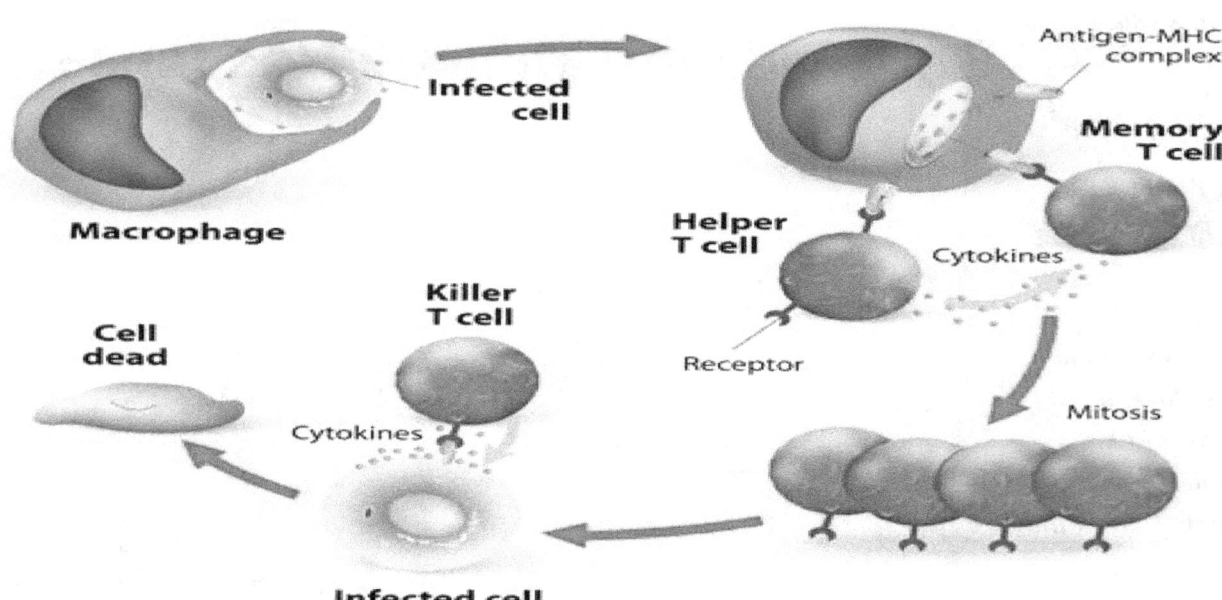

Infected cell

Macrophage

Antigen-MHC complex

Memory T cell

Helper T cell

Cytokines

Receptor

Mitosis

Killer T cell

Cell dead

Cytokines

Infected cell

The Immune System
Our Ultimate Line of Defence

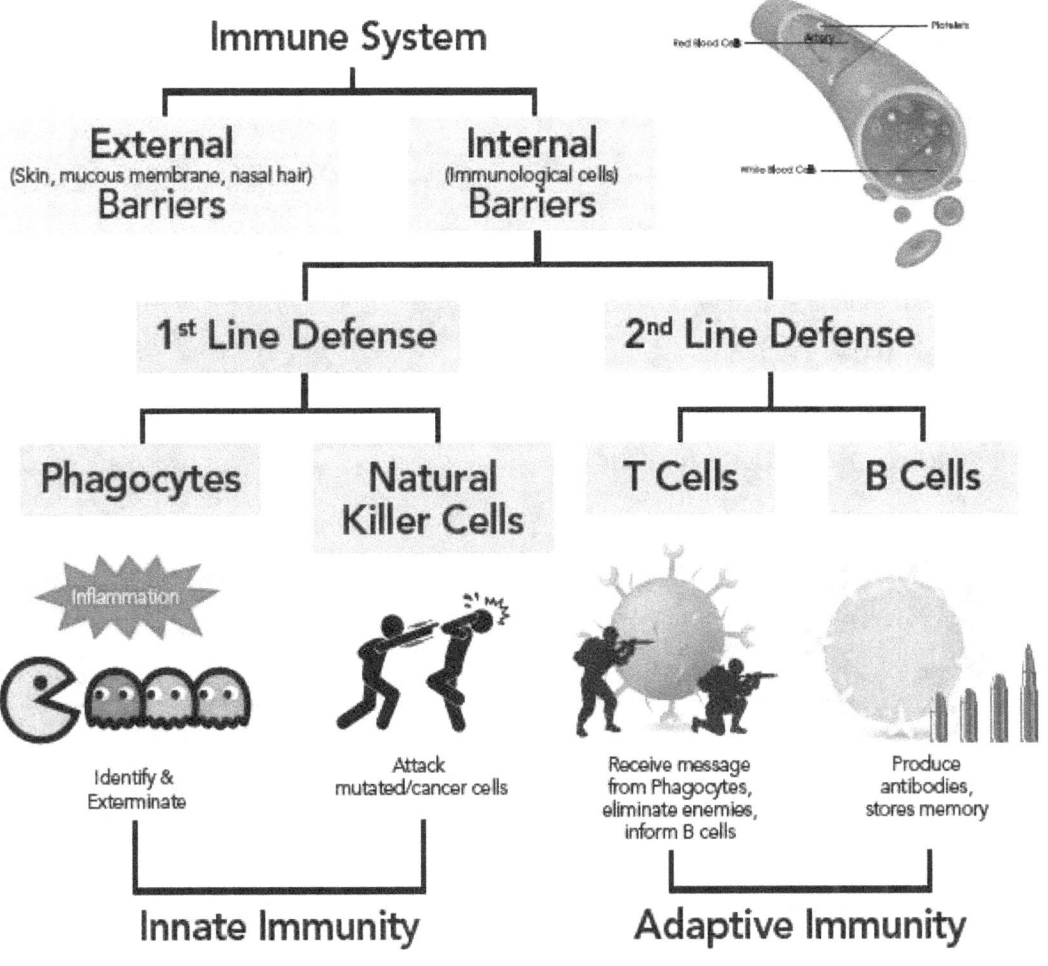

Immune System

External Barriers
(Skin, mucous membrane, nasal hair)

Internal Barriers
(Immunological cells)

Red Blood Cells — Artery — Platelets

White Blood Cells

1st Line Defense

2nd Line Defense

Phagocytes

Natural Killer Cells

T Cells

B Cells

Inflammation

Identify & Exterminate

Attack mutated/cancer cells

Receive message from Phagocytes, eliminate enemies, inform B cells

Produce antibodies, stores memory

Innate Immunity

Adaptive Immunity

Natural Killer Cell

White Blood Cell

Function: These immune cells can recognize and kill the cells of someone's body that have been infected with a pathogen. Natural killer cells can also recognize and destroy tumor cells.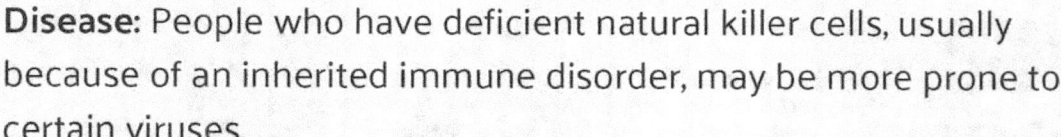

Disease: People who have deficient natural killer cells, usually because of an inherited immune disorder, may be more prone to certain viruses.

Location: Natural killer cells, or NK cells, are present in the blood and can move into other tissues to find targets.

PAGE 55

Supreme Health & Fitness!   Health & Wellness Series Volume 1

i - Capture of EVs by APCs: modulating the immune response

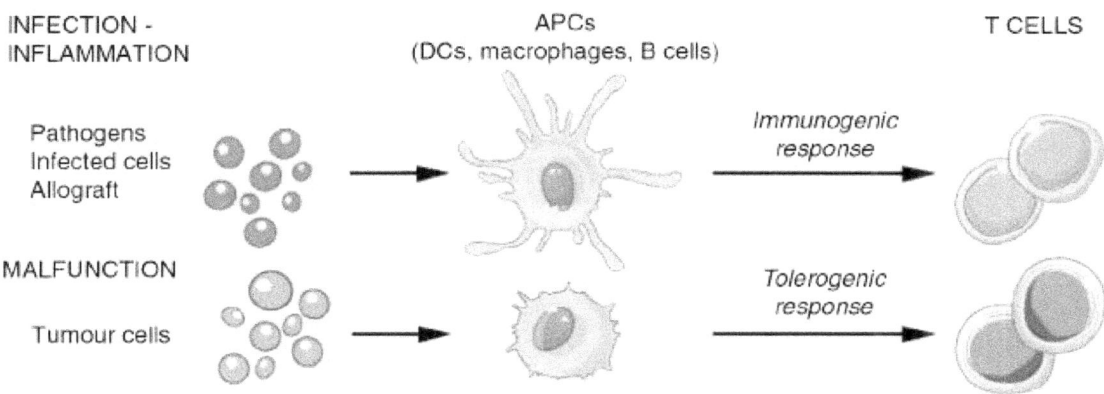

ii - Release of EVs by APCs: another way to present antigens

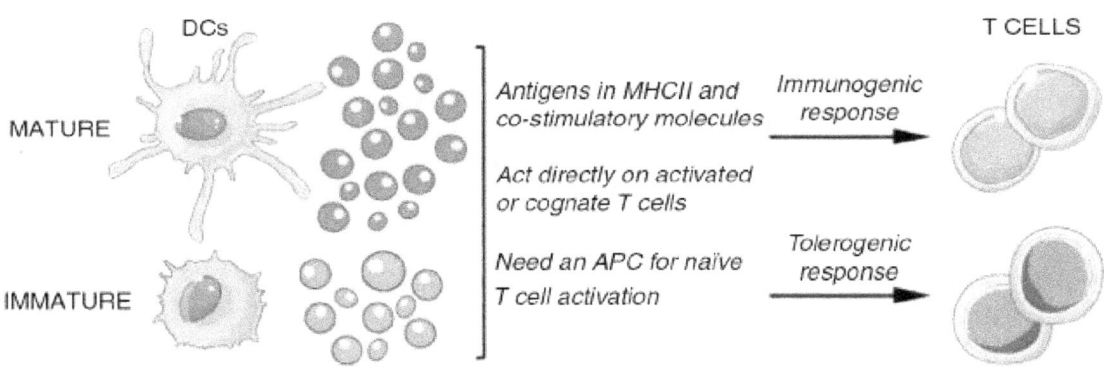

iii - T-cell-derived EVs

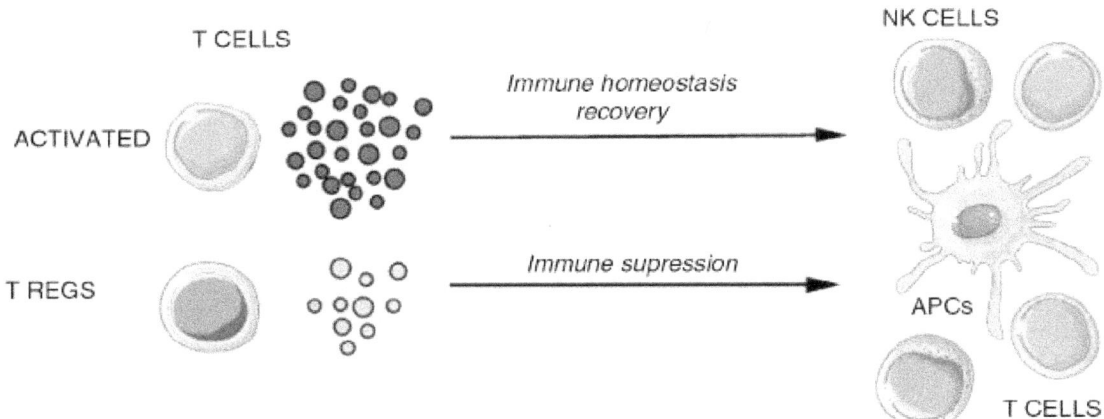

IMMUNE RESPONSE

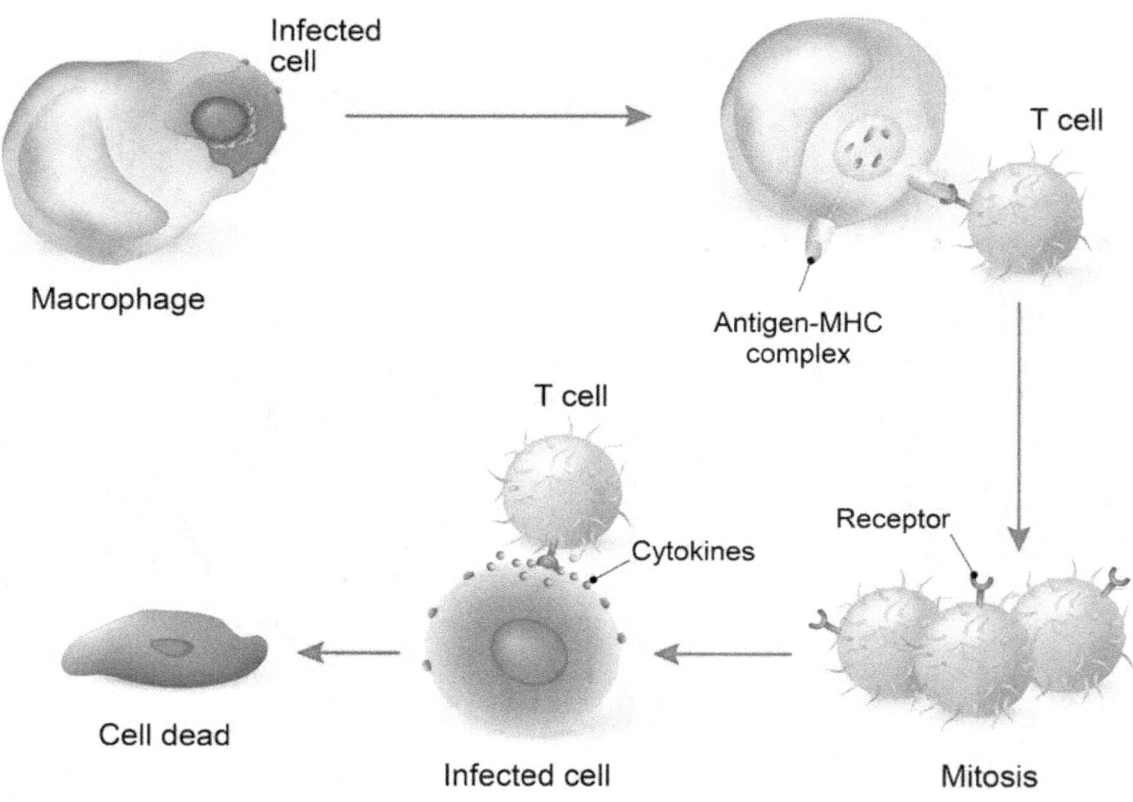

IMMUNE SYSTEM
Skin is the 1st line of defense

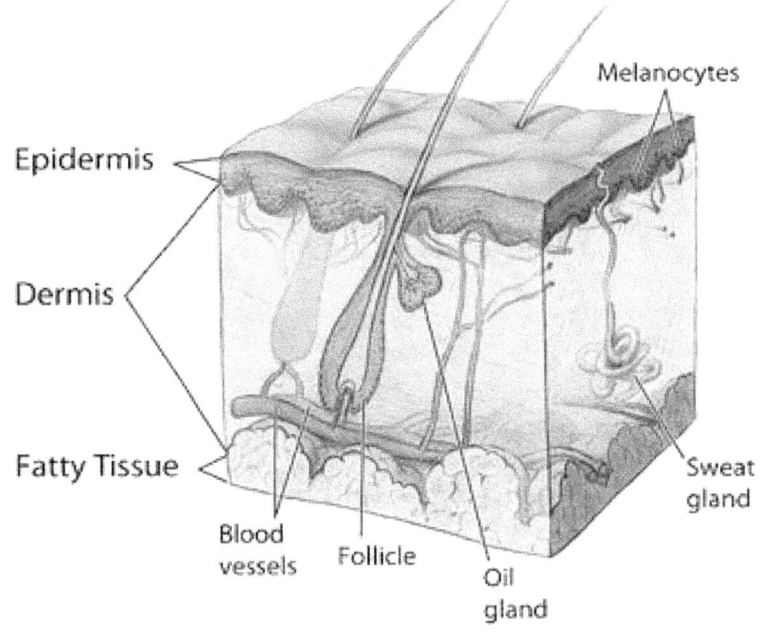

Epidermis

Dermis

Fatty Tissue

Blood vessels

Follicle

Oil gland

Sweat gland

Melanocytes

*****

Chapter 3 ... 1st Line of Defense – Skin Immunity

*****

We can think of GAS as a set of behavioral defenses—activities that the body undertakes to cope with prolonged stresses. In addition, the body has other innate, or inborn, defenses. The most obvious of these is our skin. This outer layer of epithelium is a Cutaneous Membrane that is often called our first line of defense.

The skin is our first line of defense against pathogenic invasions, but mucous membranes also serve as physical barriers against invasion.

The skin functions as a barrier between the body and its external environment, protecting the body from injury by external forces and preventing excessive loss of body fluids. The skin also constitutes a major sense organ; cutaneous sensations of touch, temperature, pressure, and pain are essential to maintain orientation in the environment.

In addition, the skin plays a vital role in regulation of body temperature, both by controlling the amount of blood brought near the surface for heat exchange and through the process of sweating, which lowers skin temperature through vaporization.

1st Line of Defense- Skin and mucous
(The outer wall)

- Skin:

- Made up of 3 layers:

  -Epidermis

  -Dermis

  -Hypodermis

- Includes hair and sweat glands

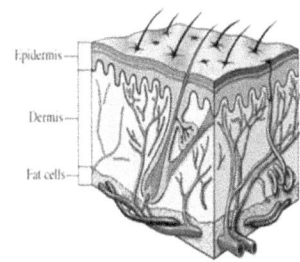

Function: Blocks most microbes from entering the body.

Our Skin is food dependent and sensitive. In fact, our food choices are immediately manifested through our skin – Clear, Smooth, Lubricated and Wrinkle-free Skin ... OR .... Blemished, Spotted, Un-even Skin Tone, Acne-filled Skin.

The strength of defense and ability to resist/fight pathogenic invaders is impaired or boosted by EVERY Liquid or Food we consume.

A Membrane is a simple organ composed of a layer of simple or stratified epithelium supported by connective tissue.

A mucous membrane lines any cavity open to the exterior, including the mouth, digestive, respiratory, urinary, and reproductive tracts. The skin and mucous membranes are physical barriers.

Skin – Primary Physical Barrier

The skin is the largest organ of the human body. It encases the body, protecting it from desiccation (drying out) and preventing the entry of disease-causing microbes.

Histologically, our skin consists of an outer covering of stratified squamous epithelium (**epidermis**); an underlying layer of fibrous connective tissue (**dermis**), which contains the hair follicles, sebaceous and sweat glands, blood vessels, and sensory nerves; and a deep layer of adipose tissue (**subcutis** or subcutaneous tissue).

Sensory receptors in the skin monitor the immediate environment, noting light touch, heavier pressure, and temperature. The skin also has vital homeostatic functions, such as helping the body regulate water content and temperature.

Finally, the skin produces vitamin D, which is necessary for bone growth and development. The skin is composed of a superficial epidermis and a deeper dermis.

The epidermis is composed of stratified squamous epithelium, but most of the cells are dead.

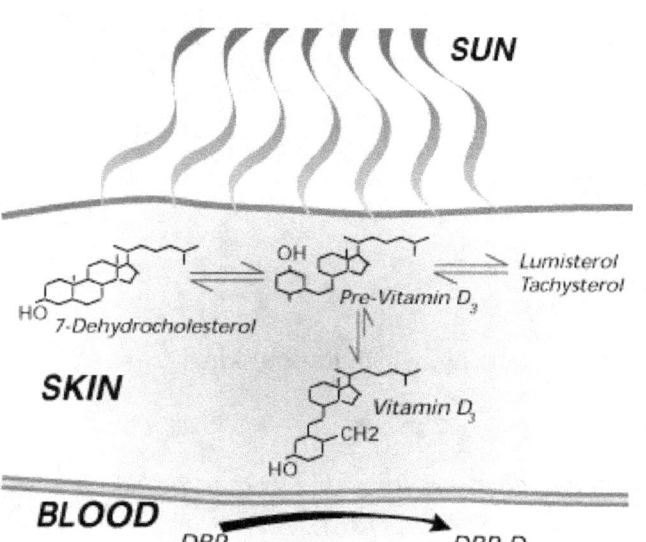

These squamous cells are produced deep within the tissue, in a layer immediately above the dermis.

The epidermis has four major morphologic divisions. The deepest, the **basal layer**, is a single layer of predominantly cuboidal germinative cells that gives rise to all other epidermal cells by mitotic division. The broad middle zone known as the **spinous layer** consists of several layers of keratinocytes undergoing progressive maturation while producing keratin fibrils.

In the **granular layer**, the keratinocytes acquire keratohyaline granules and form rows parallel to the skin surface. These cells eventually die and shed their nucleus to form the outermost layer known as the **cornified layer**.

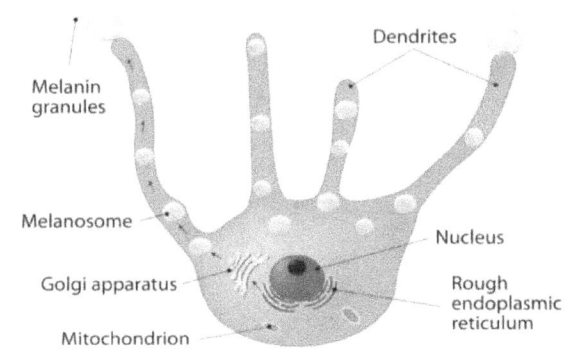

MELANOCYTE

The thickness of this layer varies greatly in different body sites; for example, it is very thick over the palm and fingers and very thin on the eyelid. Scattered throughout the basal layer are larger, pale cells that may contain brown granules.

These cells, called **melanocytes**, are embryologically derived from the neural crest and produce brown **melanin** pigment, which helps protect the skin from sunlight damage and contributes to skin color.

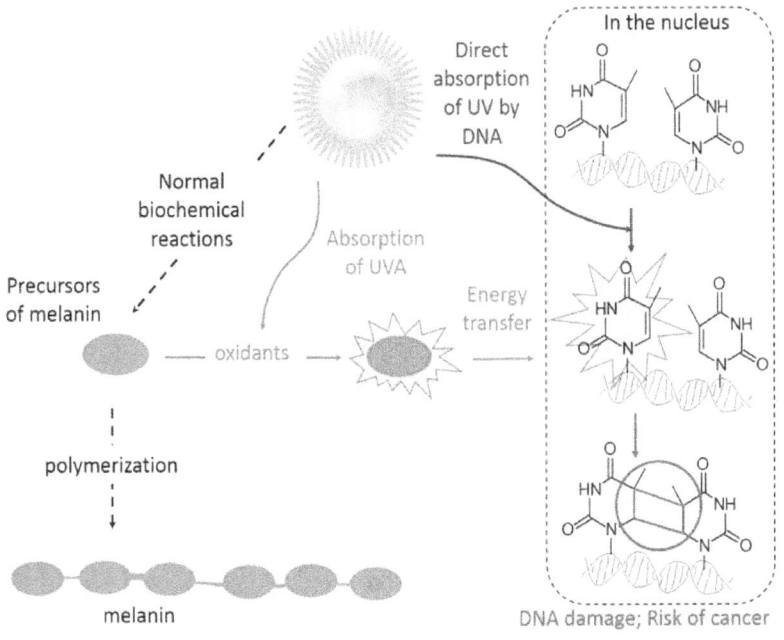

The concentration of melanocytes varies widely, with melanocytes being almost twice as numerous in the genital area as on the back.

Melanin production is increased when the skin is exposed to sunlight.

This is why fair-skinned individuals tan when exposed to sun.

As these cells divide, they continually push the daughter cells upward, away from the nutrient source in the dermis.

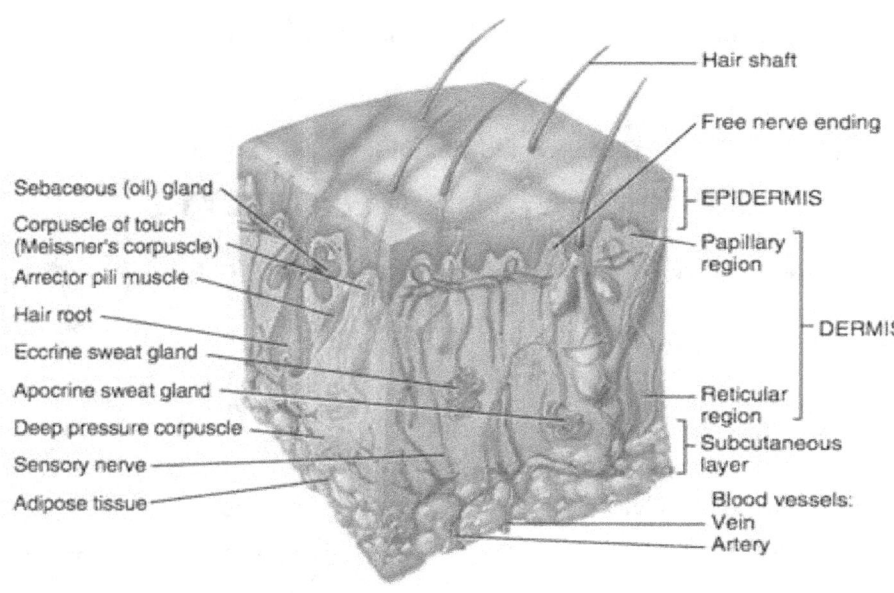

- Hair shaft
- Free nerve ending
- EPIDERMIS
- Papillary region
- DERMIS
- Reticular region
- Subcutaneous layer
- Blood vessels:
- Vein
- Artery

- Sebaceous (oil) gland
- Corpuscle of touch (Meissner's corpuscle)
- Arrector pili muscle
- Hair root
- Eccrine sweat gland
- Apocrine sweat gland
- Deep pressure corpuscle
- Sensory nerve
- Adipose tissue

Because epithelium has no blood supply, the epithelial cells are nourished by capillaries in the upper dermis.

As the epidermal cells are pushed away from these capillaries, the cells weaken and die.

This gradual dying process changes the appearance of the cells, resulting in visible layers in the epidermis.

The **dermis** consists of fibrous tissue intermixed with elastin fibers. The high collagen concentration provides great skin resistance to mechanical force and the elastin allows the skin to return to its normal form after mechanical deformation.

When elastin fibers are destroyed with aging or disease, the skin becomes loose and wrinkled. A gel-like ground substance holds the dermal fibers together.

Eccrine glands are present in the deep dermis over nearly the entire surface of the body. These Eccrine glands are sweat glands that are not connected to hair follicles. They function by

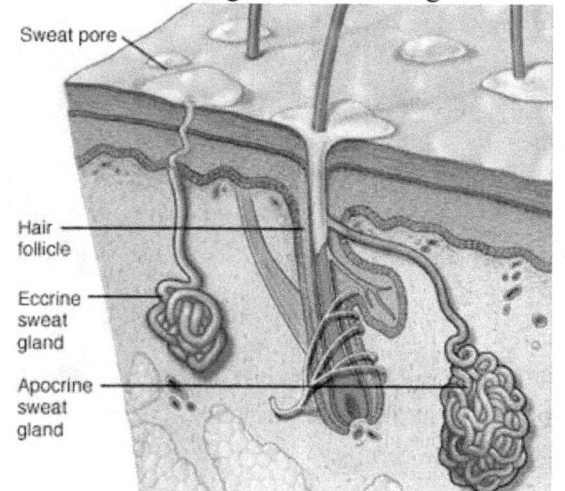

- Sweat pore
- Hair follicle
- Eccrine sweat gland
- Apocrine sweat gland

responding to elevated body temperature due to the environmental heat or physical exercise.

They produce sweat that contains electrolytes and water, which cools the body when it evaporates from the skin. Endocrine glands occur over most of your body and open directly onto the surface of the skin.

These glands are common on the forehead, neck and back. They are also responsible for the moisture that may appear on the palms and soles when a person is emotionally stressed.

Apocrine glands occur in a restricted distribution (axillae, pubis, perineum, periumbilical region, nipples, ear canal, margin of the lips) and produce a sticky proteinaceous and lipid-rich fluid in response to hormonal stimuli. These glands produce sweat that contains proteins and fatty acids, that makes perspiration thicker and more milky.

These Apocrine glands develop in areas abundant in hair follicles, such as armpits and groin, and they empty into the hair follicle just before it open onto the skin surface.

When ecrine glands produce sweat as a cooling system, apocrine glands produce sweat because of anxiety, nervousness or stress. This fluid is odorless until it combines with bacteria founded normally on your skin. Apocrine glands do not become active until we hit puberty.

Apocrine glands are largely dormant until puberty.

With the exception of palms, soles, and portions of the genitalia, the entire body surface is covered by hair.

Individual hairs are produced by division of cells lining the hair follicle. Each hair follicle, or bulb, undergoes recurring cycles of hair growth, regression, and rest. Attached to each hair follicle is a **sebaceous gland**, which secretes lipid-rich sebum.

Sebum waterproofs skin and hair and protects them from dehydration.

Epidermis: The outermost, nonvascular layer of the skin.

Dermis: The underlying, vascularized, connective tissue layer of the skin.

Melanocytes: Cells that produce melanin, a brown, light-absorbing pigment.

GLANDS OF THE SKIN

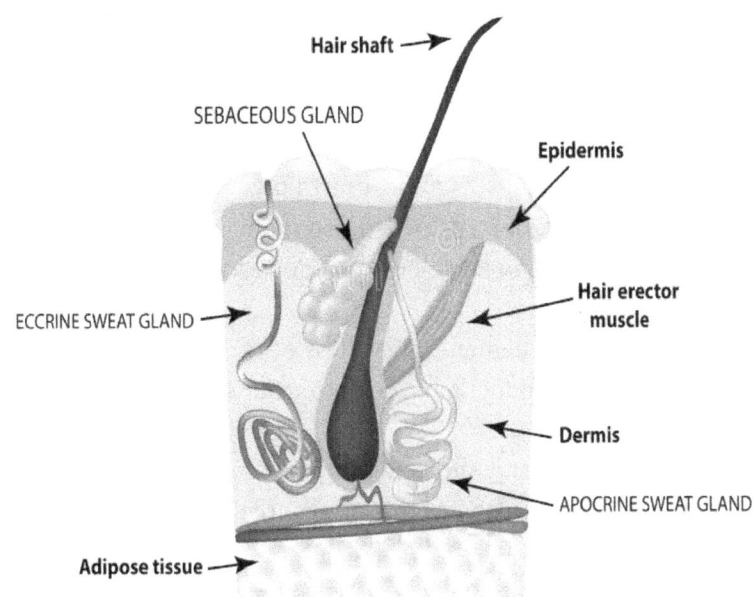

Hair shaft

SEBACEOUS GLAND

Epidermis

ECCRINE SWEAT GLAND

Hair erector muscle

Dermis

APOCRINE SWEAT GLAND

Adipose tissue

PAGE 64

Supreme Health & Fitness!　　　　Health & Wellness Series Volume 1

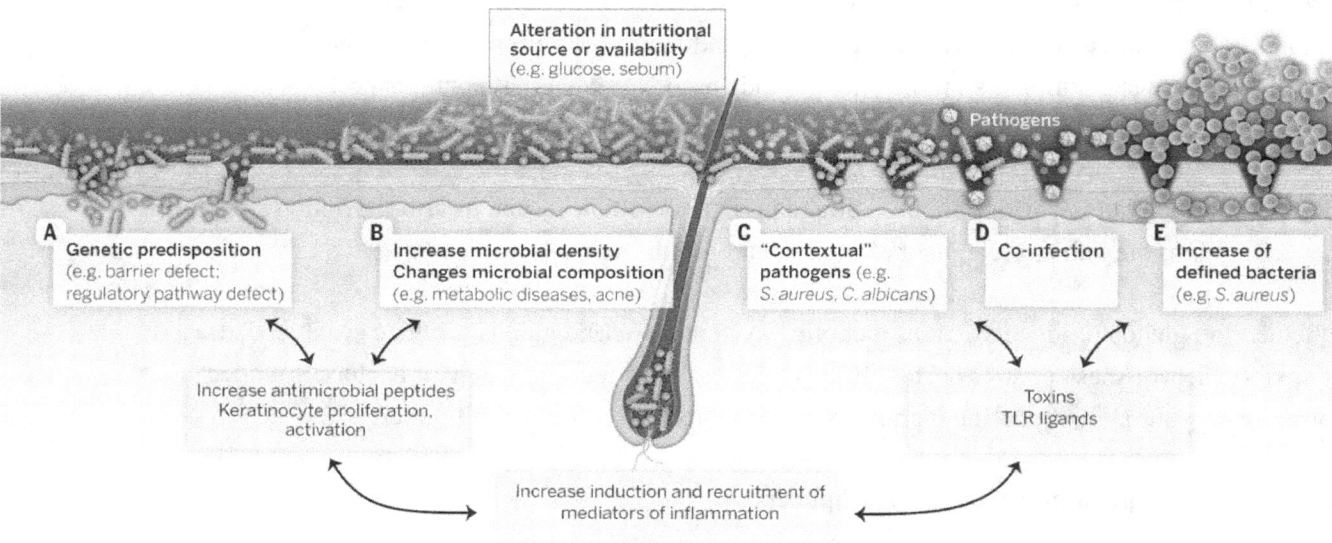

The top layer of the epidermis is composed of dead cells joined by strong cell-to-cell junctions.

The cells are filled with **Keratin**, a waterproof substance that accumulates in the epidermal cells as they progress toward the skin surface. Because of the quantity of keratin held within these cells, they are called **keratinocytes**. This layer of dead keratinocytes provides the skin's nonspecific defense against invasive pathogens. Few pathogens are attracted to dead cells, and keratin repels waterborne pathogens along with water.

Skin color results from the brown pigment melanin, which is produced by melanocytes in the deepest epidermis, demonstrated in the next Figure. UV light stimulates production of a hormone that in turn stimulates the melanocytes to produce more melanin, resulting in a tan.

Interestingly, humans, regardless of race, have the same number of melanocytes; different levels of melanin production account for our different skin colors.

Melanin is a large molecule formed from potentially damaging precursors. It is produced and stored in melanosomes that protect the cell from these dangerous chemicals.

Melanocytes are less active in people with pale skin. In those with dark skin, highly active melanocytes produce lots of melanin, even with low sunlight exposure.

In evolutionary terms, dark skin is an adaptation that protects tropical people from the intense sun. White skin is adaptive closer to the Poles because it allows the entry of enough ultraviolet light to produce vitamin D.

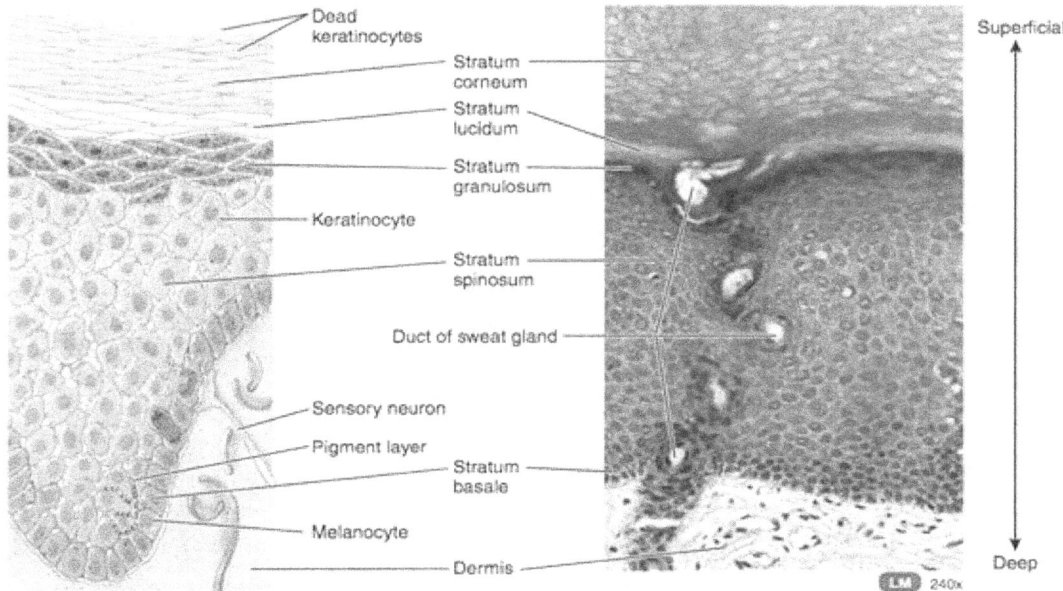

Skin cancer is a concern for anyone who has exposed his or her skin to sunlight. Skin cancer occurs in the epidermis. Skin cancer is common in the United States. In 2012, slightly more than 81,000 Americans were diagnosed with melanoma, the most lethal skin cancer.

The good news is that skin cancer occurs in the obviously visible epidermal cells and is easily detected at an early stage. As with all other cancers, these tumor cells eventually begin to multiply rapidly and uncontrollably.

Skin cancer is related to sun exposure because the ultraviolet radiation in sunlight damages the DNA in skin cells.

Basal Cell Carcinoma (BCC) is the most common cancer in humans, accounting for over 1 million cases per year in the United States. This cancer develops in the basal or deepest cells of the epidermis, usually in places that are routinely exposed to the sun. The appearance can vary, but the tumor is usually a slow-growing, shiny or scaly bump.

A wound that repeatedly heals and opens may be a form of BCC. These cancers rarely metastasize, or spread to other tissues, but dermatologists still recommend that they be removed.

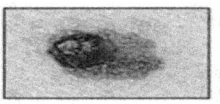

Asymmetry

If you draw a line through this mole, the two halves will not match, meaning it is asymmetrical, a warning sign for melanoma.

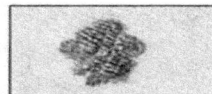

Border

The borders of an early melanoma tend to be uneven. The edges may be scalloped or notched.

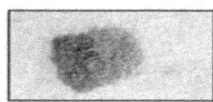

Color

Having a variety of colors is another warning signal. A number of different shades of brown, tan or black could appear. A melanoma may also become red, white or blue.

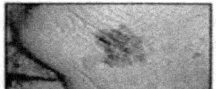

Diameter

Melanomas usually are larger in diameter than the size of the eraser on your pencil (1/4 inch or 6 mm), but they may sometimes be smaller when first detected.

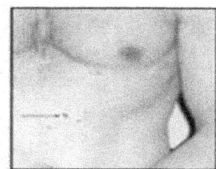

Evolving

When a mole is evolving, see a doctor. Any change — in size, shape, color, elevation, or another trait, or any new symptom such as bleeding, itching or crusting — points to danger.

Squamous Cell Carcinoma (SCC) is a tumor of the upper layers of the skin. These cancers usually develop a crusty or scaly covering and grow rapidly. The threat of metastasis is much higher with SCC than with basal cell carcinoma, so SCC tumors should be removed as soon as possible. Approximately 16% of skin cancer cases are SCC.

Melanomas are the most aggressive skin cancer, rapidly spreading to the lymph nodes and other tissues, but fortunately they comprise only 4% of all diagnosed skin cancers. The cancerous cells are melanocytes—ironically, the same cells that protect us from harmful UV radiation. Cancerous melanocytes divide rapidly and spread to the dermis.

Histology of squamous cell carcinoma

Variable sized groups of atypical
epithelial cells within dermis

Prominent nuclei and
abundant acidophilic
cytoplasm

Keratin 'pearl'

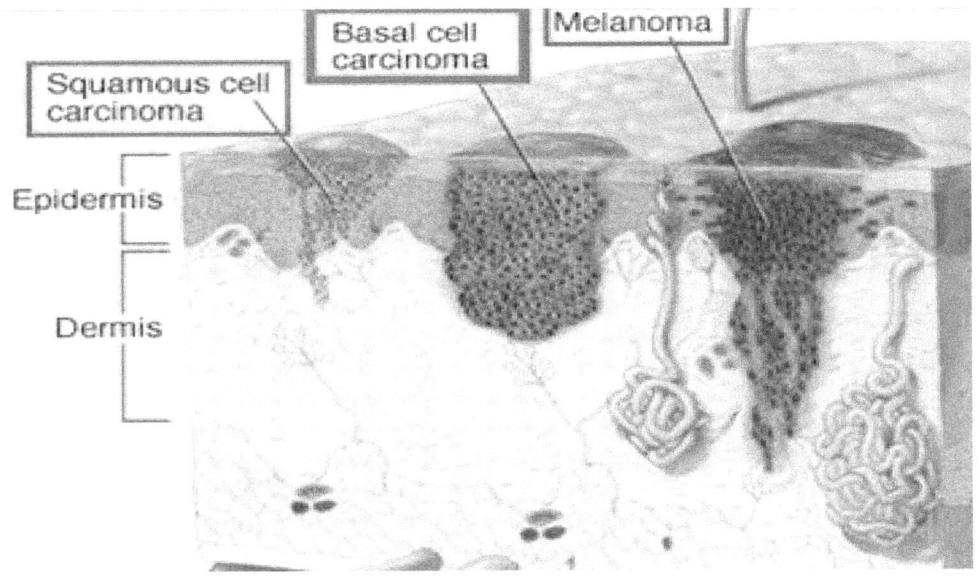

Squamous cell
carcinoma

Basal cell
carcinoma

Melanoma

Epidermis

Dermis

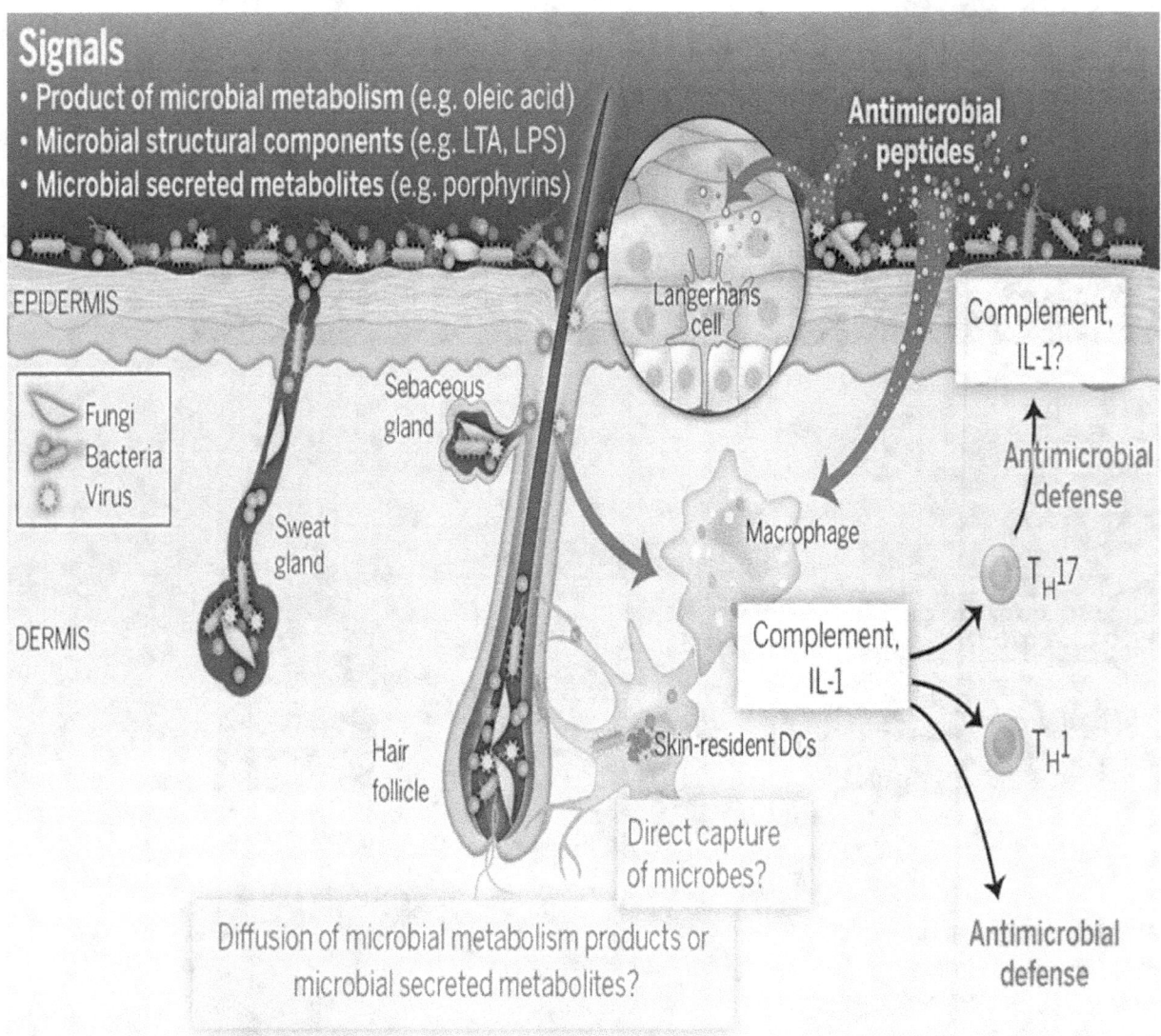

Signals
- Product of microbial metabolism (e.g. oleic acid)
- Microbial structural components (e.g. LTA, LPS)
- Microbial secreted metabolites (e.g. porphyrins)

Antimicrobial peptides

EPIDERMIS

Langerhans cell

Complement, IL-1?

Fungi
Bacteria
Virus

Sebaceous gland

Antimicrobial defense

Sweat gland

Macrophage

T_H17

DERMIS

Complement, IL-1

T_H1

Hair follicle

Skin-resident DCs

Direct capture of microbes?

Antimicrobial defense

Diffusion of microbial metabolism products or microbial secreted metabolites?

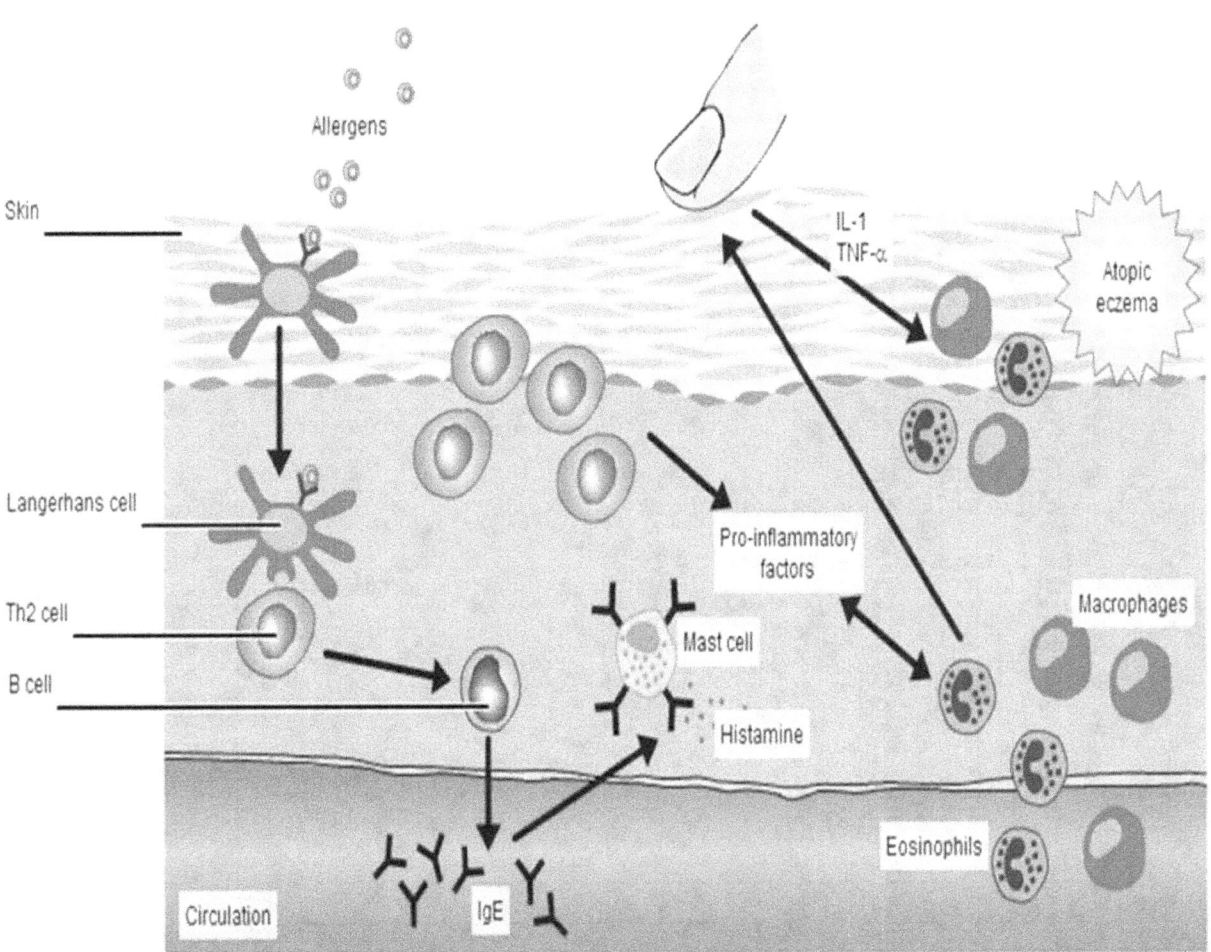

Integumentary System:
Skin and Accessory Organs

- **Accessory Organs**
  - Nails
  - Hair follicles
  - Oil glands
  - Sweat glands

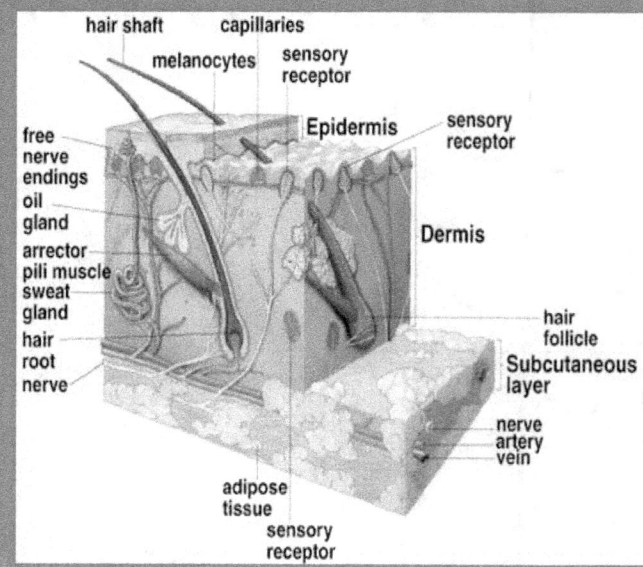

*****

Chapter 4 ... Accessory Organs – Hair, Nails & Glands

*****

The Dermis is the **source** of nutrition for the Epidermal Cells. The **bottom layer** of skin, the Dermis, is composed of loose, irregular Connective Tissue. The dermis has a large blood supply and extensive innervation.

The accessory organs of the skin (hair, glands, and nails) lie in the dermis, as do all of the sensory organs of the skin. Free (ex-posed) nerve endings register the sensation of pain (nociceptors), whereas specialized structures attached to cutaneous nerves respond to light touch and pressure.

- The skin and its accessory organs
  - Sebaceous glands
  - Sudoriferous glands
  - Sensory perceptors
  - Hair
  - Nails

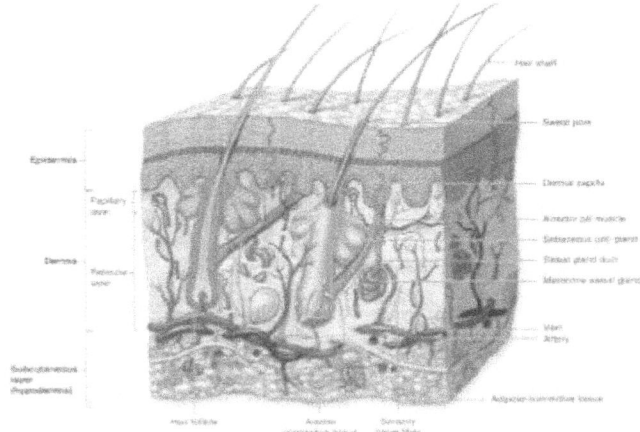

When you put on a shoe in the morning, corpuscles in the skin of your foot register the shoe's pressure. During the day, the pressure from that shoe doesn't change, and you are no longer aware of the presence of your shoes. If the pressure becomes painful, however, pain receptors remind you of your shoes. Because it would be counterproductive to do so, pain receptors do not adapt, so your discomfort will remain until you remove the source of the pain.

PAGE 72

Supreme Health & Fitness!   Health & Wellness Series Volume 1

Nociceptors: Non-adapting pain receptors in the skin (noci = pain).

Accessory Structures ~ Skin Lubrication & Protection

The accessory structures of the skin are the glands, hair, and nails. The glands produce sweat for thermal homeostasis or oils to keep the skin flexible. The hair and nails are protective structures.

Sebaceous Glands

Oil (Sebaceous) glands are found within hair follicles. Oil is secreted onto the hair shaft, helping to keep the hair and surrounding skin supple.

The hormones of puberty increase the output of these glands, often leading to acne, de- fined as a physical change in the skin because of a bacterial infection in the sebaceous glands.

Acne causes the development of lesions, cysts, blackheads, or whiteheads, common terms for various combinations of dirt, infection, and skin oils.

These glands are always associated with hairs, lying next to the hair with their ducts opening directly onto the hair (colored purple in this figure to match the epidermal cells from which they originate). When the hair is moved, oils are secreted from these ducts.

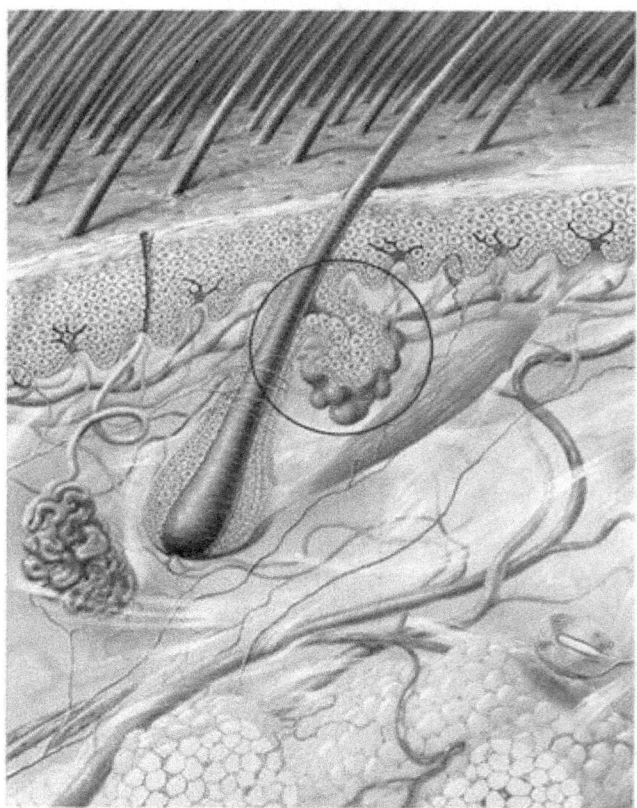

Fortunately, doctors can now treat virtually all types of acne and usually prevent scarring that can follow uncontrolled infections.

Sebaceous glands are located wherever there is hair, as shown in the accompanying Figure. This means we have oil glands everywhere on our bodies except in hairless skin, such as on the lips. The absence of oil glands explains the need for lip balms to alleviate drying and chapping in this oil-less skin.

Sudoriferous Glands

Our skin also plays a crucial role in temperature control. Sweat (Sudoriferous) glands are active in maintaining thermal homeostasis. They are found all over the body, with the exception of the lips and the tip of the penis.

A sweat gland is basically a tube from the surface of the skin into the dermis. At the base of the dermis, the tube coils into a knot. Most sweat glands open to the surface at a pore, with no hair associated.

There are two kinds of sweat glands but merocrine sweat glands are the "true" sweat glands
Sweat is a watery perspiration that helps cool the body
They are the most numerous glands of the skin
Merocrine sweat glands have a coiled duct leading to a sweat pore in the surface
Sweat begins as a protein free filtrate of blood plasma produced by deep secretory portion of the gland
Potassium ions, urea, lactic acids ammonia and some sodium chloride are found in sweat
It's about 99% water with a pH of about 4-6

The larger sweat glands of the axillary region, the groin region, and the areolae of the breasts become active during puberty.

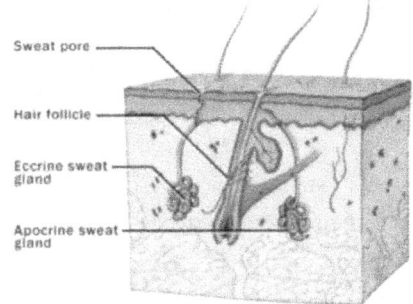

Sweat is produced in response to rising internal temperature. Blood vessels in the dermis dilate, allowing a larger volume of blood to flow from the core of the body to the skin. This blood transports excess heat to the skin, where it activates thermoreceptors that send impulses to the brain to activate the sweat glands.

The blood, having transferred its heat to the skin, returns to the heart somewhat cooler than it was previously.

During average activity, your sweat glands produce approximately a coffee cup (150 mL) of fluid per day. Athletic activity increases this volume tremendously; up to 2.5 liters of fluid per hour can be lost during strenuous activity in hot weather.

In the Tour de France, Lance Armstrong once lost a full 6% of his body weight during a hot, intense, one-hour race. This extreme fluid loss took a toll on his performance and overall health, and Armstrong needed two days to recover.

For optimal performance and general health, endurance athletes must hydrate before and during competition.

PAGE 74

Supreme Health & Fitness!   Health & Wellness Series Volume 1

Hair

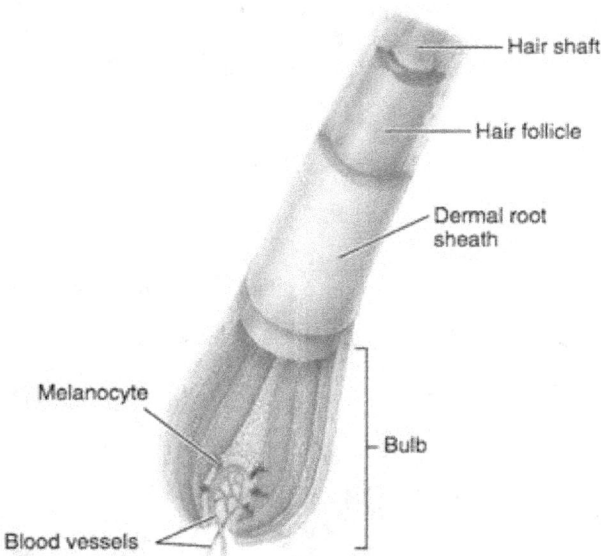

What is hair, and why does it grow where it does? Although we think of hair mainly as the coarse structures projecting from and protecting our head, hair actually covers most of our bodies, including our face, shoulders, back, and belly.

Hair is formed from the division of specialized epidermal cells in the hair follicle, located in the dermis. Just as new epidermal cells push older cells outward, the growing hair shaft pushes older cells away from the blood supply.

Follicle: A small cavity or cul-de-sac; hair originates in a hair follicle.

Hair serves as an insulator as well as protection for the eyes, nostrils, and ear openings. On our heads, hair prevents loss of heat from blood flowing beneath the scalp. On a man's face, hair indicates sexual maturity.

Beyond the epidermis, the hair shaft is composed of dead cells.

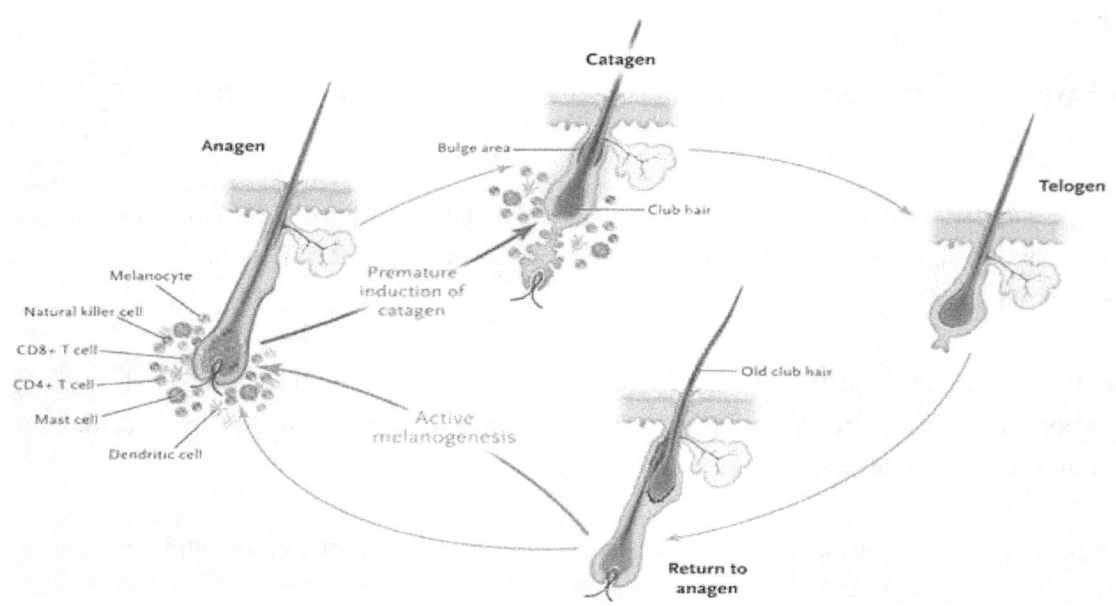

Hair is formed from pockets of epithelium that dive deep into the dermis. The hair follicle produces a hair shaft, composed of epithelial cells arranged in many layers. The innermost layer of the hair shaft contains the pigments that color our hair. The bulb of the hair follicle is what keeps the cells that form the hair shaft alive. Decreasing the blood flow through the bulb results in losing the hair shaft.

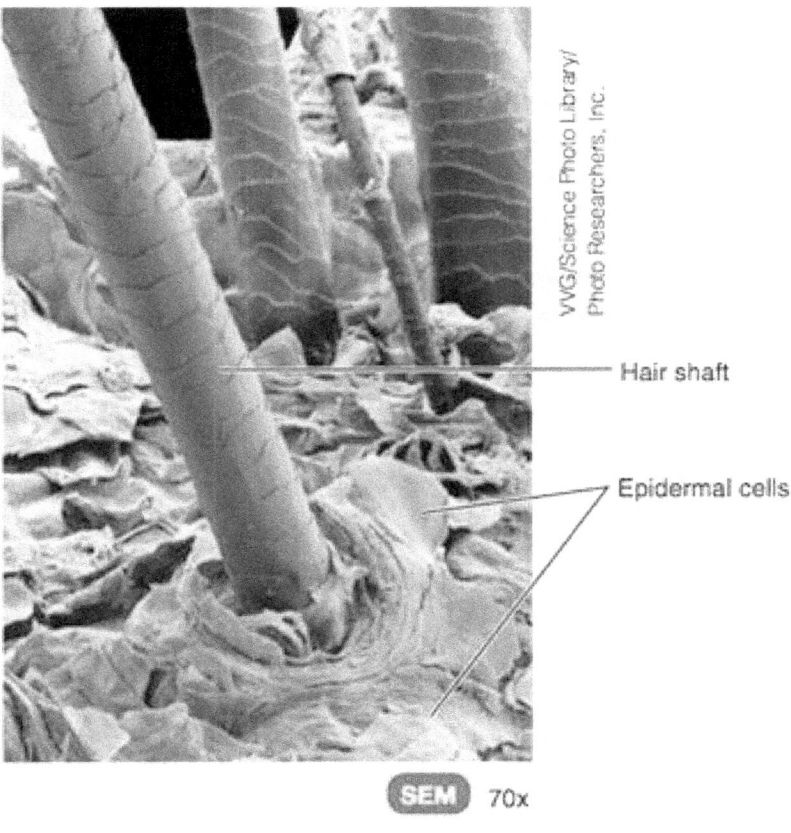

VVG/Science Photo Library/ Photo Researchers, Inc.

Hair shaft

Epidermal cells

SEM 70x

Several hair shafts showing the shingle-like cuticle cells

Nails

Nails are flattened sheets of keratinized cells that protect the ends of the digits, as shown in Figure below. Nails arise from a thick layer of specialized epithelial cells at the nail root called the lunula, located at the base of the nail bed.

The cuticle is a layer of epidermis that covers the base of the nail. Nails protect the ends of the digits from physical damage as we wave them through the environment.

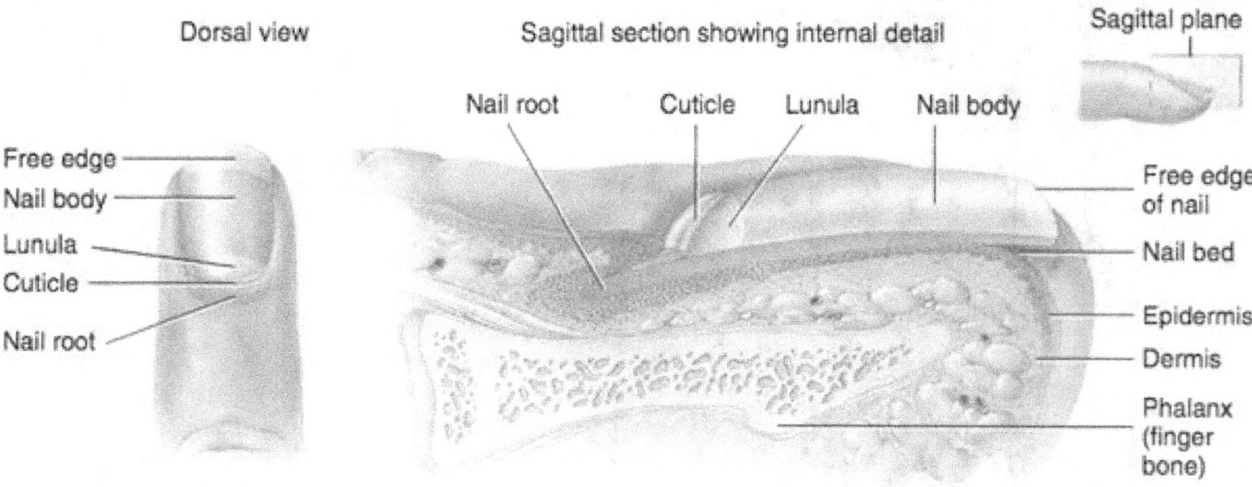

Keratinized: Filled with keratin and therefore waxy.

Physical Barriers

Like the cutaneous membrane, mucous membranes provide nonspecific immunity. This immunity is essential, because mucous membranes line any cavity open to the exterior, including the mouth and digestive tract, the respiratory tract, the urinary tract, and the reproductive tract.

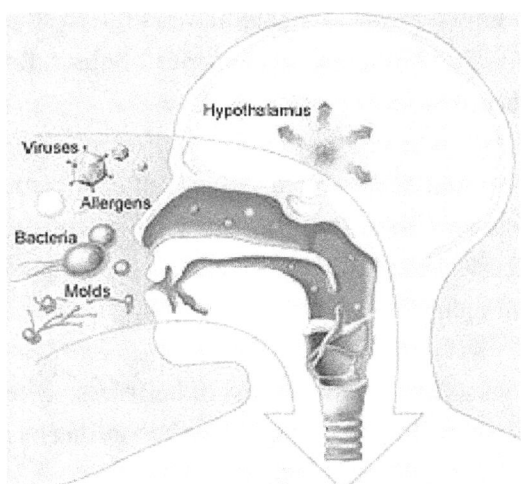

Instead of being covered in keratinized dead cells, these tracts are covered in mucus that retards pathogens.

The mucus, secreted by the epithelial cells of the membrane, constantly washes the membrane. Often, larger volumes of fluid wash these membranes as well. Urine flows across the urinary tract membrane; vaginal secretions flow out of the body across the mucous membranes of the female reproductive tract; and saliva continuously washes the oral cavity.

These "barriers" are among the chemicals that supplement our physical barriers.

Urine, mucus, saliva and our mucous membrane are all food sensitive. In fact, you can immediately notice a change in either while you are in the midst of eating and/or drinking. This change can be a positive – increase in the health and healing value change or negative – decrease in health and healing properties.

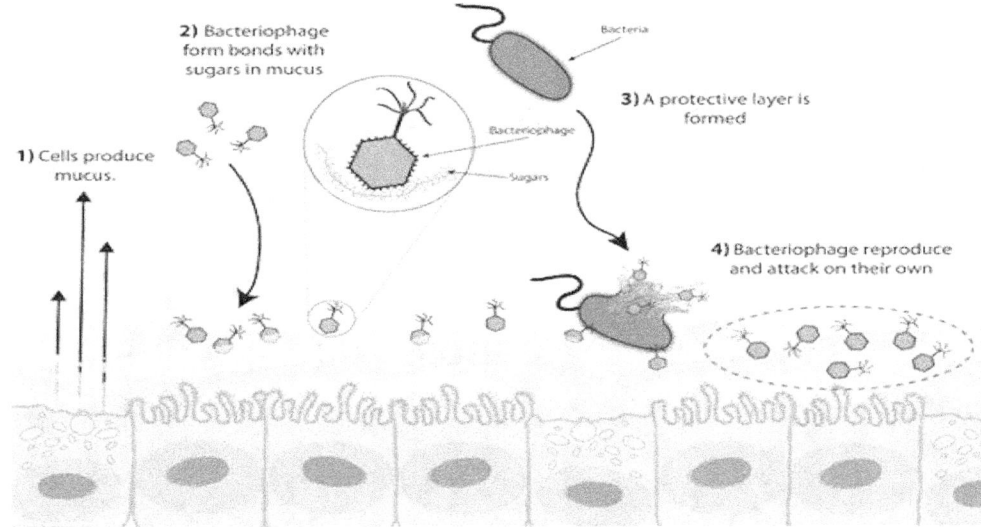

Innate Chemical Barriers Can Also Defeat Pathogens

When the physical innate barriers fail to stop a pathogen, we have another component to the first line of defense: chemical barriers. Sebum forms a protective acidic film over the skin surface that is hostile to many bacteria.

Perspiration, tears, and saliva contain an enzyme called lysozyme, which is a natural antibacterial chemical. The extremely low pH of the stomach (approximately pH 2) is a function of the gastric juices. These fluids, produced by the stomach lining, create an unfriendly environment for many pathogens.

We also have many strains of harmless bacteria that help create a hostile environment for other microbes; for example, the Lactobacillus bacteria in the vagina helps lower pH levels, which in turn kills off certain fungi and bacteria.

The First Line of Defense: Chemical Barriers

- Sweat produced by glands in the skin wash away microbes and their acidity slows bacterial growth.
- Mucous membranes produce sticky mucous that traps many microbes
- Saliva and tears contain an enzyme called lysozyme that kills bacteria by rupturing their cell walls
- Cerumen (ear wax) – produced in the ear canal and protects the canal by trapping dirt and dust particles

PAGE 79

Supreme Health & Fitness!   Health & Wellness Series Volume 1

SPECIALIZED CHEMICAL BARRIERS

Antimicrobial substances

- Both skin and mucous membranes are protected by variety of antimicrobial substances including
  - Lysozyme
    - Enzymes that degrade peptioglycan
    - Found in tears, saliva, blood and phagocytes
  - Peroxidase
    - Found in saliva, body tissues and phagocytes
    - Breaks down hydrogen peroxide to produce reactive oxygen
  - Lactoferrin
    - Sequesters iron from microorganisms
      - Iron essential for microbial growth
    - Found in saliva, some phagocytes, blood and tissue fluids
  - Defensins
    - Antimicrobial peptides inserted into microbial membrane
    - Found on mucous membranes and in phagocytes MyShared

Chemical Barriers

- Enzymes in body fluids provide a chemical barrier to pathogens, and they may include:
  - Interferons are horomone-like peptides and stimulate phagocytosis
  - Defensins are peptides produced by neutrophils and other granulocytes. They cripple microbes.
  - Collectins are proteins with broad protection against bacteria, yeast and some viruses
  - Complement is a group of proteins in plasma and other body fluids that stimulate inflammation, attract phagocytes and enhance phagocytosis

Epithelial Chemical Barriers

- Epithelial membranes produce protective chemicals that destroy microorganisms

  - Skin acidity (pH of 3 to 5) inhibits bacterial growth

  - Sebum contains chemicals toxic to bacteria

  - Stomach mucosae secrete concentrated HCl and protein-digesting enzymes

  - Saliva and lacrimal fluid contain lysozyme

  - Mucus traps microorganisms that enter the digestive and respiratory systems

4

Supreme Health & Fitness!   Health & Wellness Series Volume 1

PAGE 81

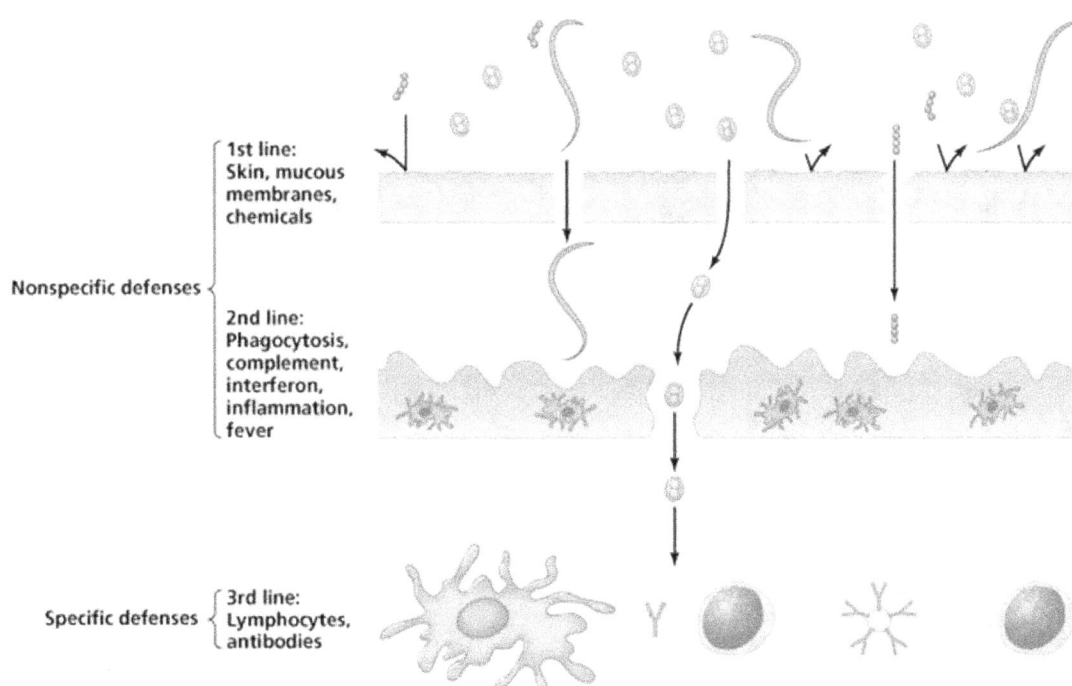

Nonspecific defenses

1st line:
Skin, mucous membranes, chemicals

2nd line:
Phagocytosis, complement, interferon, inflammation, fever

Specific defenses

3rd line:
Lymphocytes, antibodies

Specific vs. Nonspecific Immunity

Nonspecific

- Does not require any adaptation.

- We are born with these responses.

- The defenses are general (they can attack lots of different antigens).

- Act immediately, do not require time to develop.

Specific

- We "learn" these defenses via exposure to antigens.

- The defenses are meant for only one antigen.

- Takes time to build up in system, and may decrease over time with no repeat exposure.

Immune system responses to pathogens

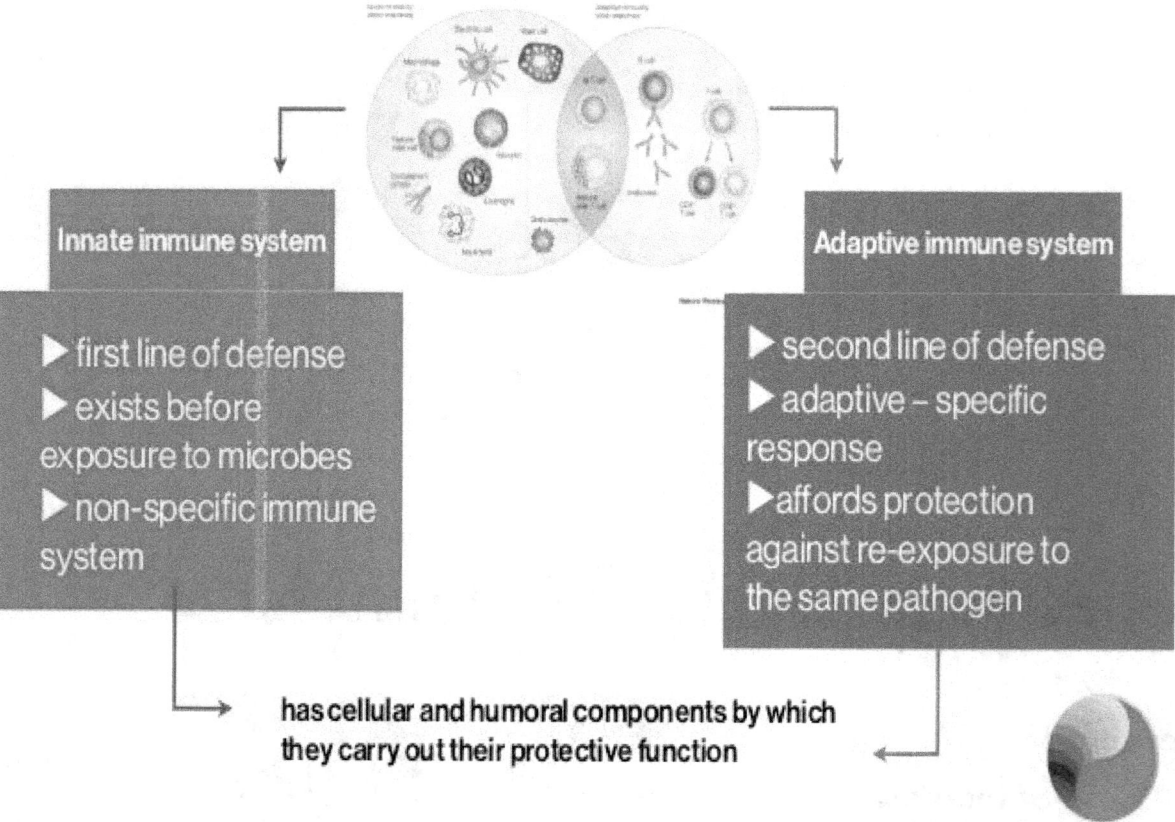

Innate immune system

▶ first line of defense
▶ exists before exposure to microbes
▶ non-specific immune system

Adaptive immune system

▶ second line of defense
▶ adaptive – specific response
▶ affords protection against re-exposure to the same pathogen

has cellular and humoral components by which they carry out their protective function

Immunity – Three Lines of Defense

- **First Line – keep pathogens <u>out</u>!**

  - HOW? Skin, Mucus, Tears (+ Lysozyme), cilia, HCl in stomach to kill bacteria, "good" symbiotic bacteria

- **Second Line – oh no, something <u>got in</u>, start pitchin' a general defense**

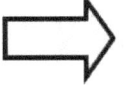

  - HOW? Phagocytes, Interferons, Complement, Histamines (red, hot, swollen), inflammatory response

Third Line – very specific <u>immune response</u> to a particular antigen

  - HOW? Macrophages, Helper T cells, B-cells, antibodies, Killer T cells

PAGE 84

Supreme Health & Fitness!   Health & Wellness Series Volume 1

\

Chapter 5 ... 2nd Line – Defense Nonspecific Immunity

*****

Despite our "fortress wall" of Skin, Mucous Membranes, and Chemical barriers, Bacteria and other Pathogens can often enter the body and cause Homeostatic **imbalances**. When this happens, we have a second line of Nonspecific defense— internal innate defenses. As with the first line of defense, these innate defenses still destroy pathogens without distinguishing between—or even recognizing—them. That is why we label them nonspecific. These nonspecific internal innate defenses include protective or antimicrobial proteins, fever, inflammation, and phagocytes.

Antimicrobial Proteins – Part of our Internal Innate Defense

One nonspecific internal defense against bacteria is called the complement system, as shown in accompanying Figure. This series of chemical reactions brings together a group of proteins that are usually floating freely in the plasma. These proteins are stacked in a specific order to create a "complement" of proteins that functions like an antibacterial missile.

When a bacterial invasion is encountered, the complement complex assembles, attaches to the bacterial walls, and impales the cell with the protein complex.

When bacteria are discovered in the body, the complement cascade is activated. These free-floating plasma proteins are brought together to form structures that pierce the bacterial wall, destroying it. (Key Process: Osmosis/diffusion)

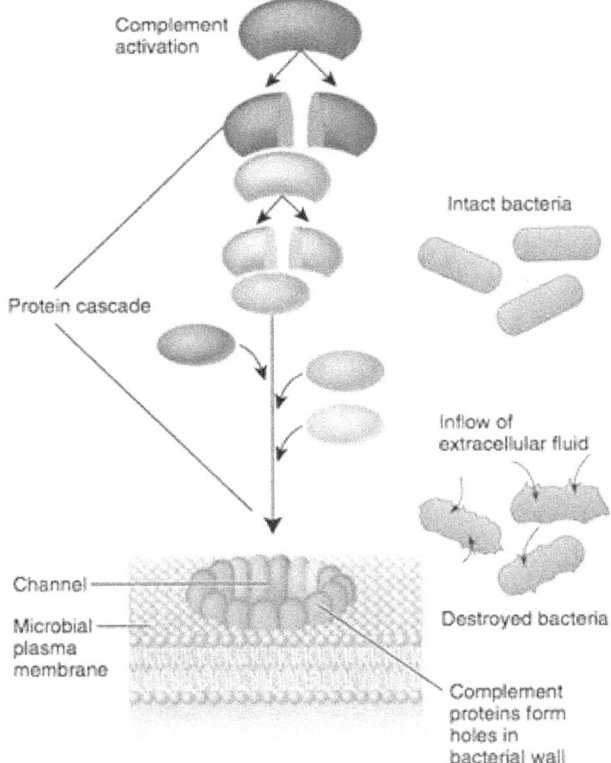

Complement activation

Intact bacteria

Protein cascade

Inflow of extracellular fluid

Destroyed bacteria

Channel

Microbial plasma membrane

Complement proteins form holes in bacterial wall

With the bacterial wall breached, osmotic pressure forces water into the bacterium, destroying its chemistry and killing it.

The complement system is effective against bacteria but not viruses. When cells are infected with a virus, another defensive protein response is needed. The chemical answer to viral infection is interferon, as illustrated in the Figure below.

Interferon is a "local" hormone that is secreted to affect nearby cells. It is a chemical warning, similar to the tornado warning sirens of the Midwest or the tsunami warnings in coastal communities. When cells detect interferon in the extracellular fluid, they prepare for viral invasion. Ideally, the viral infection can then be limited to a small area, allowing it to run its course with little effect on overall body functioning.

Cells produce interferon to help ward off a viral infection.
(Key Process: Osmosis/diffusion)

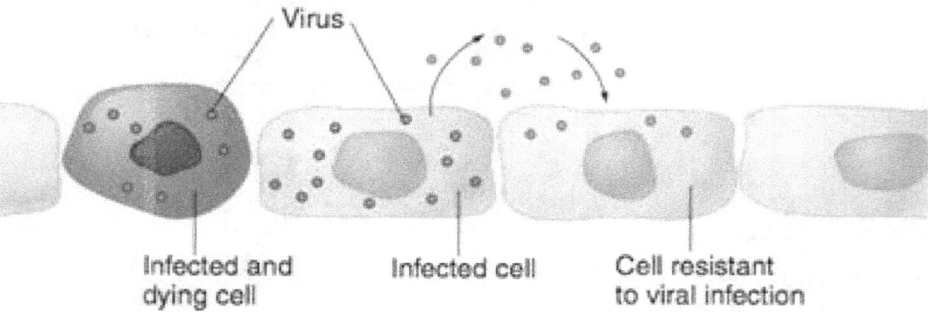

Additionally, some body cells assist in the internal innate defense system. Keratinocytes of the epidermis and both macrophages and neutrophils secrete antimicrobial peptides.

These peptides are small proteins that are effective against bacterial infection. In the laboratory, these cells secrete their defense peptide when they come into contact with viruses or fungi, too. The skin cells secrete antimicrobial proteins in response to bacterial invasion during wound healing.

Neutrophils and macrophages wander blood and tissues, phagocytosing pathogens and debris. These two cells not only remove pathogens directly, they also secrete an antimicrobial compound to aid in ridding the body of infection.

PAGE 87

Supreme Health & Fitness!   Health & Wellness Series Volume 1

Fever Harms Pathogens Directly and Indirectly

Fever is defined as a change in the body's temperature set point, resulting in an elevation in basal body temperature above 37.0°C (98.6°F). Proteins called pyrogens reset the body's thermostat to a higher temperature. Fever may harm the pathogen directly, but more likely it aids defensive mechanisms by raising the metabolic rate.

For every 1°C rise in body temperature, your metabolic rate increases by 10%. At elevated temperatures, enzymes and repair processes work faster, cells move more quickly, and specific immune cells are mobilized more rapidly.

In addition, your spleen sequesters (holds) more iron at higher temperatures, which many bacteria require to reproduce.

Fever

- **When a local response is not enough**
  - system-wide response to infection
  - activated macrophages release <u>interleukin-1</u>
    - triggers <u>hypothalamus in brain</u> to readjust body thermostat to raise body temperature
  - higher temperature helps defense
    - inhibits bacterial growth
    - stimulates phagocytosis
    - speeds up repair of tissues
    - causes liver & spleen to store iron, reducing blood iron levels
      - bacteria need large amounts of iron to grow

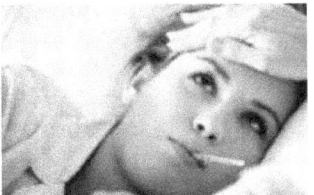

Fever elevates your basal metabolic rate, increasing your use of energy. Unless you replenish your energy supplies, you will tire quickly, which will increase the homeostatic imbalance created by the pathogen.

Ensuring proper nutrition will aid in the recovery process by providing nutrients necessary for the functioning of the immune cells, whereas not eating correctly may deplete your reserves and give the pathogen the upper hand.

Inflammation Is Localized Fever

Inflammation is similar to fever in its goal, but it is a localized, not whole-body, method for increasing enzyme function. In situ (in place) swelling, redness, heat, and pain are associated with inflammation.

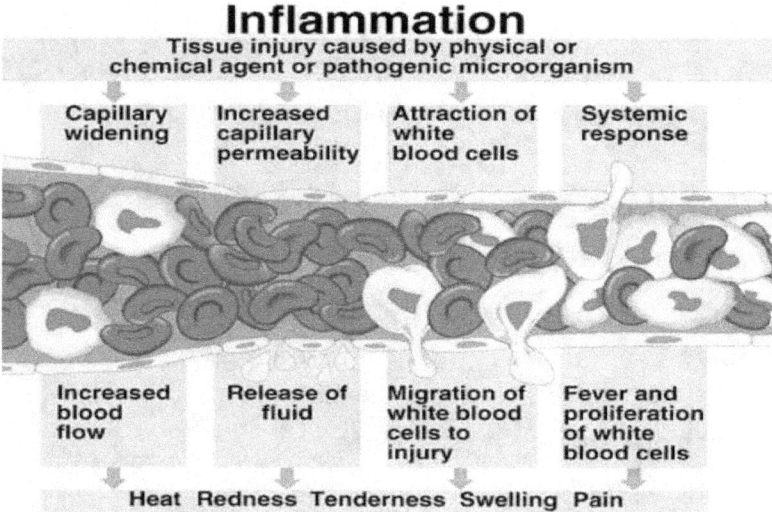

Inflammation
Tissue injury caused by physical or chemical agent or pathogenic microorganism

| Capillary widening | Increased capillary permeability | Attraction of white blood cells | Systemic response |

| Increased blood flow | Release of fluid | Migration of white blood cells to injury | Fever and proliferation of white blood cells |

Heat Redness Tenderness Swelling Pain

Damaged or irritated cells release prostaglandins, proteins, and potassium, which trigger inflammation when released into the interstitial fluid.

Mast cells, found in most tissues, release histamines that encourage blood flow to the damaged area and promote fluid buildup.

The benefits of inflammation include temporary tissue repair, blockage of continued pathogen entry, slowing of pathogen spreading, and quicker repair of the damaged tissue.

The redness associated with inflammation of the skin indicates extra blood flow to the capillaries, bringing immune-system cells and various compounds to injured or diseased tissues.

Inflammation can be triggered by many factors, including pathogen entry, tissue abrasion, chemical irritation, or even extreme temperature.

For example, mosquito bites stimulate inflammation in almost everyone. The red, hot, itchy welt actually represents a local inflammation resulting from the lady mosquito's poor table manners. As she completes her meal and withdraws her proboscis, she spits into the skin, releasing cellular debris and salivary chemicals that initiate an inflammatory response.

PAGE 89

Supreme Health & Fitness!   Health & Wellness Series Volume 1

Phagocytes – Cell Eaters

Phagocytes are a final nonspecific defense for dealing with stressors. Phagocytes are cells that protect the body by ingesting (phagocytosing) harmful foreign particles, bacteria, and dead or dying cells. Their name comes from the Greek ***phagein*** - "to eat" or "**devour**", and "-***cyte***", the suffix in biology denoting "**cell**", from the Greek ***kutos*** - "**hollow vessel**".

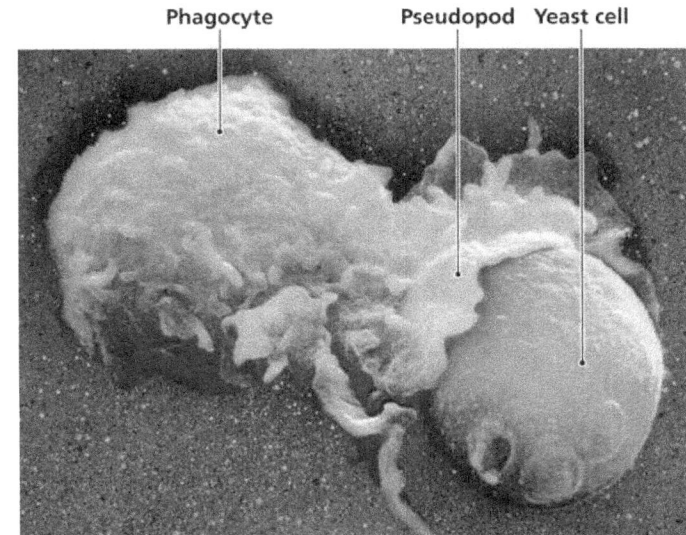

Phagocyte   Pseudopod   Yeast cell

Phagocytes, therefore, are eating cells, or cells that wander through the tissues, engulfing and removing anything that does not belong there.

Phagocytes, which are our 1st cellular line of defense against pathogens, remove all dead or dying cells, cellular debris, and foreign material. This "**clean sweep**" action classifies them as a nonspecific defense.

Phagocytes of humans and other animals are called "professional" or "non-professional" depending on how effective they are at phagocytosis. The professional phagocytes include many types of white blood cells (such as neutrophils, monocytes, macrophages, mast cells, and dendritic cells).

During an infection, chemical signals attract phagocytes to places where the pathogen has invaded the body. These chemicals may come from bacteria or from other phagocytes already present. The phagocytes move by a method called chemotaxis.

When phagocytes come into contact with bacteria, the receptors on the phagocyte's surface will bind to them. This binding will lead to the engulfing of the bacteria by the phagocyte. Some phagocytes kill the ingested pathogen with oxidants and nitric oxide.

After phagocytosis, macrophages and dendritic cells can also participate in antigen presentation, a process in which a phagocyte moves parts of the ingested material back to its surface.

This material is then displayed to other cells of the immune system.

Some phagocytes then travel to the body's lymph nodes and display the material to white blood cells called lymphocytes. This process is important in building immunity and many pathogens have evolved methods to evade attacks by phagocytes.

Microphages are quite small and are mainly found in the nervous system. Macrophages are large, actively patrolling cells. They arise from blood cells and travel through every tissue looking for foreign material.

Some tissues have resident, or "**fixed**," macrophages, whereas other tissues get patrols of wandering macrophages passing through, like security guards making the rounds at a mall.

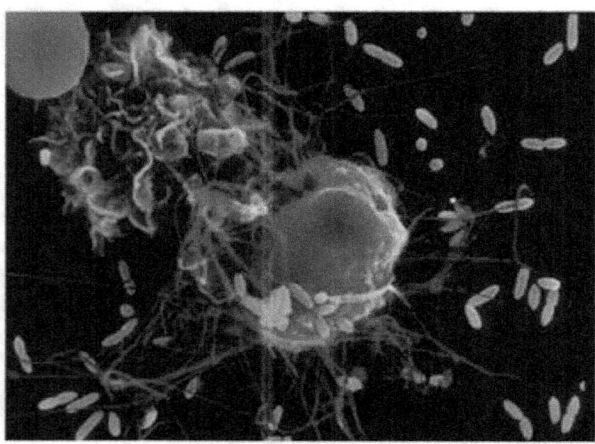

Both microphages and macrophages are attracted to pathogens and damaged cells via chemical messengers. Once they locate a pathogen or damaged cell, they surround, engulf, and destroy it. Some phagocytes are capable of continuous removal of pathogens and cellular debris, whereas others have a limit on how much they can ingest. Once they reach that limit, the phagocytes die and must be removed. Pus is actually dead phagocytes, filled with cellular debris from the wound they were helping to clean. In this colorized micrograph, the macrophage is blue, the bacteria are golden, and a damaged cell is seen in green.

Neutrophils are white blood cells that are among the first phagocytes to arrive at any damaged tissue. As they begin to clean the area, they recruit macrophages to join. Sometimes, this is all it takes to rid the body of an impending infection.

Activation of Phagocytes

All phagocytes, and especially macrophages, exist in degrees of readiness. Macrophages are usually relatively dormant in the tissues and proliferate slowly. In this semi-resting state, they clear away dead host cells and other non-infectious debris and rarely take part in antigen presentation. But, during an infection, they receive chemical signals—usually interferon gamma—which increases their production of MHC II molecules and which prepares them for presenting antigens. In this state, macrophages are good antigen presenters and killers.

PAGE 91

Supreme Health & Fitness!   Health & Wellness Series Volume 1

However, if they receive a signal directly from an invader, they become "hyperactivated", stop proliferating, and concentrate on killing. Their size and rate of phagocytosis increases—some become large enough to engulf invading protozoa.

In the blood, neutrophils are inactive but are swept along at high speed. When they receive signals from macrophages at the sites of inflammation, they slow down and leave the blood. In the tissues, they are activated by cytokines and arrive at the battle scene ready to kill.

Neutrophil

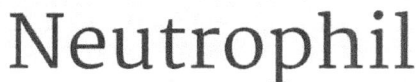

White Blood Cell

Function: Neutrophils engulf and destroy bacteria and other pathogens. They are the most abundant type of white blood cell in most people's bloodstreams and play a large role in fighting many types of infection.

Disease: Because of genetic anomalies, some people are born with too few neutrophils, a condition known as neutropenia, or with neutrophils that do not function properly. This causes people to be more prone to infections.

Location: Neutrophils circulate in the blood and quickly move to sites of infection or injury to fight off pathogens.

Migration of Phagocytes

Neutrophils move from the blood to the site of infection

When an infection occurs, a chemical "SOS" signal is given off to attract phagocytes to the site. These chemical signals may include proteins from invading bacteria, clotting system peptides, complement products, and cytokines that have been given off by macrophages located in the tissue near the infection site. Another group of chemical attractants are cytokines that recruit neutrophils and monocytes from the blood.

To reach the site of infection, phagocytes leave the bloodstream and enter the affected tissues. Signals from the infection cause the endothelial cells that line the blood vessels to make a protein called selectin, which neutrophils stick to on passing by. Other signals called vasodilators loosen the junctions connecting endothelial cells, allowing the phagocytes to pass through the wall. Chemotaxis is the process by which phagocytes follow the cytokine "scent" to the infected spot.

Neutrophils travel across epithelial cell-lined organs to sites of infection, and although this is an important component of fighting infection, the migration itself can result in disease-like symptoms.

PAGE 92

Supreme Health & Fitness!   Health & Wellness Series Volume 1

An example is like a person feels when they have a 'cold'. They aren't 'sick', they are actually feeling the effects of the Neutrophils and other Immune defense mechanisms FIXING them.

During an infection, millions of neutrophils are recruited from the blood, but they die after a few days.

PHAGOCYTOSIS

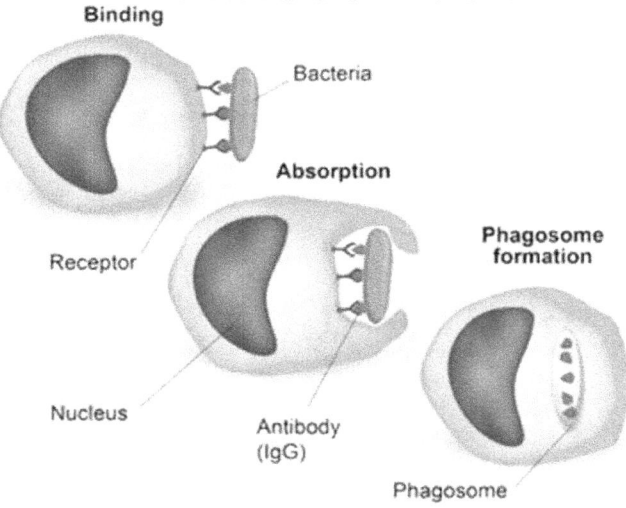

Binding

Bacteria

Receptor

Absorption

Nucleus

Antibody
(IgG)

**Phagosome
formation**

Phagosome

Phagocytes

This is a group of immune cells specialized in finding and "eating" bacteria, viruses, and dead or injured body cells. There are three main types, the granulocyte, the macrophage, and the dendritic cell.

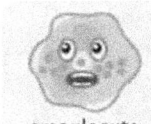

granulocyte

The granulocytes often take the first stand during an infection. They attack any invaders in large numbers, and "eat" until they die. The pus in an infected wound consists chiefly of dead granulocytes. A small part of the granulocyte community is specialized in attacking larger parasites such as worms.

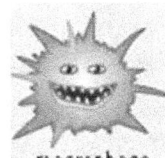

macrophage

The macrophages ("big eaters") are slower to respond to invaders than the granulocytes, but they are larger, live longer, and have far greater capacities. Macrophages also play a key part in alerting the rest of the immune system of invaders. Macrophages start out as white blood cells called monocytes. Monocytes that leave the blood stream turn into macrophages.

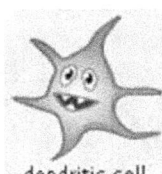

dendritic cell

The dendritic cells are "eater" cells and devour intruders, like the granulocytes and the macrophages. And like the macrophages, the dendritic cells help with the activation of the rest of the immune system. They are also capable of filtering body fluids to clear them of foreign organisms and particles.

"Every time you eat or drink, you are either feeding disease or fighting it."

— Heather Morgan, MS, NLC

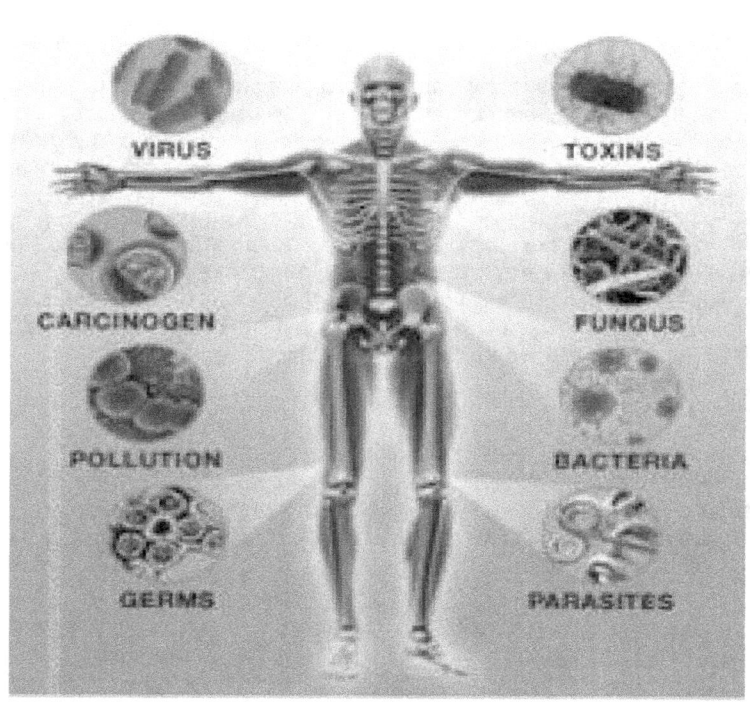

VIRUS

TOXINS

CARCINOGEN

FUNGUS

POLLUTION

BACTERIA

GERMS

PARASITES

What is specific immunity?

- Third line of defense
- Pathogen specific
- Involves antigens and antibodies

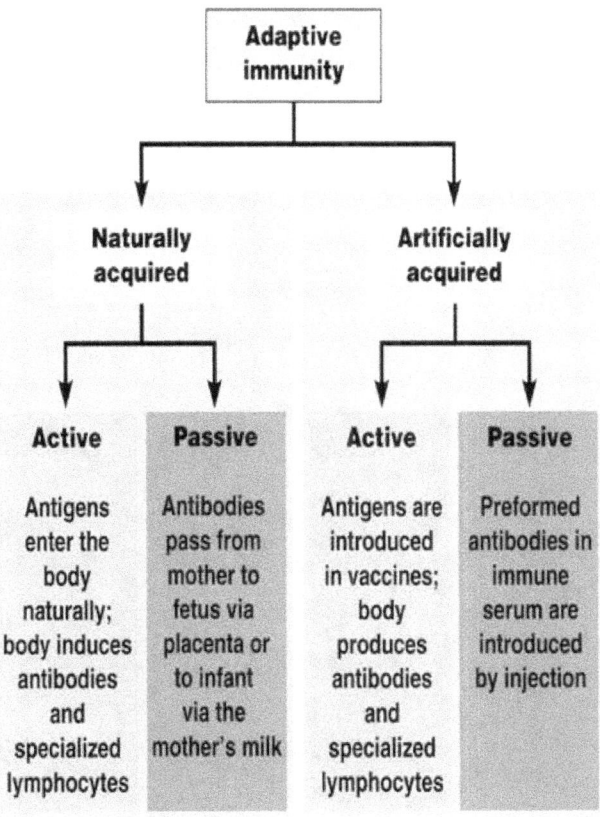

*****

Chapter 6 ... 3rd Line of Defense - Specific Immunity

*****

When Nonspecific defenses, prove inadequate, our body can begin to create and employ more selective defenses against disease. This **3rd line of defense**, called our **Acquired** or **Specific** Immune response, is governed by our **Lymphatic System**. The immune response is acquired, not innate, meaning that it is a conditioned, or "learned," reaction of the lymphatic system. Whereas the innate defenses function the same way regardless of the pathogen, the acquired immune response is specific. Each pathogen triggers a slightly different reaction, and the immune system must "learn" to identify each pathogen through experience.

The lymphatic system helps explain why we rarely need medical help to combat infectious disease as well as how DANGEROUS vaccinations are. The lymphatic system is complicated but lovable. Without its Awesome Healing and Health value, you likely would not be reading this book today. Instead, you would be long gone.

**Immune response**: The disease-fighting activity of an organism's immune system.

**Lymphatic system**: The tissues, vessels, and organs that produce, transport, and store cells that fight infection.

Adenoids
Tonsils
Right
Lymphatic
Duct
Thymus
Lymph Nodes
Thymus
Lymphatic
Vessel
Blood
Capillary
Spleen
Tissue Cells
Interstitial
Fluid
Lymphatic
Capillary
Masses of
Lymphocytes
and
Macrophages
Bone
Marrow
Lymph
Vessel
Lymph Node

Our **Lymphatic System** reaches most of our Body. The lymphatic system is composed of lymph, lymphatic vessels, and lymphatic organs and tissues. The organs of the lymphatic system include the Tonsils, Spleen, Thymus, Lymph Nodes, and the Peyer's Patch Glands of our digestive system.

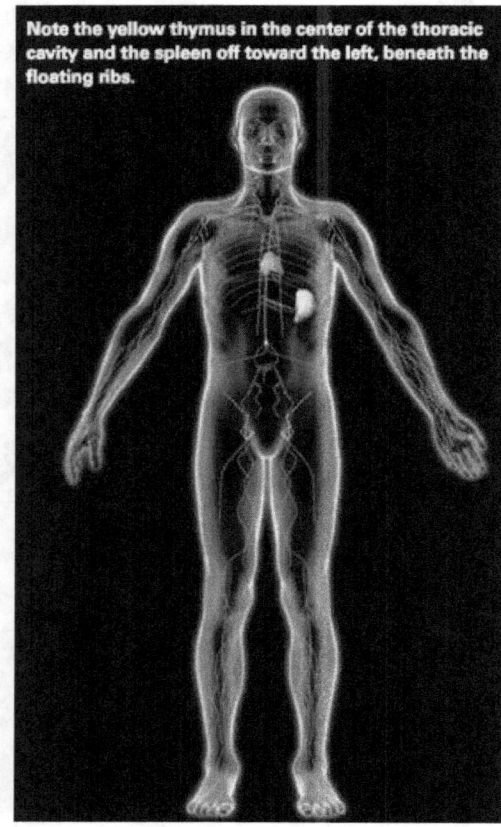

Note the yellow thymus in the center of the thoracic cavity and the spleen off toward the left, beneath the floating ribs.

Connecting these organs is a network of **lymphatic vessels** that **collect** lymph from the tissues and **deposit** it in the **bloodstream**.

Like the circulatory system, the lymphatic system touches most of the body and carries out both transportation and Homeostatic services.

You are probably familiar with the lymph nodes, those small, bean-shaped structures that you may feel alongside your Adam's apple when you have a sore throat.

You may also be surprised to learn that you have lymph nodes elsewhere, including your intestinal tract and chest.

These lymph nodes function in concert with lymphatic tissue, organs, and vessels to (1) **return** excess fluid from the tissues to the bloodstream, (2) **absorb** fats from the intestine and transport them to the blood- stream, and (3) **defend** the body against specific invaders.

Our tissues are bathed in lymph, a clear fluid that is called interstitial fluid when it is found in the interstices between cells.

Chemically, lymph is quite similar to blood plasma, which makes sense because lymph originates in fluid that diffuses from the capillaries into the tissue.

If you scrape your epidermis—say, when you "skin your knee"— clear interstitial fluid will bead-up on the exposed dermis.

Normally, lymphatic vessels collect this fluid for return to the bloodstream. When interstitial fluid is inside lymph vessels, we call it lymph.

Interstices: The small fluid-filled spaces between tissue cells.

The flow of interstitial fluid into lymphatic capillaries, where it is called lymph

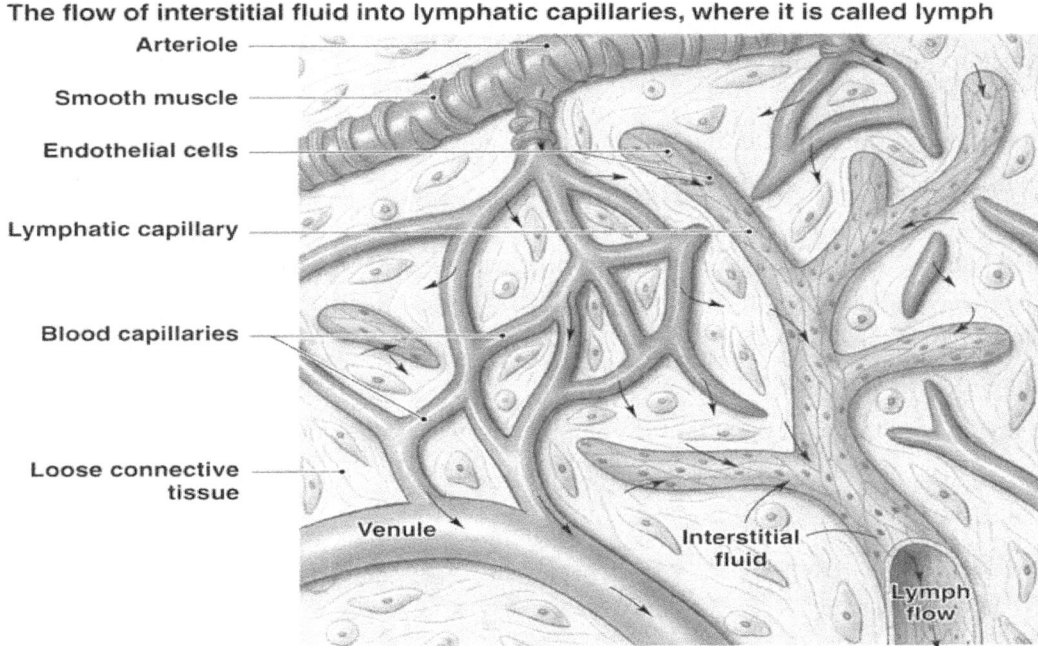

Lymphatic Capillaries and Vessels – Immune Circulatory System

The lymphatic system has many similarities to the circulatory system because both systems reach almost every cell in the body. Because interstitial fluid is so widespread, lymphatic capillaries (very small vessels) are also found throughout the body.

Often, the lymph in these capillaries is filled with ingested fats, turning the vessel milk white.

In the circulatory system, capillaries are part of a closed system that takes blood from the heart to the body and back to the heart. Larger vessels attach to either side of a capillary.

In contrast, lymphatic capillaries are small tubes with one closed end and one end leading to a larger lymphatic vessel. They are part of an open system in which vessels lead from the tissues to the bloodstream but not in the opposite direction.

Open System: A system with a starting point and an ending point rather than a continuous circular flow.

 Unlike our circulatory system, the lymphatic system has no central pump. Lymph flows through tissues and into lymphatic capillaries mainly because of the squeezing action of skeletal muscles.

PAGE 100

Supreme Health & Fitness! Health & Wellness Series Volume 1

As muscles contract, they shorten and thicken, forcing excess fluid from the muscular tissue and surrounding organs into the lymphatic capillaries.

Lymphatic capillaries allow fluid to enter but not to exit, because their walls are composed of cells positioned with slight overlaps.

Pressure from outside the vessel parts the cells so that fluid can enter the lumen (center) of the capillary. Fluid pressure inside the capillary presses the cells shut so that the fluid cannot escape. This action is rather like your front door.

If you push on one side, the door will open, but if you push from the other side, it will only close tighter.

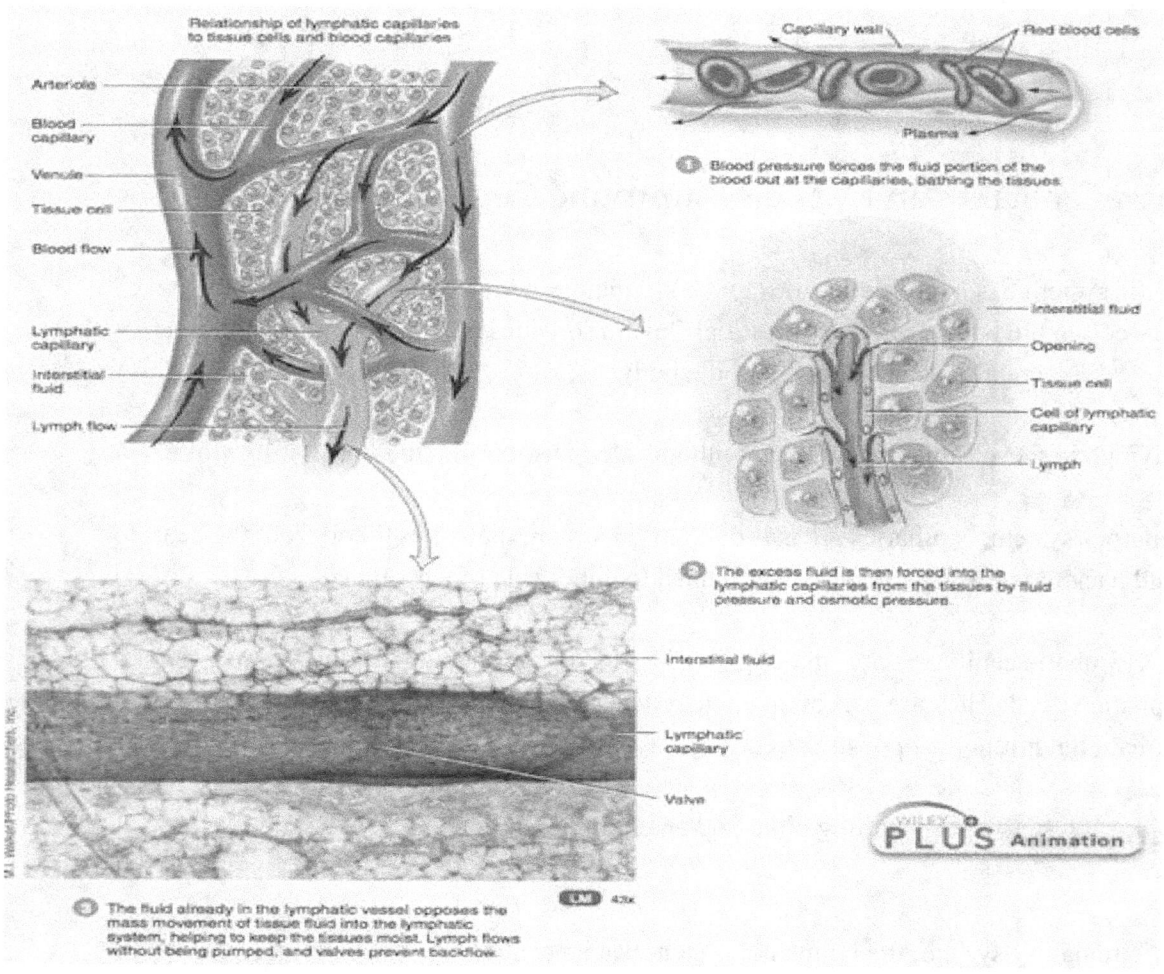

Lymphatic vessels are similar to the veins, which are thin-walled, flexible, and not built to withstand much pressure. Because lymph flows through the lymphatic system without being pumped, larger lymphatic vessels require valves to prevent backflow.

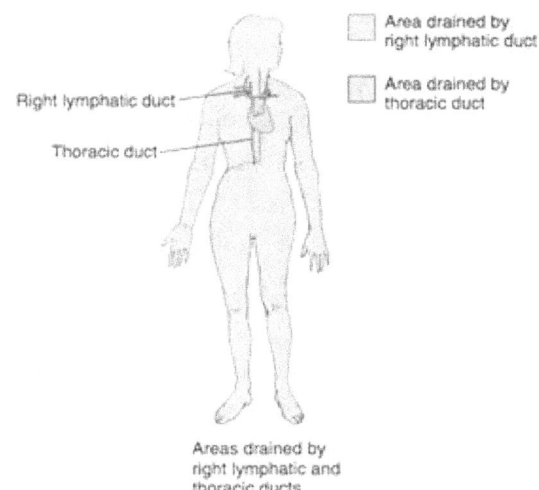

Lymphatic vessels transport their lymph to either the thoracic duct or the right lymphatic duct, just posterior to the right clavicle. Both ducts drain into the subclavian veins, allowing lymph to return to the bloodstream. The right lymphatic duct drains the right side of the head, the right shoulder, and the upper portion of the right chest.

Lymph collected from the rest of the body is drained into the thoracic duct. This arrangement causes concern for breast cancer patients, whose cancer may metastasize into the lymph.

If this happens, it is easy to see how quickly those cells can be spread throughout the body via the lymphatic system.

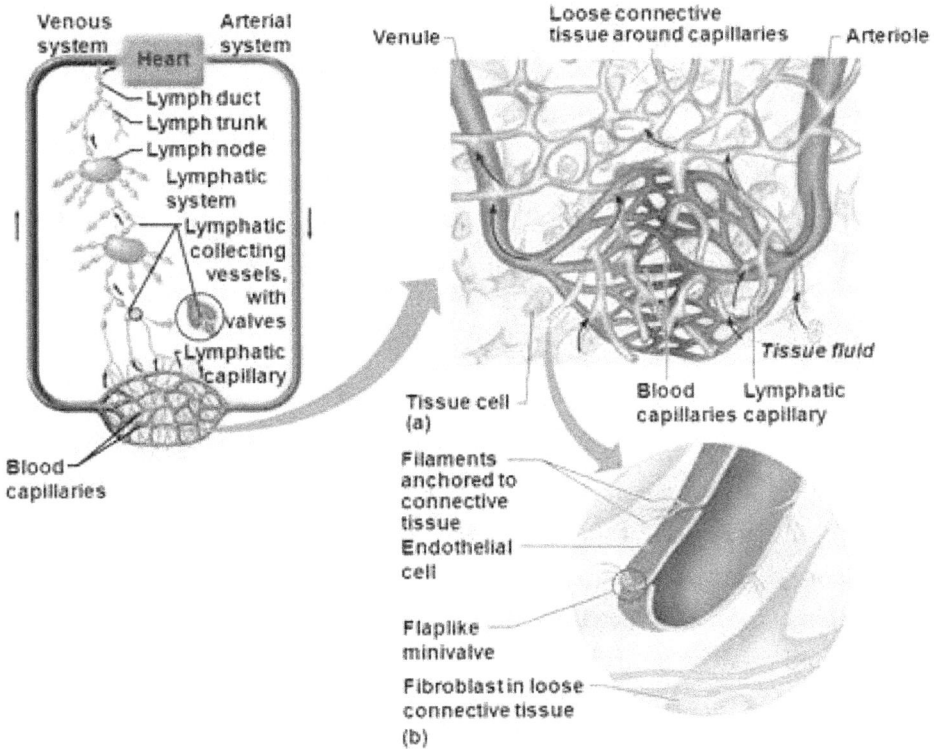

Lymphatic Organs – Filter and Protect

Before lymph returns to the bloodstream, it must be filtered and cleaned. Otherwise, the lymph would dump into the bloodstream the cellular debris and waste products it has picked up while traveling through the tissues. This cleaning occurs in the lymphatic organs—the Lymph nodes, Tonsils, and Spleen. The spleen cleans whole blood, not just the lymph. Two other lymphatic organs, the thymus and the bone marrow, produce lymphatic cells.

Lymph nodes are cleansing units. Lymph nodes are small, encapsulated glands that are strategically located to filter large volumes of lymph. Some are found in the groin, some in the armpit, and some in the neck. The mesenteric lymph nodes form a chain at the center of the abdominal cavity.

Nodes are filtering stations for lymph, as shown in Figure below. Lymph enters a node via many pas- sages but can leave by only one or two exits, forcing lymph to flow through the nodes in one direction.

Lymph slowly flows through a maze inside the node, giving phagocytic cells in the lymph node time to interact with the fluid and remove and destroy infectious agents and debris.

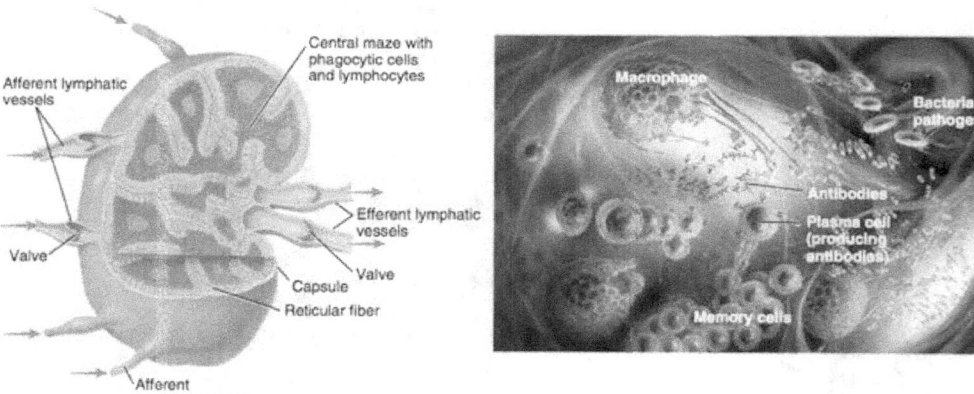

Lymph nodes filter lymph that has been collected from nearby tissues, therefore they can tell us a good deal about the health of that region of the body. "Swollen glands" are lymph nodes that are enlarged due to localized or systemic infection, abscess formation, malignancy, or other, rarer causes. A bacterial infection can often be detected in the lymph, because immune cells in lymph nodes increase in number and produce antibodies.

Mesenteric: Pertaining to the membranous fold in the abdominal cavity attaching many of the abdominal organs to the body.

Many infections can cause swollen lymph nodes, including mononucleosis, German measles, tuberculosis, mumps, ear infections, tonsillitis, an abscessed tooth, gingivitis (infection of the gums), large and untreated dental cavities, and various sexually transmitted diseases.

Immune disorders that can cause swollen lymph nodes include rheumatoid arthritis and HIV. Cancers that can cause swollen glands include leukemia, Hodgkin's disease, and non-Hodgkin's lymphoma.

Swollen lymph nodes may also be caused by certain medications or vaccinations. Cells of certain cancers, especially breast cancer, can be found in lymph nodes near the site of the primary tumor. As these cells metastasize, or migrate, to form new tumors, the number of lymph nodes containing cancer cells increases. This then is a good indicator of how advanced the cancer is.

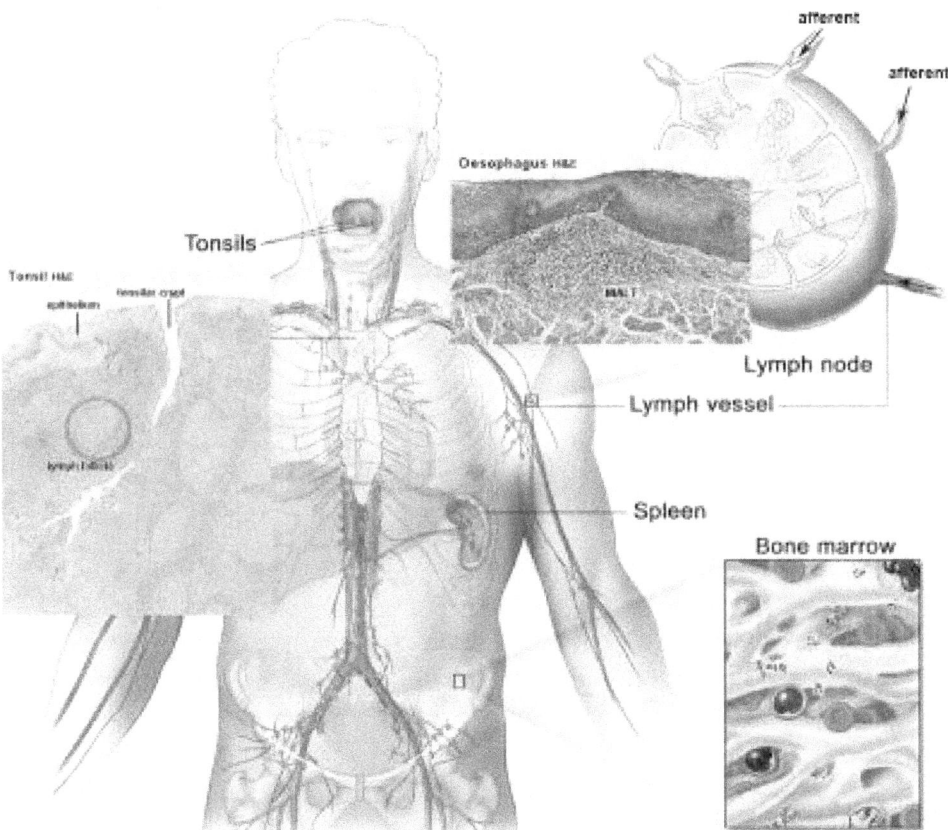

PAGE 104

Supreme Health & Fitness!   Health & Wellness Series Volume 1

Tonsils & MALT Protective Tissue

Tonsils and MALT are patches of un-encapsulated lymphatic tissue.

The tonsils are similar to lymph nodes in their organization and function. You were born with three sets of tonsils: the pharyngeal tonsils in the nasopharynx, the palatine tonsils, which are visible on either side of the pharyngeal opening, and the lingual tonsils found on the base of the tongue.

Tonsils & Adenoids

- Trap bacteria which work their way into the follicles where they are destroyed
- This helps develop memory

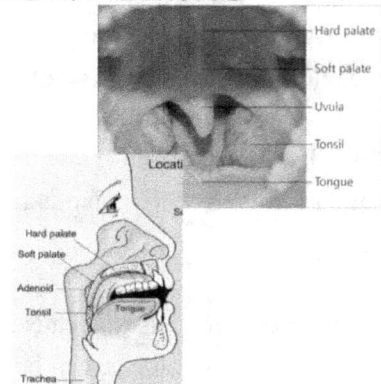

The main difference between tonsils and lymph nodes is that the tonsils are not entirely encapsulated. Instead, they are open to the fluids that pass through the throat. Infectious agents can be trapped in these organs, swelling the tonsils enough to almost shut off the throat.

Similar patches of lymphoid tissue are found in areas of the body such as the lungs, skin and eye. The largest patches of this are found in the lining of the small intestine.

These egg- shaped masses, called mucosa-associated lymphoid tissue, or MALT, help filter fluid absorbed from the intestinal lumen.

Mucosa-Associated Lymphoid Tissue (MALT)

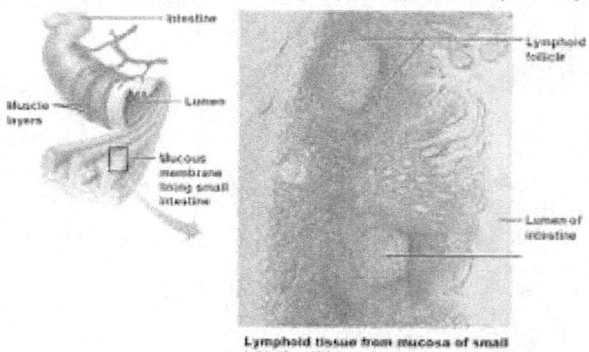

Lymphoid tissue from mucosa of small intestine (14x)

MALT

MALT – mucosa-associated lymphatic tissue:

•**GALT**- Peyer's patches, tonsils, and the appendix (digestive tract)

•**BALT**- Lymphoid nodules in the walls of the bronchi (respiratory tract)

MALT protects the digestive and respiratory systems from foreign matter

The Spleen

The largest lymphatic organ is the spleen. The largest collection of lymphoid tissue in the body is the fist-sized spleen (accompanying Figure).

The spleen has a strong outer capsule surrounding red and white pulp. Red pulp, containing red blood cells and macrophages, purifies blood by re- moving bacteria and damaged or exhausted red blood cells.

The white pulp contains lymphocytes and is involved in specific immunity. For this reason, the spleen is considered a lymphatic organ, even though it filters whole blood rather than lymph.

Lymphocytes: White blood cells that patrol the body, fight infection, and prevent disease.

The spleen is highlighted in yellow in this CT scan.

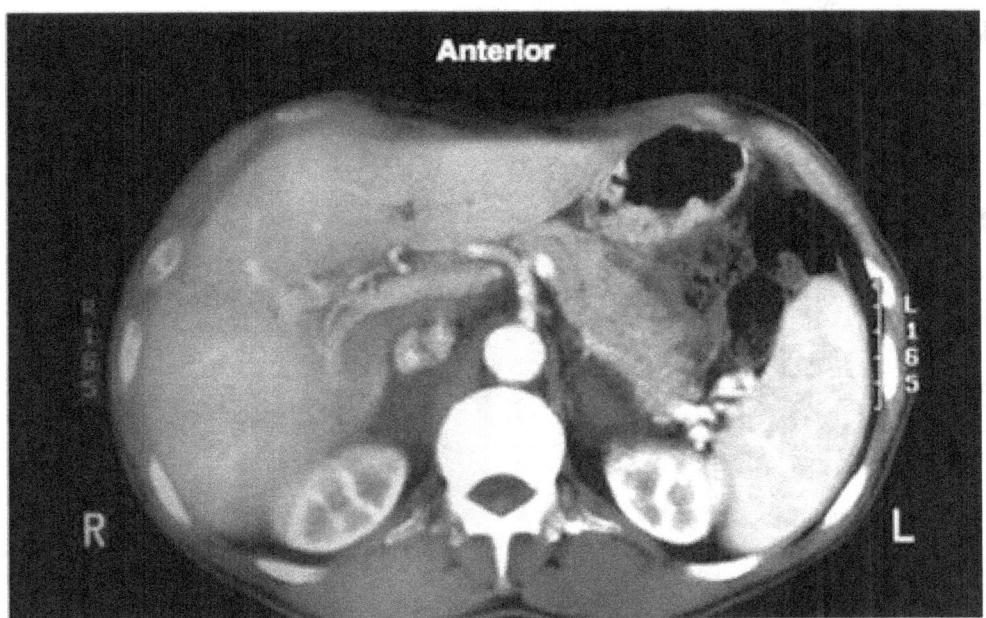

PAGE 106

Supreme Health & Fitness!   Health & Wellness Series Volume 1

Thymus - Mature Immune Cells

The thymus gland is located in the thoracic cavity, behind the sternum and draping over the upper portion of the heart. It is composed of two lobes held together by connective tissue

The primary function of the thymus is to produce mature, functional T cells, a distinct group of immune cells. The cortex of the thymus gland is involved in "*training*" T cells to distinguish self from pathogens.

It also produces thymic hormones that promote maturation of T cells.

The thymus is largest in infants and toddlers and it shrinks with age, losing function as it shrinks. This is one reason your parents or grandparents probably suffer more than you from a common cold or a passing virus.

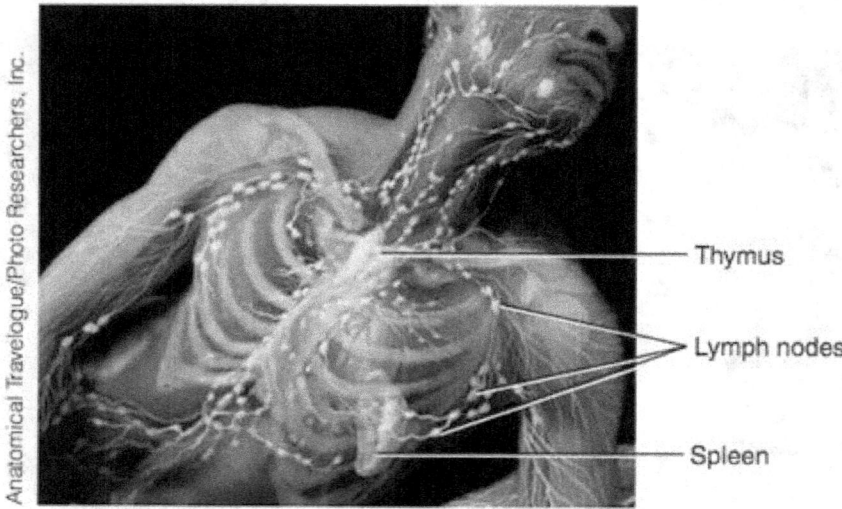

Anatomical Travelogue/Photo Researchers, Inc.

Thymus

Lymph nodes

Spleen

Bone Marrow – Stem Cells

Bone marrow is a spongy substance found in the center of the bones. It manufactures bone marrow stem cells and other substances, which in turn produce blood cells. Each type of blood cell made by the bone marrow has an important job:

- **Red blood cells** carry oxygen to tissues in the body.

- **Platelets** help blood to clot in order to stop bleeding.

- **White blood cells** fight infections.

Bone marrow also produces mature immune cells. The final type of lymphatic tissue is red bone marrow. In children, red bone marrow is found in the center of virtually all the bones. When we reach adulthood, only the skull bones, sternum, ribs, clavicle, epiphyses of the femur, pelvic bones, and the vertebral column retain red marrow.

The remaining bones contain yellow marrow in their marrow cavities. Red bone marrow includes blood stem cells that can produce both red and white blood cells. T

he cells involved in specific immunity are a subset of these white blood cells. As we now understand, the lymphatic system cleans and returns excess fluid to the circulatory system.

It is also of paramount importance in maintaining homeostasis through its role in specific immunity.

**stem cells**: Undifferentiated cells that remain able to divide and specialize into functional cells.

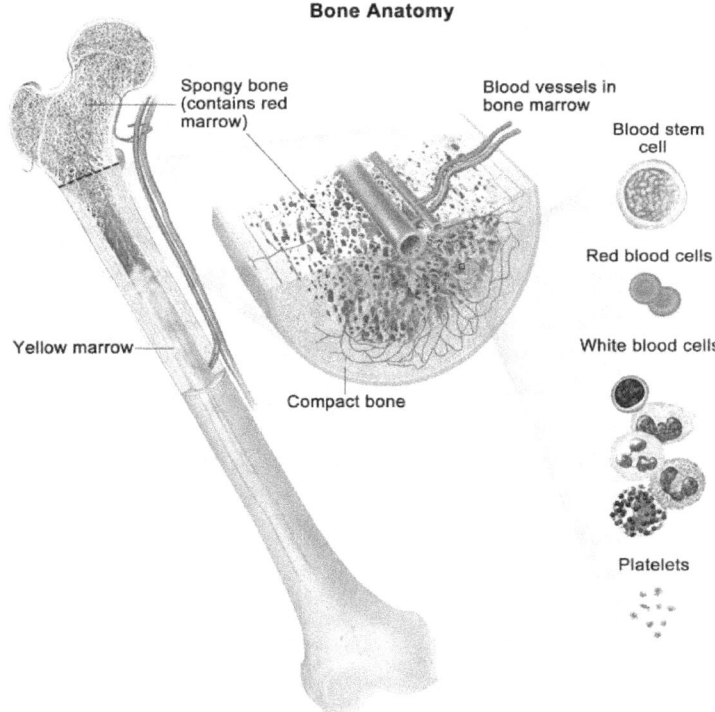

Bone Anatomy

Spongy bone (contains red marrow)

Blood vessels in bone marrow

Blood stem cell

Red blood cells

White blood cells

Yellow marrow

Compact bone

Platelets

Immune system cells

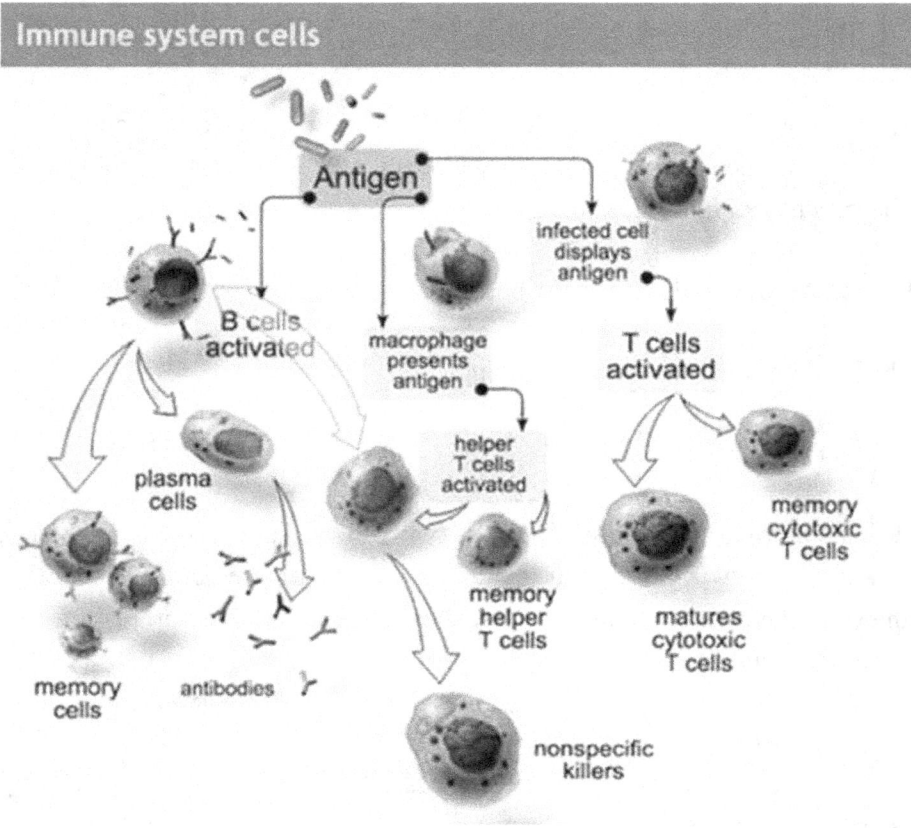

Immunity and Cancer

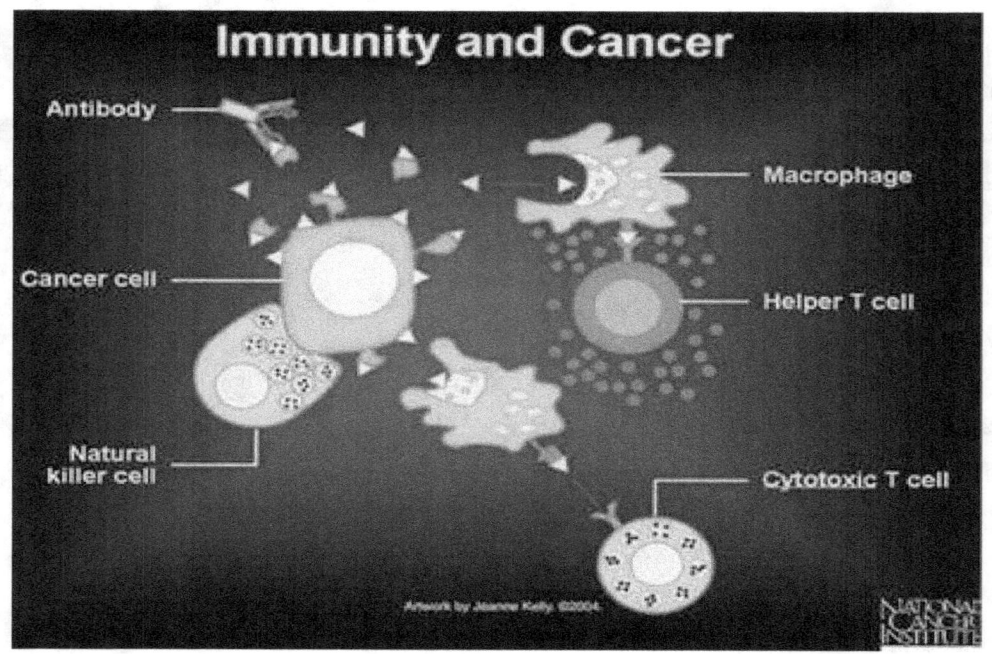

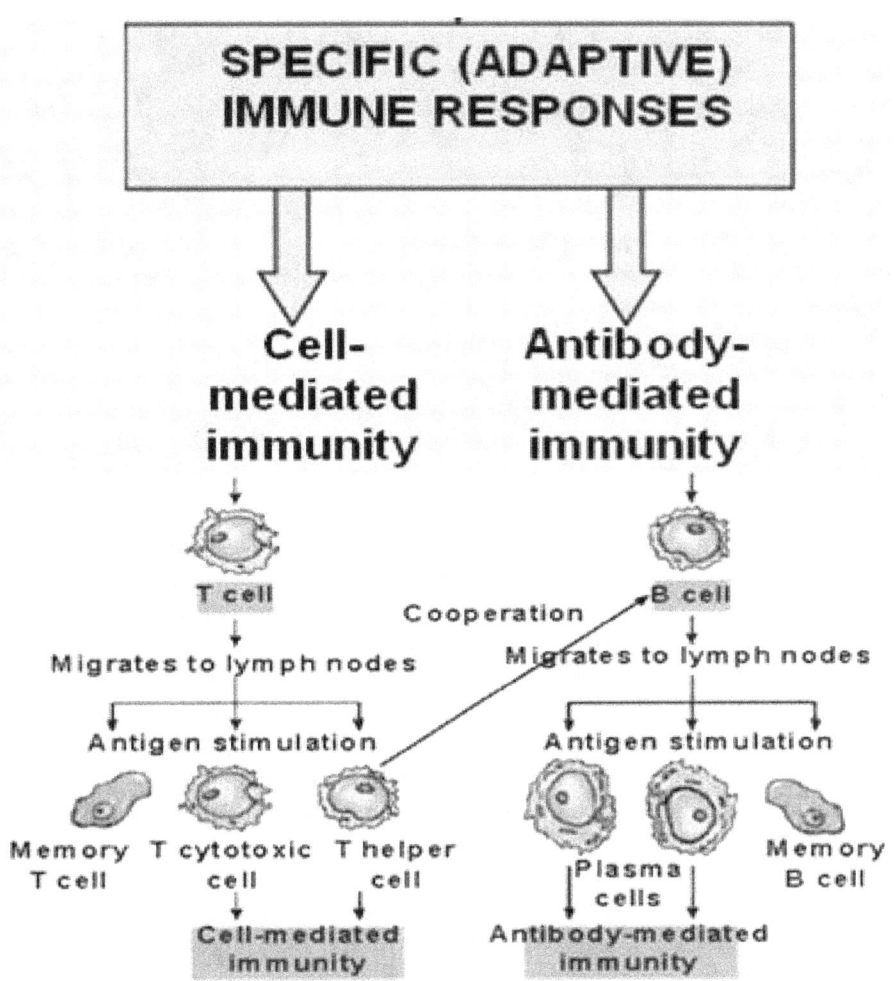

*****

Chapter 7 ... Your Body Learns to Heal Itself

*****

Specific Immunity Relies on a Series of Deadly Cells That Recognize and Remember Pathogens
When a pathogen slips past our nonspecific defenses, the battle is not over. Rather than immediately succumb to the disease, we rely on our specific defense—the immune system.

This system is composed of a set of blood cells collectively called lymphocytes. The various subtypes of lymphocytes look alike but have subtly different functions.

Immune cells share common characteristics, including:

- The ability to distinguish Self from Non-self (otherwise immune cells would destroy the very fabric on which they depend).
- Specificity, meaning each one reacts only to a specific antigen (a component of a disease-causing agent).
- The ability to remember certain pathogens and react more quickly the second or subsequent times the pathogen is encountered. This is the basis for immunization.

The specific immune system (now referred to simply as the "immune system") has two methods for combating pathogens, both of which are carried out by lymphocytes.

In one method, referred to as cell-mediated (or cellular) immunity, specialized lymphocytes function directly in any pathogen attack.

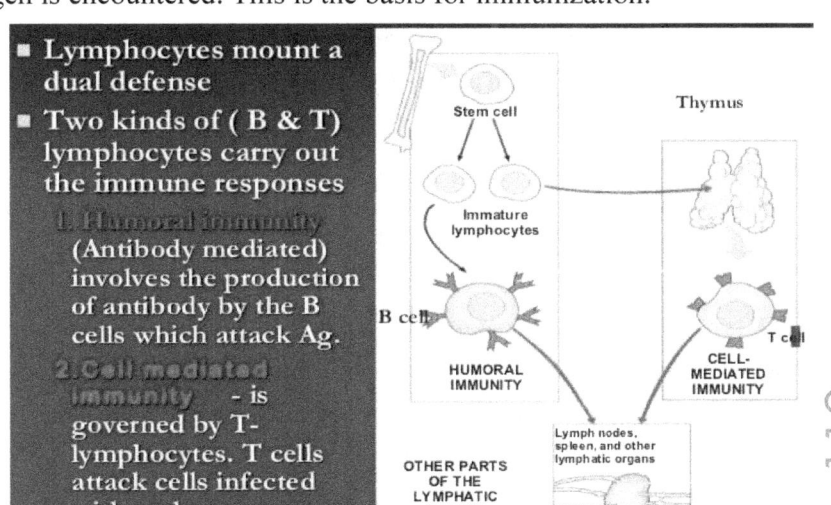

- Lymphocytes mount a dual defense
- Two kinds of (B & T) lymphocytes carry out the immune responses
  1. Humoral immunity (Antibody mediated) involves the production of antibody by the B cells which attack Ag.
  2. Cell mediated immunity - is governed by T-lymphocytes. T cells attack cells infected with pathogens

Stem cell

Thymus

Immature lymphocytes

B cell

T cell

HUMORAL IMMUNITY

CELL-MEDIATED IMMUNITY

Lymph nodes, spleen, and other lymphatic organs

OTHER PARTS OF THE LYMPHATIC SYSTEM

In the other method, called antibody-mediated (or humoral) immunity, specialized lymphocytes function indirectly by helping create disease-fighting compounds called antibodies.

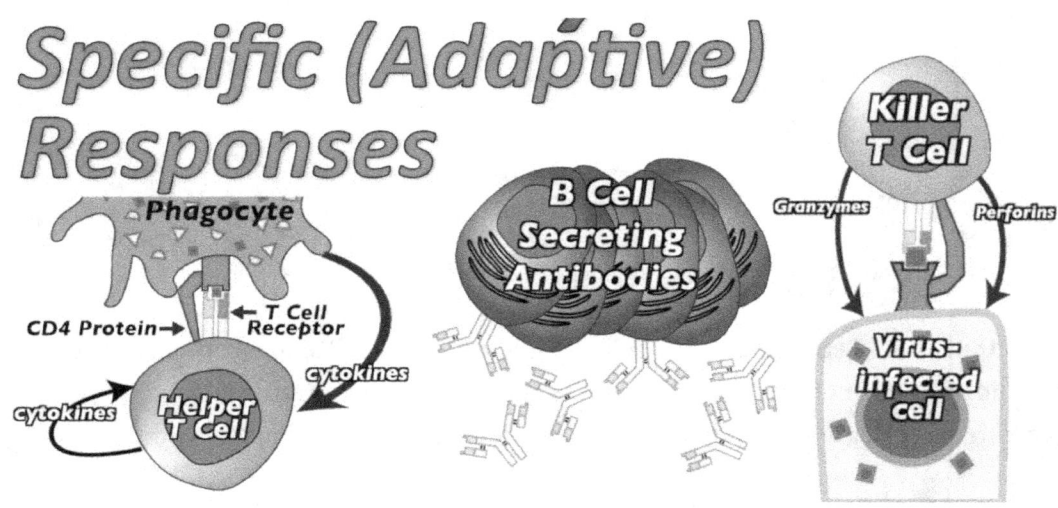

Immunization: The process of stimulating resistance to a specific disease through exposure to a non-pathogenic form of the disease- causing organism.

Antibodies: Proteins produced by lymphocytes and directed against specific pathogens or foreign tissue.

Our immune system uses two kinds of assassins. Two main classes of lymphocytes are involved in immunity: **B cells** and **T cells**.

B cells (B lymphocytes) mature in the bone marrow and spend most of their time inside lymph nodes and interstitial fluid. The B designation indicates that these cells were discovered in the bursa of fabricus in birds, but it can also remind us that B cells originate in the bone marrow of humans.

B cells produce antibodies that are specific to a particular pathogen, and so are usually considered part of antibody-mediated immunity.

T cells (T lymphocytes) mature in the thymus gland (hence the "T" name) in response to thymic hormones. T cells make up about half of the circulating lymphocytes in the blood, and they do not produce antibodies. T cells are responsible for stimulating B cells, as well as the direct destruction of antigens.

PAGE 113

Supreme Health & Fitness!   Health & Wellness Series Volume 1

T cells are most associated with cell-mediated immunity.

Lymphocytes have receptors on their cell membranes waiting to detect the exact antigen that fits the receptor like a lock and key, as shown in the Figure.

Each lymphocyte is specific to one antigen; it will ignore all others. During our lives, we are constantly exposed to antigens.

Amazingly, our lymphocytes develop a specific response to every one of them by mixing and matching the genes that create the receptor proteins of the immune system.

Small changes in receptor shape on the surface of a T cell or B cell will cause that cell to react to a different antigen.

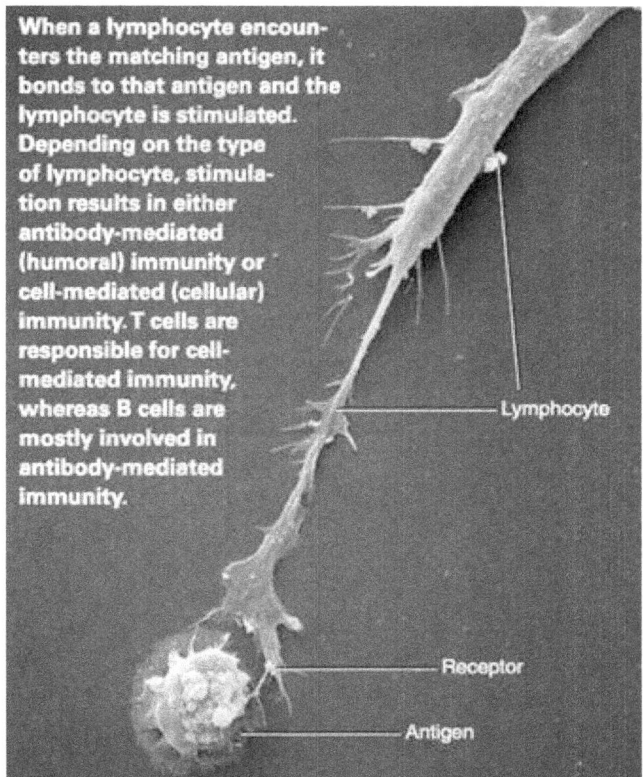

When a lymphocyte encounters the matching antigen, it bonds to that antigen and the lymphocyte is stimulated. Depending on the type of lymphocyte, stimulation results in either antibody-mediated (humoral) immunity or cell-mediated (cellular) immunity. T cells are responsible for cell-mediated immunity, whereas B cells are mostly involved in antibody-mediated immunity.

Our B Cells Antibody

Antibody-mediated immunity has an alternative name, humoral immunity, which reflects the fact that this immunity takes place in the fluids or "humors" of the body.

Antibodies are proteins that remove antigens from the bloodstream, usually by causing them to agglutinate.

Each B cell produces a different antibody that is directed toward a specific antigen. Because the B cell "wears" this antibody on its surface, the antibody is called a marker. When the surface antibody reacts with its specific antigen, the B cell is activated and begins to divide, cloning itself. Because the antigen in effect "chooses," or selects, which B cell will be cloned, this process is called clonal selection.

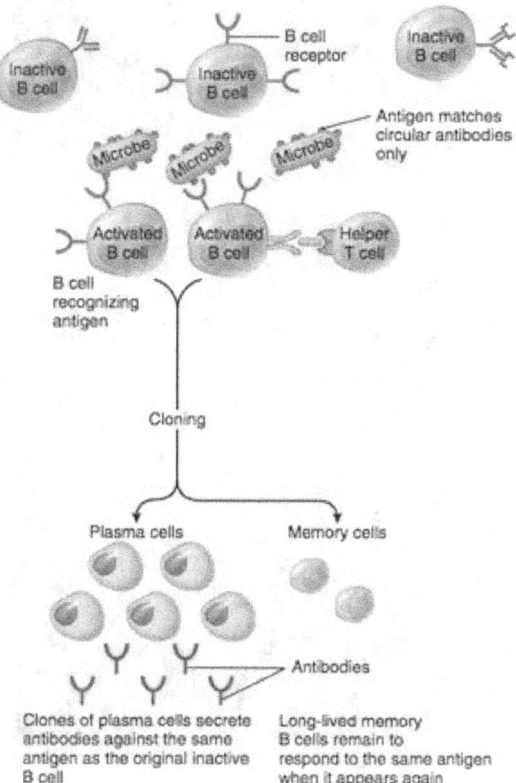

Plasma cells

Memory cells

Clones of plasma cells secrete antibodies against the same antigen as the original inactive B cell

Long-lived memory B cells remain to respond to the same antigen when it appears again

The cloned B cells produced during clonal selection are identical to the original, so they will react to the same antigen that started the cloning in the first place. As the cloned B cells are produced, two populations are created: **Plasma** cells and **Memory** cells.

Mature antibody-producing B cells, called plasma cells, pump out an arsenal of antibodies directed against the specific antigen that stimulated the original B cell, ensuring that the antigen is removed from the body, as shown in accompanying Figure.

When the antigen is gone, the plasma cells undergo apoptosis and die.

The second variety of cloned B cells, called memory cells, contributes to a library of long-term immunity that we call the secondary immune response.

For as long as 10 years, memory cells stand ready to go into action. If the pathogen reappears within that period, the memory cells quickly produce antibodies, ready to combat the pathogen before it can cause harm.

Vaccinations and booster shots are attenuated pathogens, designed to carry the "look and feel" of a harmful pathogen, but without the ability to cause disease. Supposedly your body will respond as if the attenuated pathogen were still capable of causing illness, cloning the proper B cell and producing both plasma and memory cells.

Importantly and Unfortunately, these shots CAN NOT trigger the formation of memory cells, but you are injected with memory cells for a disease whose symptoms we have never actually experienced or possibly never experience.

This is a dangerous process. Because these vaccines and boosters DON"T create Memory Cells they have to be repeatedly given. After consecutive shots, they can interfere with our natural ability to fight an invader and produce our own naturally occurring Memory Cells.

PAGE 115

Supreme Health & Fitness!   Health & Wellness Series Volume 1

Agglutinate: To clump with other cells due to the adhesion of surface proteins.

Apoptosis: Programmed cell death.

Attenuated: Having reduced capability to cause disease.

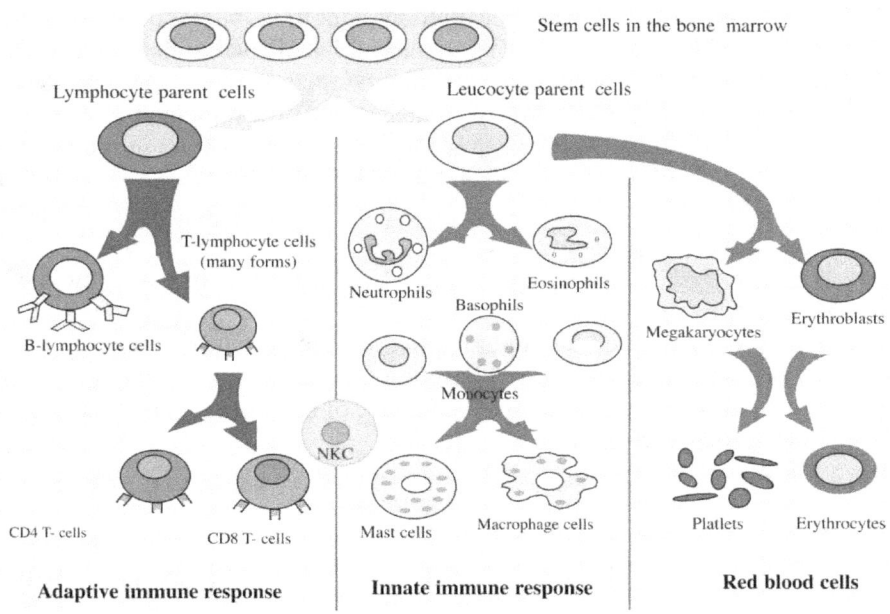

Antibodies

Antibodies are more specific than your social security number. Antibodies are proteins secreted by plasma cells in response to antigen binding. Antibodies all have the same general shape: a doubled, Y-shaped protein with one heavy chain and one light chain polypeptide.

The upper tips of the heavy chain and the corresponding tips on the light chain identify each antigen, and because they change so much, they are called the variable region. It is the variable region that interacts with the antigen and causes agglutination. A large conglomeration of antigen and anti- body marks the antigens for destruction by the macrophages.

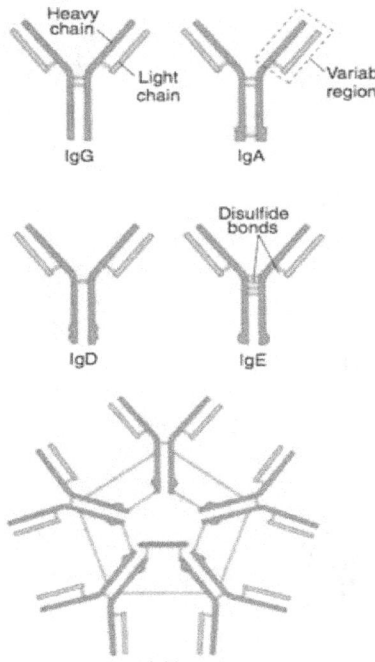

The five classes of antibodies (also called Immuno- Globulins) are IgG, IgM, IgA, IgD, and IgE.

- **_IgG1_** - the most common of our antibodies, and manifests in our circulating blood, lymph, and extracellular fluid. IgG immunoglobulins bind directly to an antigen, inactivating it almost immediately.
- **_IgM_** - our 1st immunoglobin that is released in any immune response and is also the predominant immunoglobulin produced in infants. IgM is a large polymer of 5 Y-shaped molecules that causes infected or foreign cells to clump together when IgM binds to them. Like IgG, IgM also aids in the release of complement.
- **_IgA_** - can manifest as a Monomer, Dimer (2 subunits), or larger molecule composed again of Y-shaped units. One form of IgA, found in secretions such as saliva, can bind to pathogens before they enter the bloodstream.
- **_Igd_** - found in mature B Cells, binds Antigens that stimulate B cell activation.
- **_IgE_** – the immunoglobulin that is responsible for allergic reactions, binds to the surface of basophils and mast cells. When it also binds to its antigen, IgE causes the release of histamines and other chemicals

implicated in allergic symptoms.

In our body, natural antibody-mediated immunity results when many different plasma cells are simultaneously stimulated to form antibodies. Each clone of plasma cells originates from a different B cell.

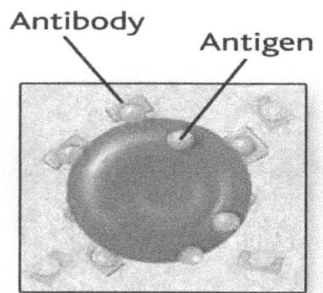

Antibody   **Antigen**

Red blood cell

An antibody is a protein produced by the immune system in response to the presence of an antigen

Each of these plasma cells produces an antibody that responds to a slightly different portion of the invading pathogen. The resulting soup of antibodies is polyclonal, meaning that the antibodies are produced by many different plasma cells.

Polyclonal antibodies are directed against one specific antigen, but they link to many different antigenic sites on that antigen. Directing so many slightly different antibodies against differing portions of the same antigen ensures that no antigen will be left in the bloodstream.

Because antibodies are specific, they are an interesting source of precisely targeted drugs. Most of these cutting-edge medical treatments propose to use "monoclonal antibodies." As the words imply, monoclonal antibodies are antibodies that are formed from clones of a single activated cell. The idea is to deliver the death knell directly to the diseased cells without harming healthy cells.

The specificity of monoclonal antibodies is often used in medical tests. The pregnancy tests sold in drugstores use a monoclonal antibody directed against a protein found only in the urine of pregnant women. Because monoclonal antibodies are so specific, any reaction in the test proves that the woman is pregnant. (If there is no reaction, the test should be repeated within a few days because the protein level could be too low to detect on the first test.)

Antibody Molecule

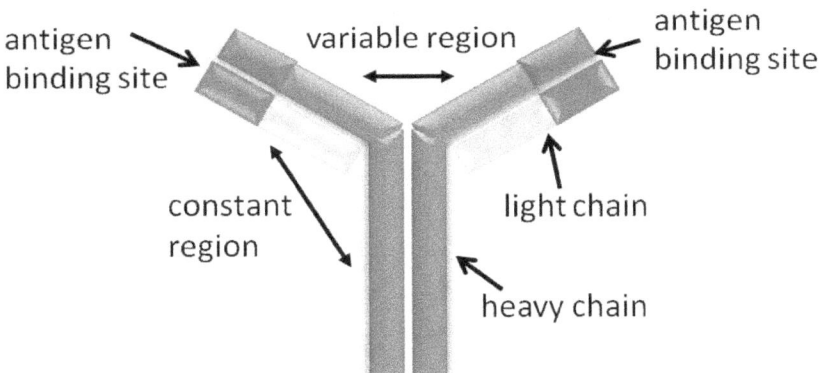

ATP is exploring amino acid substitutions in the antibody structure to improve stability and control affinity

T Cells & Immunity

Cell-mediated immunity involves two kinds of T cells. **Cell-mediated immunity** is governed by the T cells that are carried through the tissues of the blood. There are two large populations of T cells: **Helper T Cells** and **Cytotoxic T Cells.**

Unlike B cells, which can directly detect the presence of an antigen using the antibodies on their surface, T cells must have the antigen presented to them. This is done by **Antigen-Presenting Cells** (APCs), which are usually macrophages. The APC encounters an antigen, phagocytoses it, and "**presents**," or wears, a portion of that antigen on its surface.

APCs present their ingested pathogens using a specific membrane protein complex. Just like B Cells, T Cells carry receptors on their surface that will bind to specific antigens. However, these T cell receptors only recognize antigens presented on the surface of an APC. T cells that recognize the APC- presented pathogen are stimulated to differentiate into either helper T cells or cytotoxic T cells.

The Cytotoxic T cell will seek out and destroy the stimulating pathogen wherever it occurs in the body.

HOW CAN YOU GET SICK WITH THIS SOLDIER CELL PRESENT?

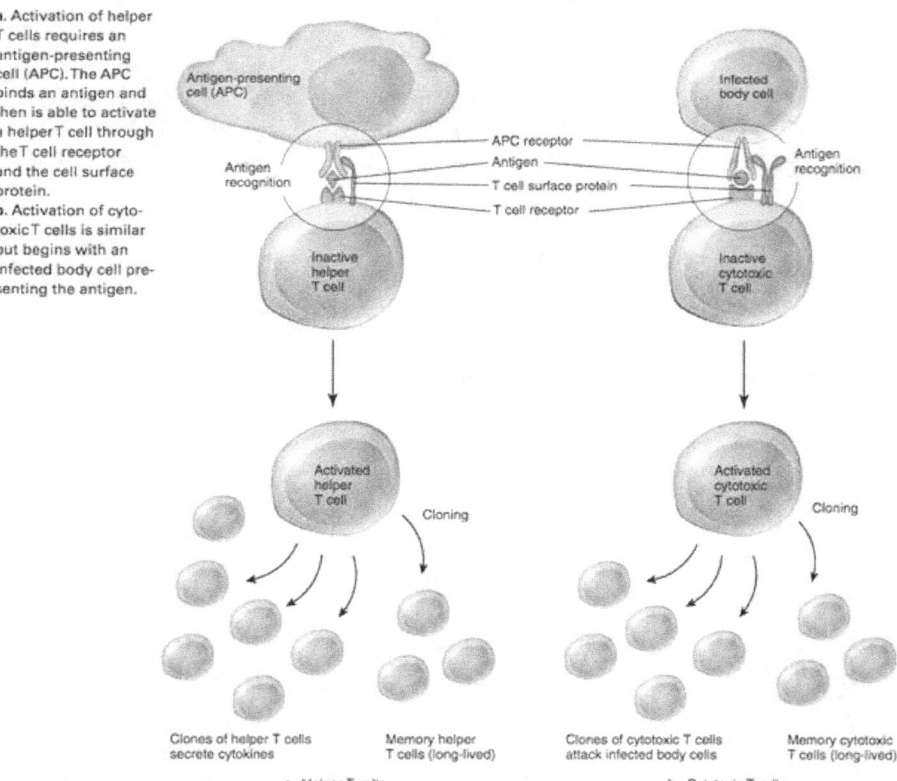

a. Activation of helper T cells requires an antigen-presenting cell (APC). The APC binds an antigen and then is able to activate a helper T cell through the T cell receptor and the cell surface protein.
b. Activation of cyto-toxic T cells is similar but begins with an infected body cell pre-senting the antigen.

Cytotoxic T cells: A subset of T lymphocytes responsible for killing virally infected cells.

Stimulated helper T cells will travel through the blood and lymph to the lymph nodes, where they will in turn stimulate the matching B cell. In this way, they are helping to bring the antigen to the specific B cell equipped to produce antibodies to destroy it. When activated, both kinds of T cells make copies of themselves to fight pathogens and also produce memory cells for fighting future invasions. These memory cells lie in wait in the blood, ready to jump quickly into action should the same antigen again threaten the body.

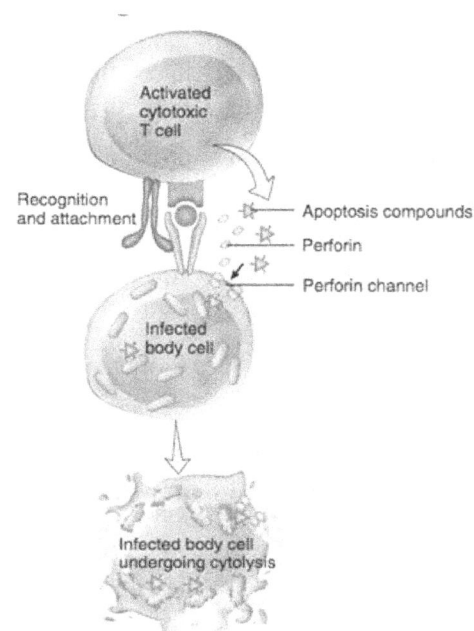

Cytotoxic T cells are stimulated to divide by cytokines released from helper T cells. Cytotoxic T cells respond specifically to altered HLA (human leukocyte antigen) proteins. The HLA com- plex is a marker that identifies the cell as belonging to the body and is what we identify when we "tissue type" a person to find a matching organ before an organ transplant. During organ transplants, HLA mismatches can trigger a rejection reaction by cytotoxic T cells. Incorrectly matched tissue types can lead to complete destruction of foreign HLA-carrying transplanted organs.

Cytotoxic T cell destruction of infected cell by release of perforins that cause cytolysis; microbes are destroyed by other released chemicals.

Most cells in the body with foreign HLA complexes are not introduced during organ transplants but rather are cancerous or virally infected. Cytotoxic T cells will remove any cell without the proper HLA antigens, whether cancerous, infected, or beneficial to the body.

Cytotoxic T cells, or killer cells, physically attach to the foreign HLA-carrying cell and release perforin molecules from their vacuoles. Perforin molecules are like little molecular darts that poke through the plasma membrane of the infected cell. A pore forms in the cell membrane, allowing salts and water to enter the cell, causing it to swell and burst.

Some T Lymphocytes differentiate into natural killer cells. Natural killer (NK) cells are actually part of our innate defense system. They are introduced here because they are produced exactly like the helper T cells of our specific immune defenses.

**NK cells function as a natural cancer screen, patrolling the body and identifying virally infected cells and tumor cells. After detection, NK cells kill the diseased cell via cell-to-cell contact.**

With this Powerful Cell that is designed by God to Protect us from everything – including the incurable CANCER – HOW DO WE STILL SUFFER AND DIE FROM CANCER?

This contact is carried out by proteins. As with the cytotoxic T cell, Perforin is released by the NK cell, creating pores in the doomed cell. Along with perforin, other proteins are released that induce apoptosis when taken into the target cell.

These apoptosis- inducing proteins are absorbed by the target cells once perforin has punctured their membranes. NK cells are not part of the specific immune response because they remove all foreign or infected cells in exactly the same way. They do not respond to immunization, and they do not seem to produce clones of memory cells.

There is some evidence that our emotions and thoughts can affect our immune systems, possibly by suppressing the T cells when we are stressed and enhancing our T cells when we are particularly upbeat.

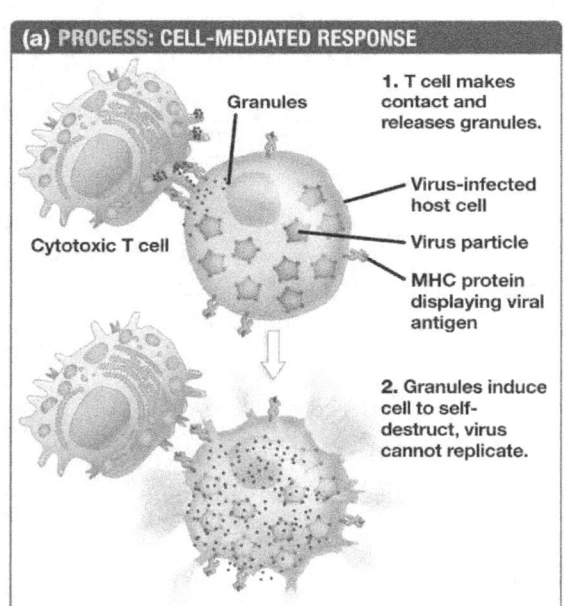

(a) PROCESS: CELL-MEDIATED RESPONSE

Granules

Cytotoxic T cell

1. T cell makes contact and releases granules.

Virus-infected host cell

Virus particle

MHC protein displaying viral antigen

2. Granules induce cell to self-destruct, virus cannot replicate.

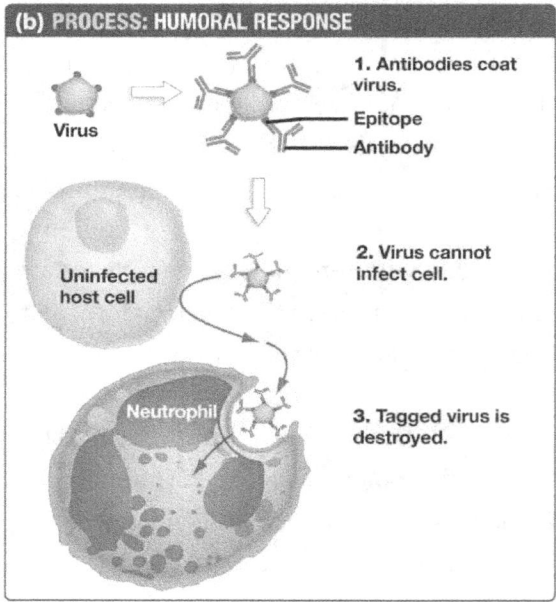

(b) PROCESS: HUMORAL RESPONSE

Virus

Uninfected host cell

Neutrophil

1. Antibodies coat virus.

Epitope

Antibody

2. Virus cannot infect cell.

3. Tagged virus is destroyed.

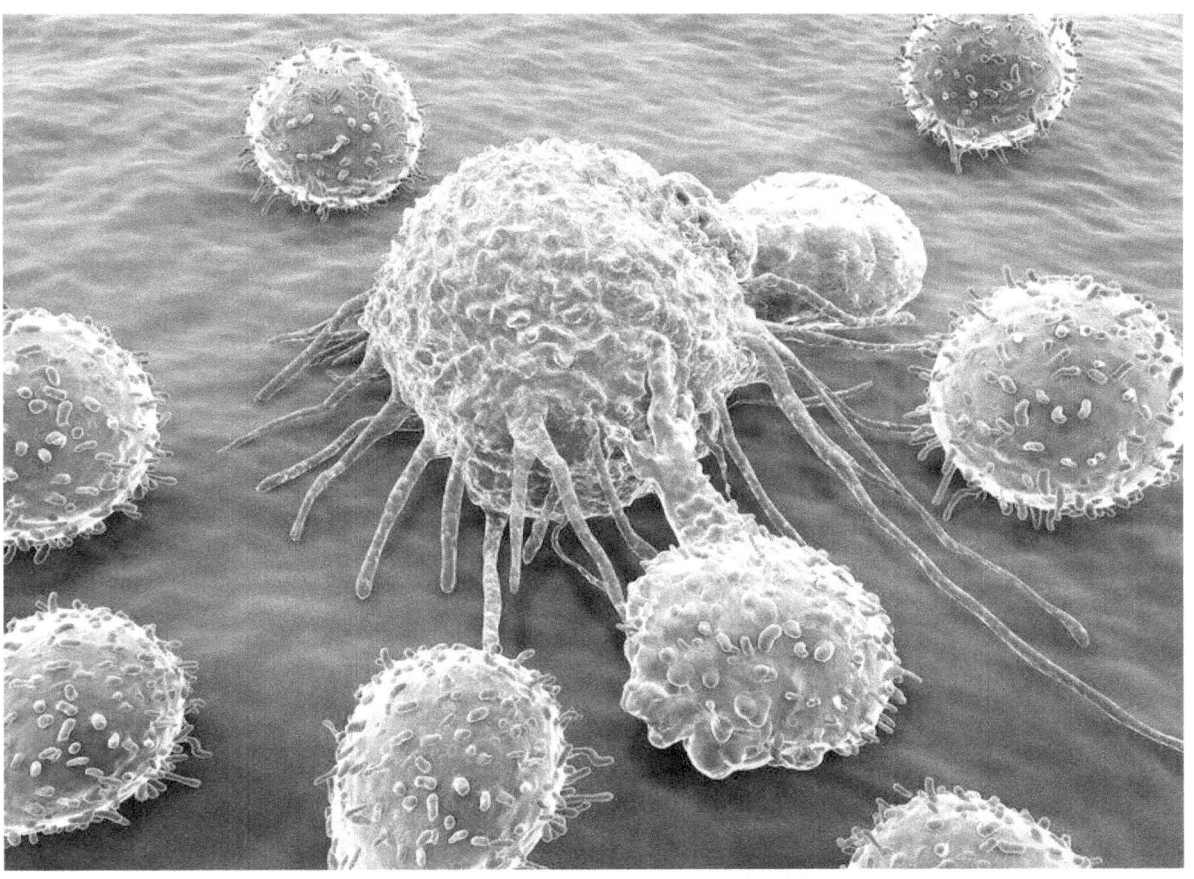

Lymphocytes DETECT and ATTACK a Foreign Cell!

How Do Thoughts and Emotions Affect Our T Cells and Immune Systems?

Are you happy? Sad? Sleep deprived? Stressed out? Worried sick?

There is evidence that your mind can have a large impact on your health. From your general demeanor to how you handle the slings and arrows of life—job loss, death of a loved one, breakup of a relationship—your emotional and mental health has a subtle yet pronounced effect on your immune system.

The earliest evidence was anecdotal. Doctors noticed that people who suffered from depression as well as another physiological illness, such as heart disease, diabetes, or AIDS, needed more intense medical treatment and often experienced higher rates of disability and death than people with the same illnesses but no depression. Also, people who were convinced that they were going to get sick actually got sick at a higher rate than those who believed that they would be healthy. These observations led to clinical studies and basic scientific research on how the mind affects the body.

One study involved 34 college students who were told that an electric current would be passed through their heads and that they might feel headaches as a result. No current was actually used, but more than two-thirds of the students reported headaches. The nocebo effect (*nocebo* is Latin for "I will harm") is the opposite of the better-known placebo effect, in which a drug or treatment makes a patient feel better merely because the patient *believes* that it is going to work. The nocebo effect occurs when patients think that their health will worsen because of a drug or treatment, and as a result their health deteriorates despite the absence of an immediate physical cause.

What could link the mind to the body and the immune system? We have seen that the release of hormones is a natural reaction to stress. Some studies have shown that releasing excess stress hormones makes the immune system work less efficiently by lowering the number and activity level of some kinds of T cells, and there is some evidence that thinking positively actually may raise the killer T cell count over time.

Critical Reasoning Issues Unlike placebo-based experiments, experiments testing the nocebo effect are usually unethical, since a doctor or an experimenter should not deliberately cause harm or illness. Hence, there are no large studies of the nocebo effect with large samples of patients. Small studies and anecdotes have provided all the available evidence so far.

*****

Chapter 8 ... Active & Passive Immunity

*****

Most of us acquire immunity from experience. We are exposed to a pathogen, it invades our tissues, and our immune system counterattacks by making antibodies (as just described).

This is natural active immunity: Your immune system is exposed to the antigen in the natural course of your life; your immune cells respond and actively combat the pathogen.

Passive immunity, in contrast, occurs when antibodies are transferred without stimulating the immune system.

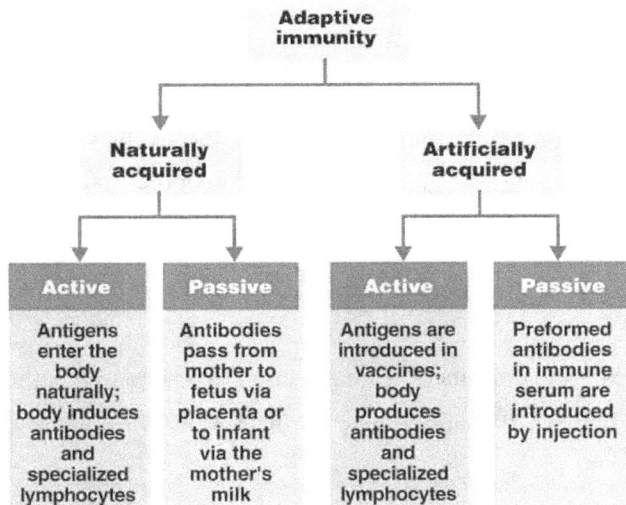

Active Immunity - Our "Trainable" Immune System

The primary advantage of active immunity comes from the creation of memory cells, which arise many hours after the initial reaction to the pathogen.

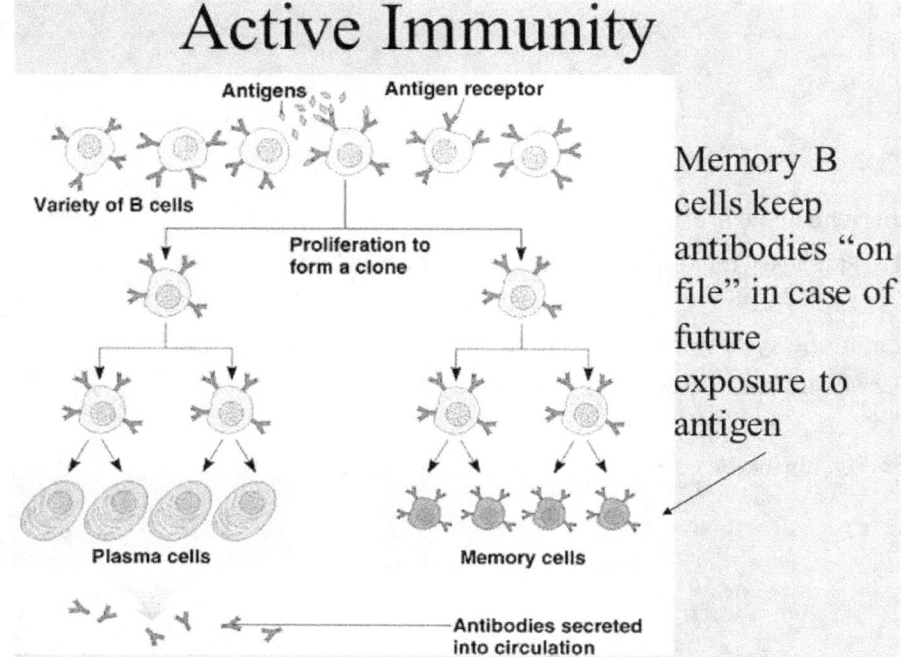

Active Immunity

Antigens — Antigen receptor

Variety of B cells

Proliferation to form a clone

Plasma cells

Memory cells

Antibodies secreted into circulation

Memory B cells keep antibodies "on file" in case of future exposure to antigen

Initially, the body needs days to respond to the pathogen, stimulate the proper cells, and follow the chain through helper T cells to B cells to plasma cells to antibody production.

Then our body needs a few more days of antibody production to elevate the antibody titer to an effective level.

Memory cells produced during the primary response remain in the body for years, lying dormant until the same antigen reappears, when they will start the secondary response. This secondary response to a particular antigen happens far faster than the first response because the immune system needs to stimulate and clone only the memory cells.

These Secondary responses also require less energy from the body.

Although active immunity can prevent illness from a second exposure to a pathogen, the process we have described requires that you have previously been exposed to the pathogen, gotten sick, and recovered.

It's preferable to prevent illness from the outset, so we never get the disease; some pathogens, after all, are fatal!

Vaccines are modern medicines attempts to train the immune system. In this case, they intentionally introduce a pathogen to the body rather than allow you to contract the pathogen naturally.

These pathogens are attenuated so that they can stimulate a primary immune response without causing disease.

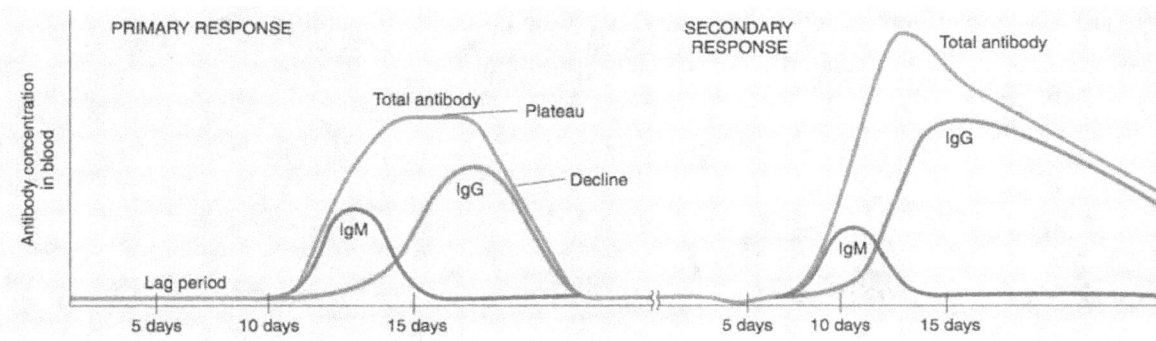

Activity immunity comes from exposure to a pathogen. Surface markers on the pathogen surface act as antigens, which are binding sites for antibodies. Antibodies are Y-shaped protein molecules, which can exist on their own or attached to the membrane of special cells. The body doesn't keep a store of antibodies on hand to take down an infection immediately. A process called clonal selection and expansion builds up sufficient antibodies.

An example of natural activity immunity is fighting off a cold. An example of artificial active immunity is building up a resistance to a disease due to an immunization. An allergic reaction is an extreme response to an antigen, resulting from active immunity.

Features of Active Immunity

- Active immunity requires exposure to a pathogen or to the antigen of a pathogen.

- Exposure to the antigen leads to the production of antibodies. Antibodies essentially mark a cell for destruction by special blood cells called lymphocytes.

- Cells involved in active immunity are T cells (cytotoxic T cells, helper T cells, memory T cells, and suppressor T cells), B cells (memory B cells and plasma cells), and antigen-presenting cells (B cells, dendritic cells, and macrophages).

- There is a delay between exposure to the antigen and acquiring immunity. The first exposure leads to what is called a primary response. If a person is exposed to the pathogen again later, the response is much faster and stronger. This is called a secondary response.

- Active immunity lasts a long time. It can endure for years or the entire life.

- There are few side effects of active immunity. It can be implicated in autoimmune diseases and allergies, but generally doesn't cause problems.

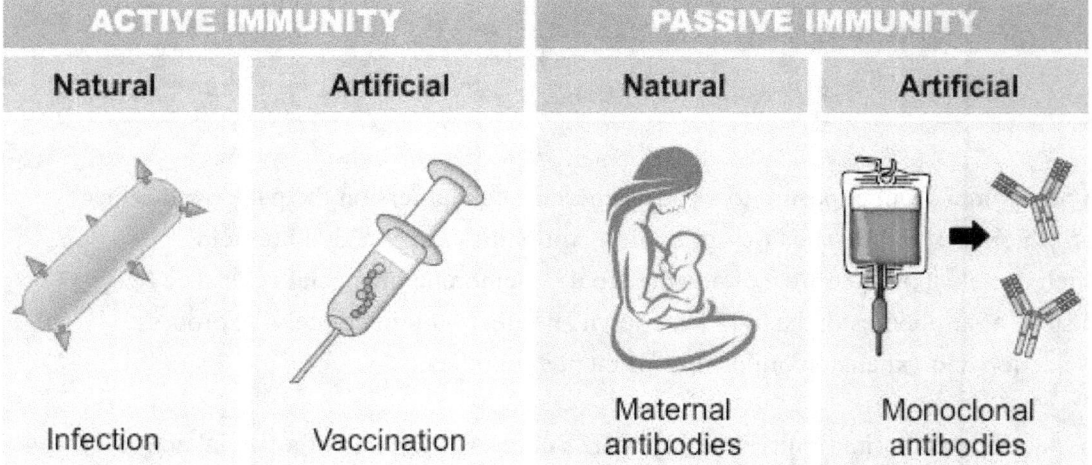

ACTIVE IMMUNITY		PASSIVE IMMUNITY	
Natural	Artificial	Natural	Artificial
Infection	Vaccination	Maternal antibodies	Monoclonal antibodies

Passive Immunity - Help from the Outside

As noted in the previous section, passive immunity is the transfer of antibodies without stimulating the immune system. Although active immunity is helpful because the memory cells can launch a quick secondary response, passive immunity is also beneficial because you do not expend energy creating antibodies or producing clones.

However, passive immunity is like giving an infantryman a gun with only one magazine. Introduced antibodies provide the recipient with immediate resistance to specific antigens.

Once the antibodies are used or broken down, however, the body cannot create more, and the immune protection is lost. There are no memory cells, because the antibodies were not created by active stimulation of the immune system.

La Leche League is a nonprofit organization that promotes healthy prenatal and postnatal care for both the infant and the mother. Their best-known campaign is designed to educate women on the advantages of breastfeeding until at least age 6 months. The antibodies received by the baby from the maternal blood in utero

Passive immunity can be acquired naturally, when maternal antibodies pass through breast milk to an infant, which is one reason La Leche League and many doctors encourage breastfeeding.

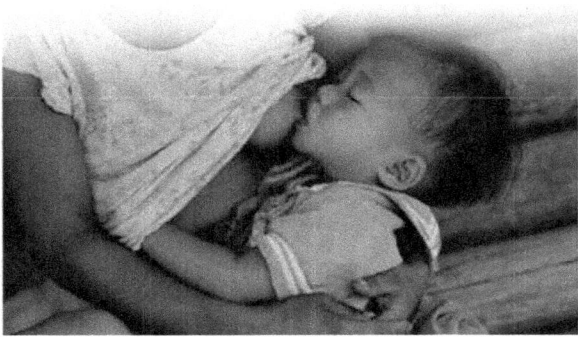

sustain the infant for approximately 2 to 3 months. Soon after, these antibodies begin to break down, and the infant must either produce antibodies via active immunity or receive maternal antibodies via breast milk.

Breastfed infants continue to gain passive immunity from their mothers and are therefore more able to resist disease. Infant formula may have a nutrient content similar to that of human milk, but it does not contain any antibodies.

Passive immunity can be used to fight diseases that cannot be fought in any other way. Horses, goats, rats, mice, and rabbits have all been used to generate antibodies against specific human diseases. These animals are given vaccines that cause them to produce antibodies, just as we do. The antibodies in the animals' blood are harvested, purified, and administered to hu- mans for treating diseases, such as diphtheria, botulism, and tetanus.

Passive immunity can also be administered artificially in gamma globulin shots, which are mixtures of many antibodies designed to match the pathogens the patient may contact.

These are often given before travel to foreign countries, where new diseases may be encountered. Passive immunity generally lasts three to six months, long enough for most foreign vacations.

Passive Immunity

In passive immunity, individuals do not have the antibodies, but rather, are passed down to them naturally or through human intervention. This is a temporary fix. Lasting only a few months.

Antibodies are passed from mother to fetus during the last month of pregnancy or through breastfeeding after birth.

Antibodies are introduced directly into the blood stream.

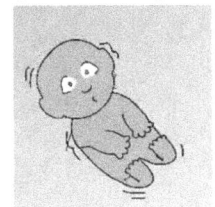

OR

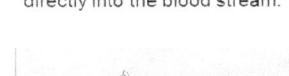
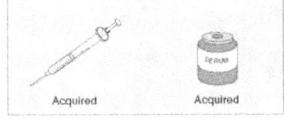

Acquired

Acquired

An example of natural passive immunity is a baby's protection against certain infections by getting antibodies through colostrum or breast milk. An example of artificial passive immunity is getting an injection of antisera, which is a suspension of antibody particles. Another example is the injection of snake antivenom following a bite.

Features of Passive Immunity

- Passive immunity is conferred from outside the body, so it doesn't require exposure to an infectious agent or its antigen.

- There is no delay for the action of passive immunity. Its response to an infectious agent is immediate.

- Passive immunity is not as long-lasting as active immunity. It's typically only effective for a few days.

- A condition called serum sickness can result from exposure to antisera.

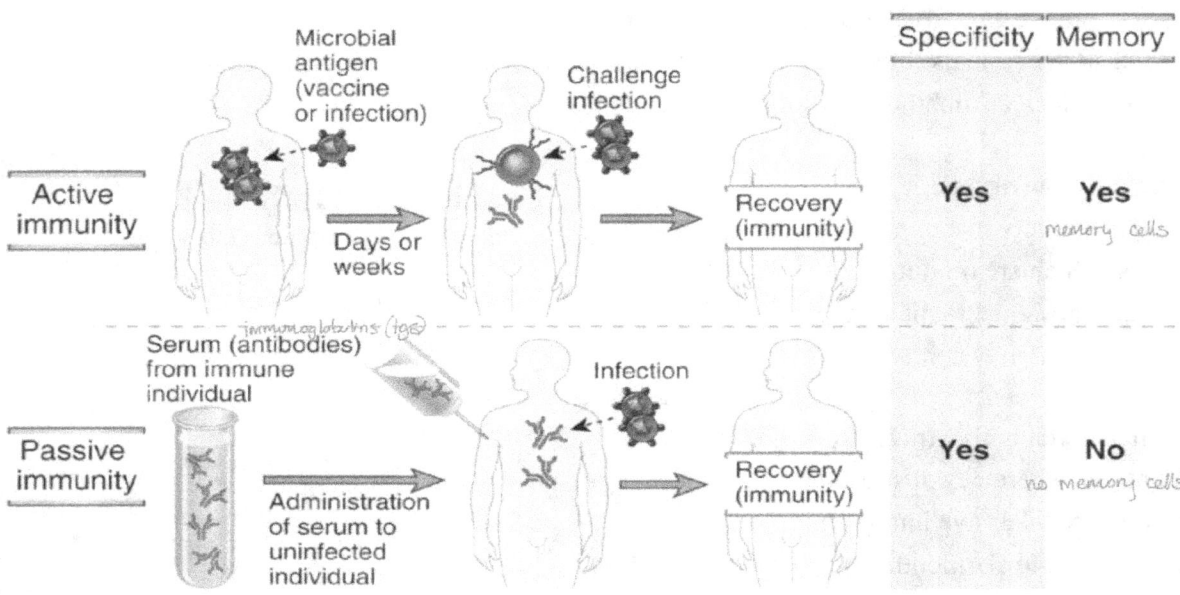

PAGE 129

Supreme Health & Fitness!   Health & Wellness Series Volume 1

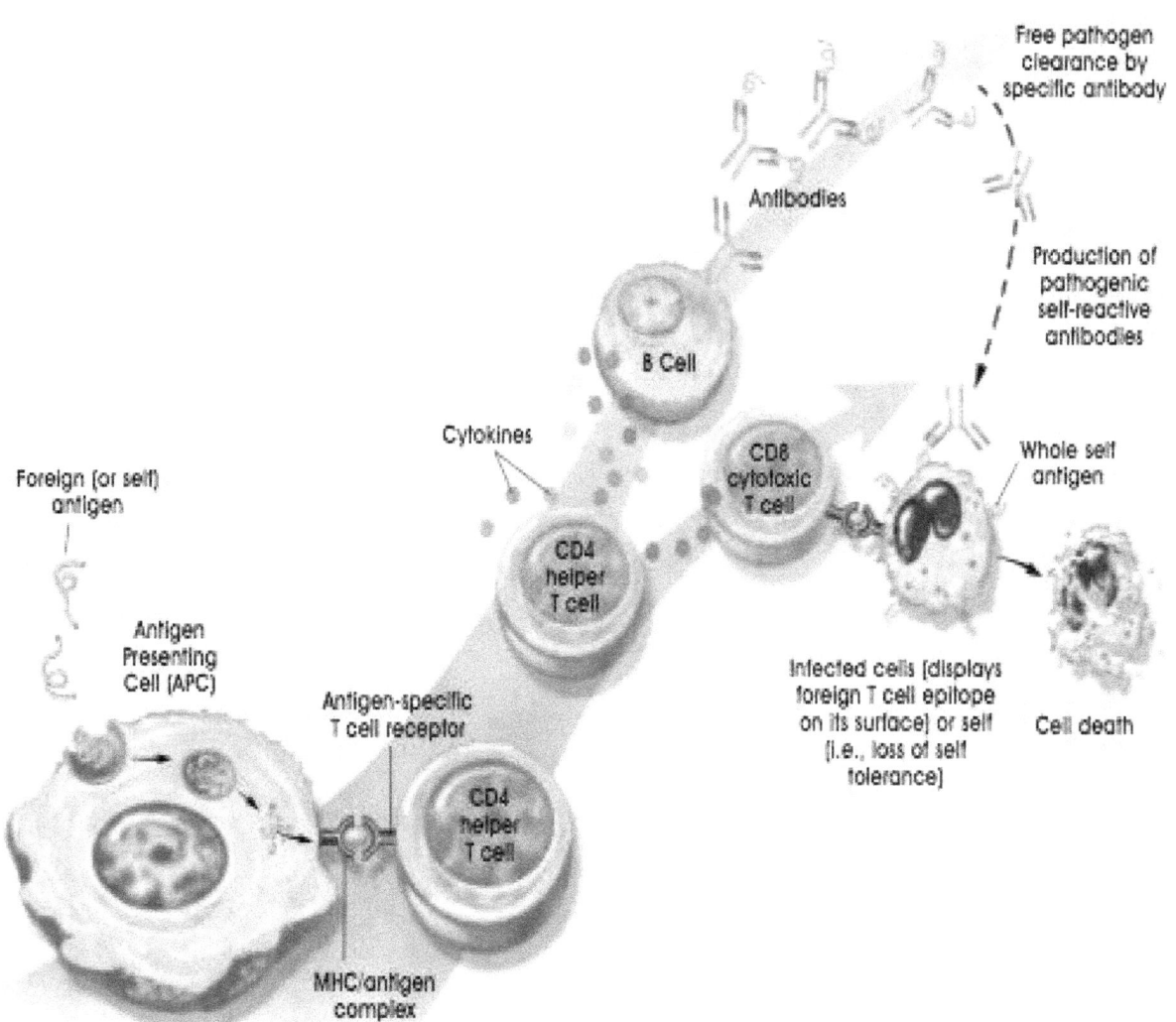

Free pathogen clearance by specific antibody

Antibodies

Production of pathogenic self-reactive antibodies

B Cell

Whole self antigen

Cytokines

CD8 cytotoxic T cell

Foreign (or self) antigen

CD4 helper T cell

Infected cells (displays foreign T cell epitope on its surface) or self (i.e., loss of self tolerance)

Cell death

Antigen Presenting Cell (APC)

Antigen-specific T cell receptor

CD4 helper T cell

MHC/antigen complex

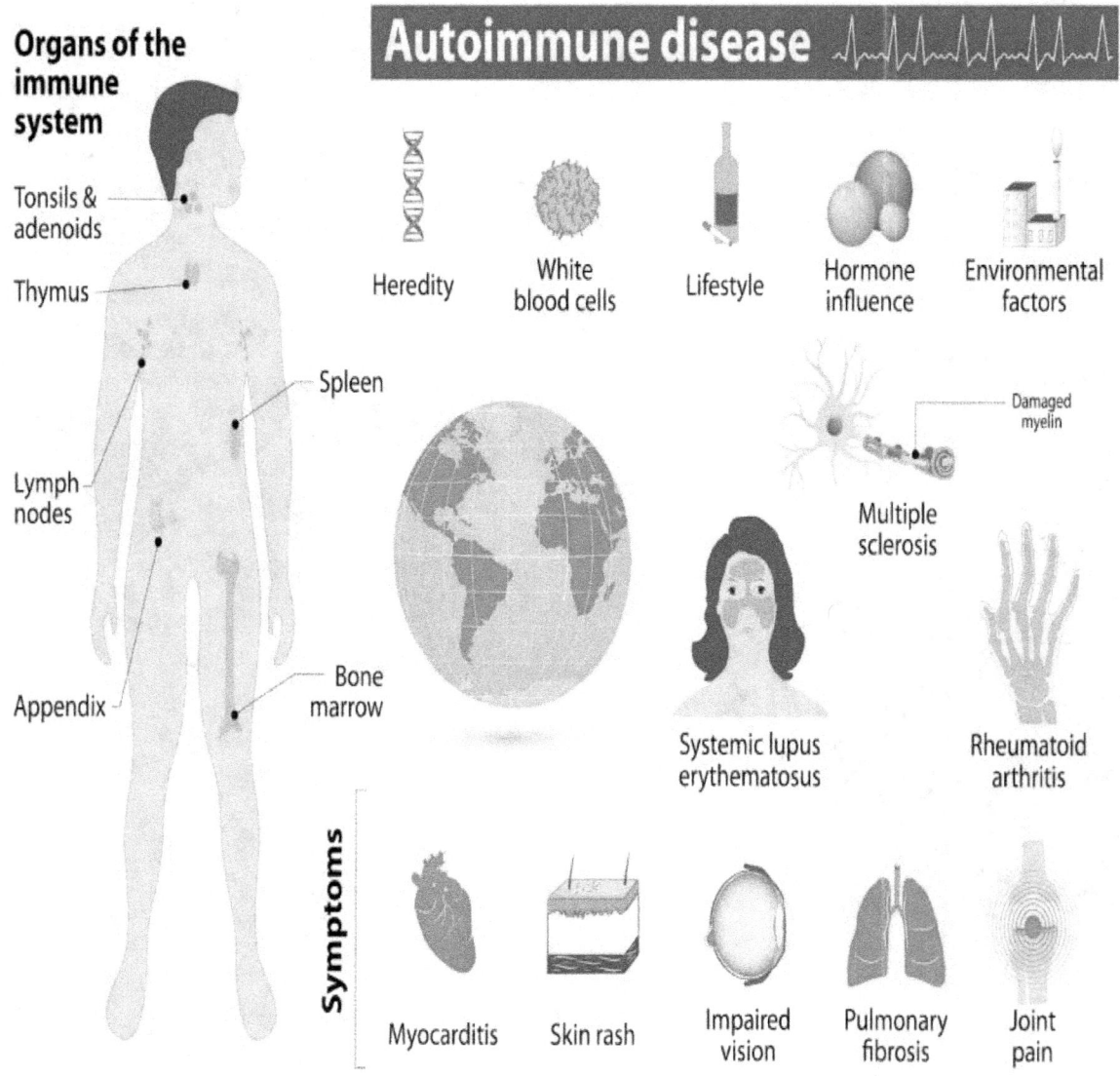

Organs of the immune system

Tonsils & adenoids

Thymus

Spleen

Lymph nodes

Appendix

Bone marrow

Autoimmune disease

Heredity

White blood cells

Lifestyle

Hormone influence

Environmental factors

Damaged myelin

Multiple sclerosis

Systemic lupus erythematosus

Rheumatoid arthritis

Symptoms

Myocarditis

Skin rash

Impaired vision

Pulmonary fibrosis

Joint pain

AUTOIMMUNE DISEASES

Brain
Multiple Sclerosis
Guillain-Barre Syndrome
Autism

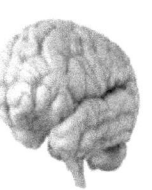

Thyroid
Thyroiditis
Hashimoto's Disease
Graves' Disease

Blood
Leukemia
Lupus Erythematosus
Hemolytic Dysglycemia

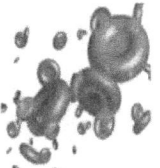

Bones
Rheumatoid Arthritis
Ankylosing Spondylitis
Polymyalgia Rheumatica

Over 100
Different Types of
AutoImmune
Disorders

GI Tract
Celiac's Disease
Crohn's Disease
Ulcerative Colitis
Diabetes Type I

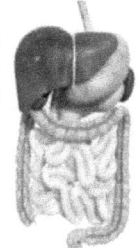

Muscles
Rheumatoid Arthritis
Ankylosing Spondylitis
Polymyalgia Rheumatica

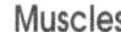

Nerves
Peripheral Neuropathy
Diabetic Neuropathy

Skin
Psoriasis
Vitiligo
Eczema
Scleroderma

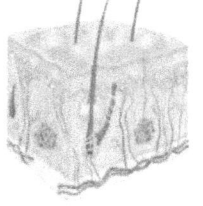

Lung
Fibromyalgia
Wegener's Granulomatosis

*****

Chapter 9 ... Autoimmune Dis-ease

*****

Our immune system is a complicated network of cells and cell components that normally defend the body and eliminate bacterial, viral, and other pathogenic infections. This sophisticated mechanism goes awry in autoimmune disease, when the immune system mistakenly attacks the body's own cells, tissues, and organs.

Auto is Greek for "self," so an autoimmune response is an immune response in which the body attacks itself.

Your body's immune system protects you from disease and infection. But if you have an autoimmune disease, your immune system attacks healthy cells in your body by mistake.

Autoimmune diseases can affect many parts of the body.

No one is sure what causes autoimmune diseases.

They do tend to run in families. Women - particularly African-American, Hispanic-American, and Native-American women - have a higher risk for some autoimmune diseases.

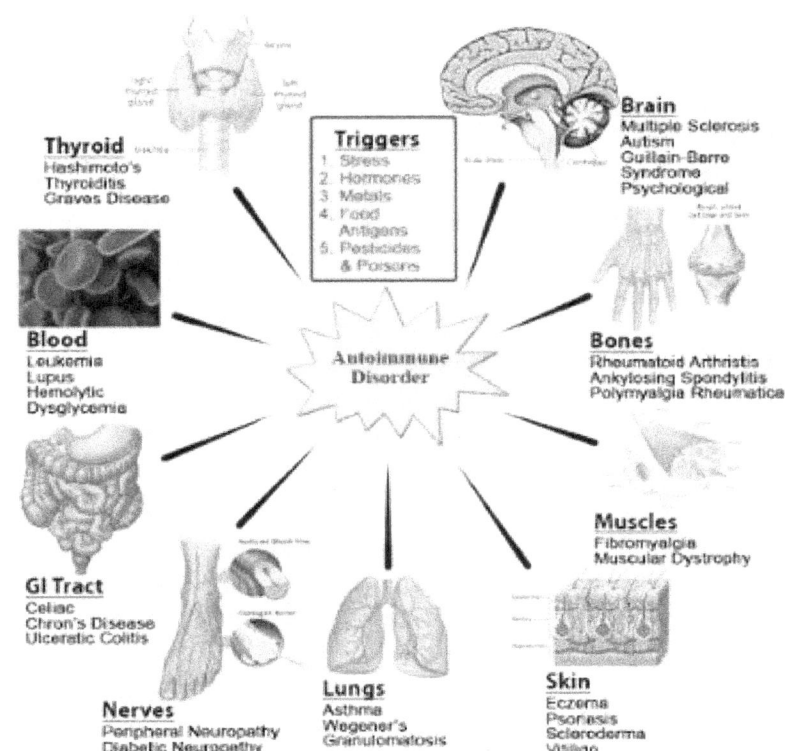

Tissues of The Body Affected By Autoimmune Attack

Thyroid
Hashimoto's
Thyroiditis
Graves Disease

Blood
Leukemia
Lupus
Hemolytic
Dysglycemia

GI Tract
Celiac
Chron's Disease
Ulcerative Colitis

Nerves
Peripheral Neuropathy
Diabetic Neuropathy

Triggers
1. Stress
2. Hormones
3. Metals
4. Food Antigens
5. Pesticides & Poisons

Autoimmune Disorder

Brain
Multiple Sclerosis
Autism
Guillain-Barre Syndrome
Psychological

Bones
Rheumatoid Arthritis
Ankylosing Spondylitis
Polymyalgia Rheumatica

Muscles
Fibromyalgia
Muscular Dystrophy

Lungs
Asthma
Wegener's
Granulomatosis

Skin
Eczema
Psoriasis
Scleroderma
Vitiligo

PAGE 134

Supreme Health & Fitness!   Health & Wellness Series Volume 1

Autoimmune Disease Root Causes & Risk Factors

Infections

Pathogens
Bacteria, Virus
Fungi, Parasites

Other Diseases

Food Intolerance
Gluten, Grains,
Dairy, Soy

Oxidative Stress

Chronic Inflammation

Leaky Gut Syndrome

Nutrient Deficiencies

Vaccines (Immunizations)

Environmental Toxins

Autoimmune System Dysfunction

Chronic Stress/ Psychological Factors

Hormonal Imbalances

Lifestyle, Trauma/ Surgery Events

Genetics, Gender, Age, Ethnicity

Thyroid, Other Glandular Dysfunctions

Medical/Dental Practices

Weakened Immunity

Prescription/ OTC Drugs

Tobacco, Alcohol, Other Drugs

There are more than 100 types of autoimmune diseases, and some have similar symptoms. This makes it hard for your health care provider to know if you really have one of these diseases, and if so, which one.

Getting a diagnosis can be frustrating and stressful. Often, the first symptoms are fatigue, muscle aches and a low fever.

The classic sign of an autoimmune disease is inflammation, which can cause redness, heat, pain and swelling.

The diseases may also have flare-ups, when they get worse, and remissions, when symptoms get better or disappear. Treatment depends on the disease, but in most cases one important goal is to reduce inflammation. Sometimes doctors prescribe corticosteroids or other drugs that reduce your immune response.

Autoimmunity: What it is and How it Occurs

Hidden allergens, infections, environmental toxins, an **inflammatory** diet, and stress are the real causes of these **inflammatory** conditions.

We are facing an epidemic of allergic (60 million people), asthmatic (30 million people), and autoimmune disorders (24 million people).

Autoimmune diseases include rheumatoid arthritis, lupus, multiple sclerosis, psoriasis, celiac disease, thyroid disease, and the many other hard-to-classify syndromes in the 21st century.

Type 1 Diabetes Autoimmune Disease Pathogenesis

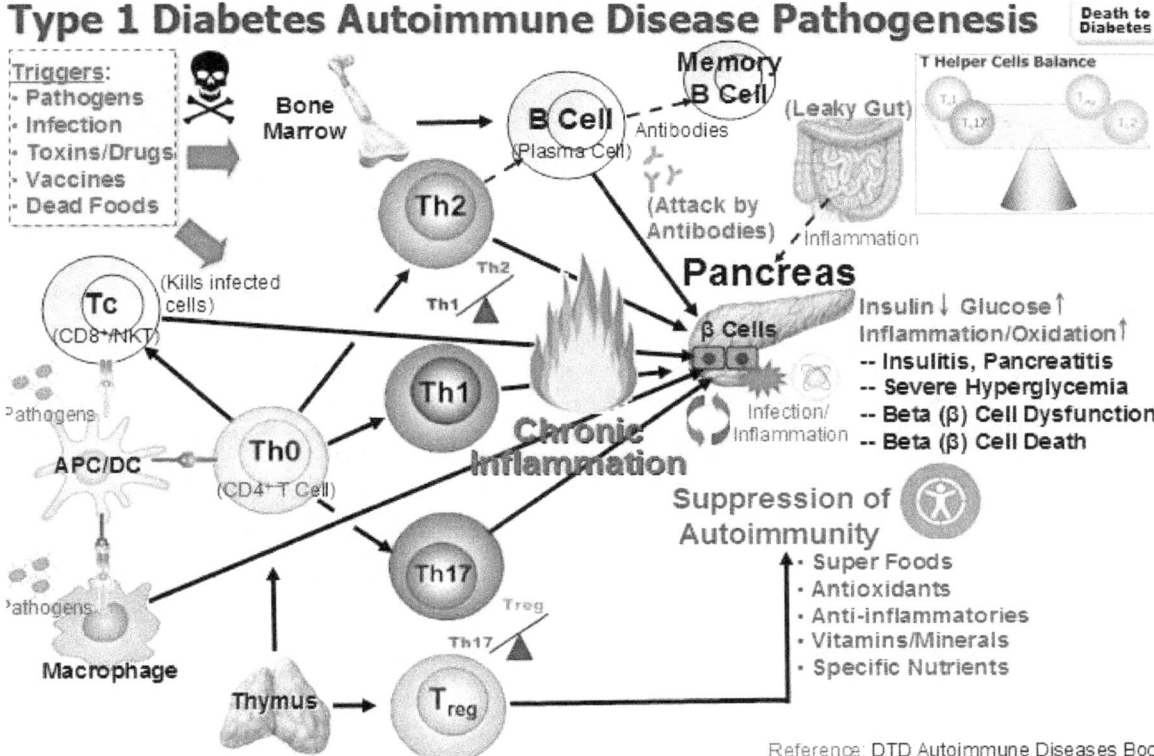

Reference: DTD Autoimmune Diseases Boo

These are all autoimmune conditions, and at their root they are connected by one central biochemical process: A runaway immune response also known as systemic inflammation that results in your body attacking its own tissues.

Your immune system is your defense against invaders. It is your internal army and has to clearly distinguish friend from foe — to know you from others. Autoimmunity occurs when your immune system gets confused and your own tissues get caught in friendly cross-fire.

Your body is fighting something — an infection, a toxin, an allergen, a food or the stress response — and somehow it redirects its hostile attack on your joints, your brain, your thyroid, your gut, your skin, or sometimes your whole body.

This immune confusion results from what is referred to as molecular mimicry. Conventional approaches don't have a method for finding the insult causing the problem. Functional medicine provides a map to find out which molecule the cells are mimicking.

The many autoimmune diseases have different effects, depending on what tissue is under attack.

In multiple sclerosis, for example, the autoimmune attack is directed against nervous tissue.

Pick an organ, any organ . . .

Autoimmunity can affect ANY organ/organ system in the human body

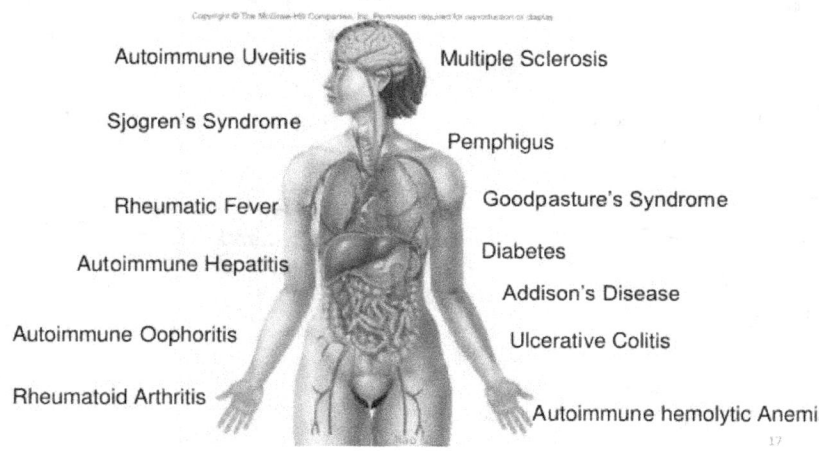

Copyright © The McGraw-Hill Companies, Inc. Permission required for reproduction or display

Autoimmune Uveitis

Sjogren's Syndrome

Rheumatic Fever

Autoimmune Hepatitis

Autoimmune Oophoritis

Rheumatoid Arthritis

Multiple Sclerosis

Pemphigus

Goodpasture's Syndrome

Diabetes

Addison's Disease

Ulcerative Colitis

Autoimmune hemolytic Anemia

Immune cells break down the myelin surrounding neurons of the CNS, resulting in the buildup of scar tissue that impedes normal impulse transmission.

Crohn's disease is an autoimmune disease directed against the absorptive portion of the gut.

Type I diabetes mellitus is an autoimmune disease that attacks the pancreas. If the pancreas is not functioning properly, cells of the body **cannot** absorb glucose as they should, resulting in the myriad symptoms of diabetes.

In diseases like systemic lupus erythematosus (lupus), the site of the attack may vary. In one person, lupus may affect the skin and joints, and in another it may affect the skin, kidney, and lungs.

Rheumatoid arthritis is an extremely common autoimmune disease, attacking the joint capsules of the body, causing painfully deformed joints. Although this type of arthritis is usually considered a disease of older people, 1 in 1,000 children under age 16 show signs of juvenile rheumatoid arthritis.

The damage of autoimmune disease may be permanent. For example, once the insulin-producing cells of the pancreas are destroyed in Type I diabetes, they do not regenerate. Autoimmune diseases afflict millions of Americans, and for reasons not understood, they strike more women than men. Some autoimmune diseases are also more frequent in certain minority populations.

For example, lupus is more common in African American and Hispanic women than in Caucasian women of European ancestry.

Rheumatoid arthritis and scleroderma, another autoimmune disease, affect a higher percentage of some Native American communities than the general U.S. population.

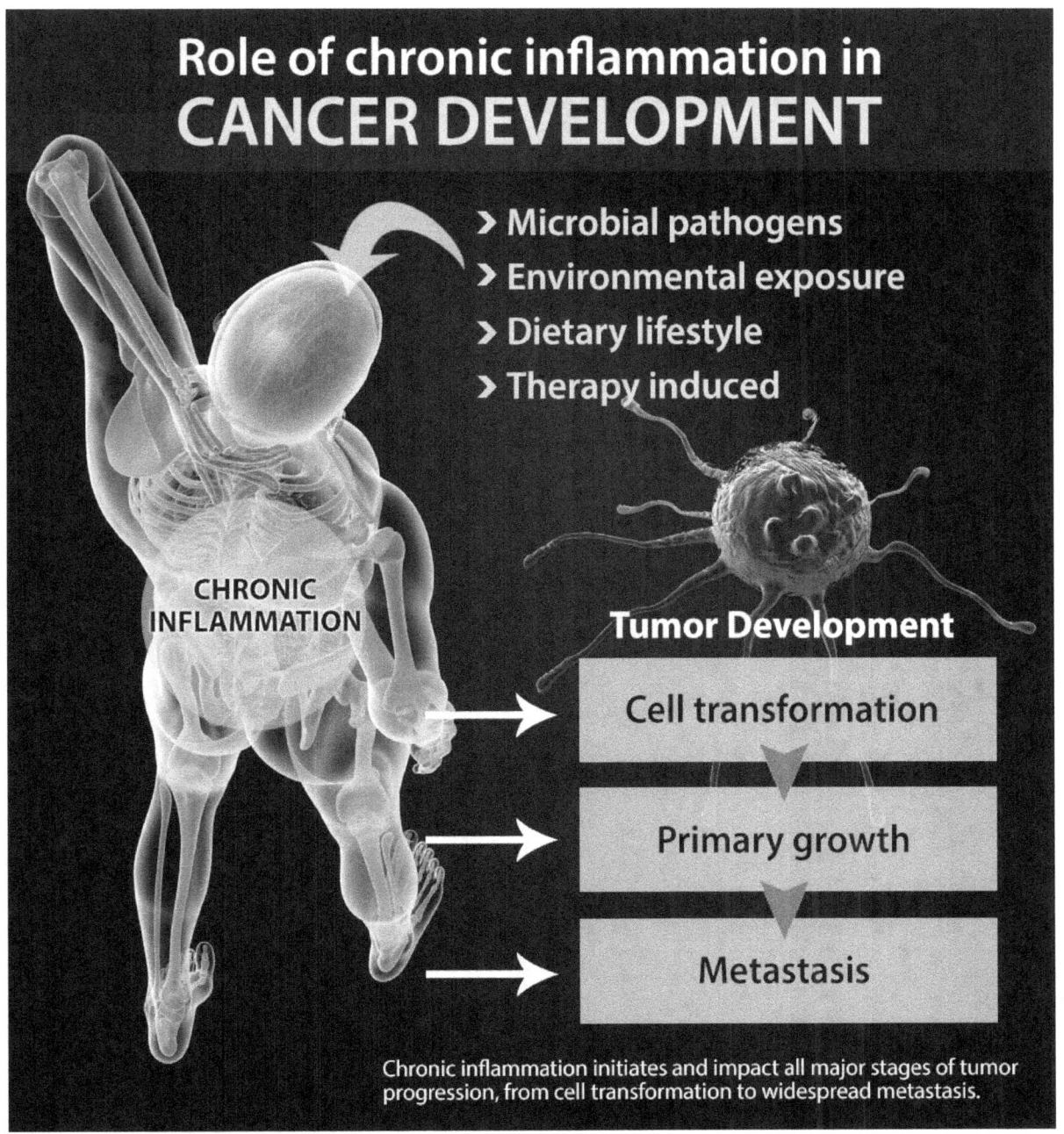

Role of chronic inflammation in
CANCER DEVELOPMENT

> Microbial pathogens
> Environmental exposure
> Dietary lifestyle
> Therapy induced

CHRONIC
INFLAMMATION

Tumor Development

Cell transformation

Primary growth

Metastasis

Chronic inflammation initiates and impact all major stages of tumor progression, from cell transformation to widespread metastasis.

AUTOIMMUNE DISEASE

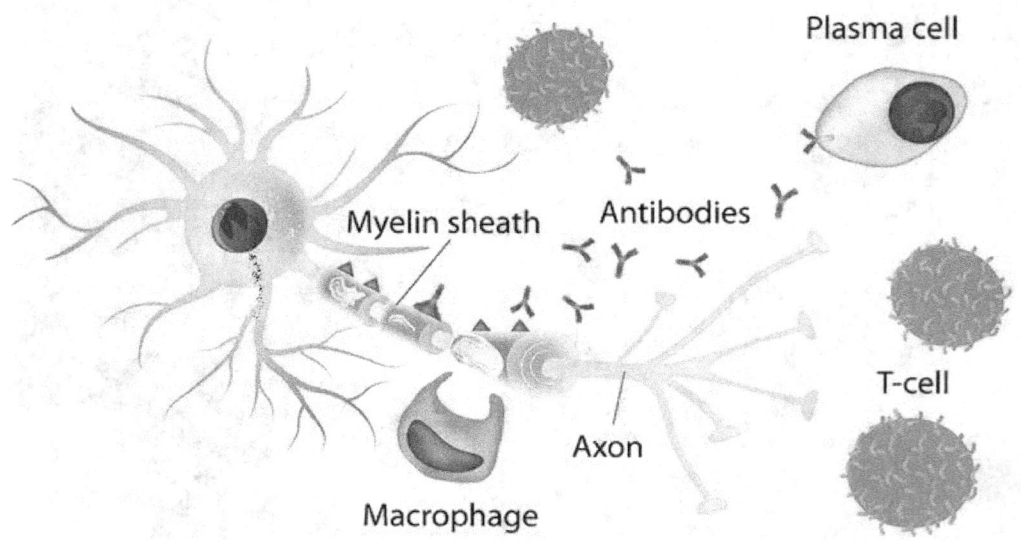

Plasma cell

Myelin sheath   Antibodies

Axon

T-cell

Macrophage

THE MECHANISM OF ALLERGY

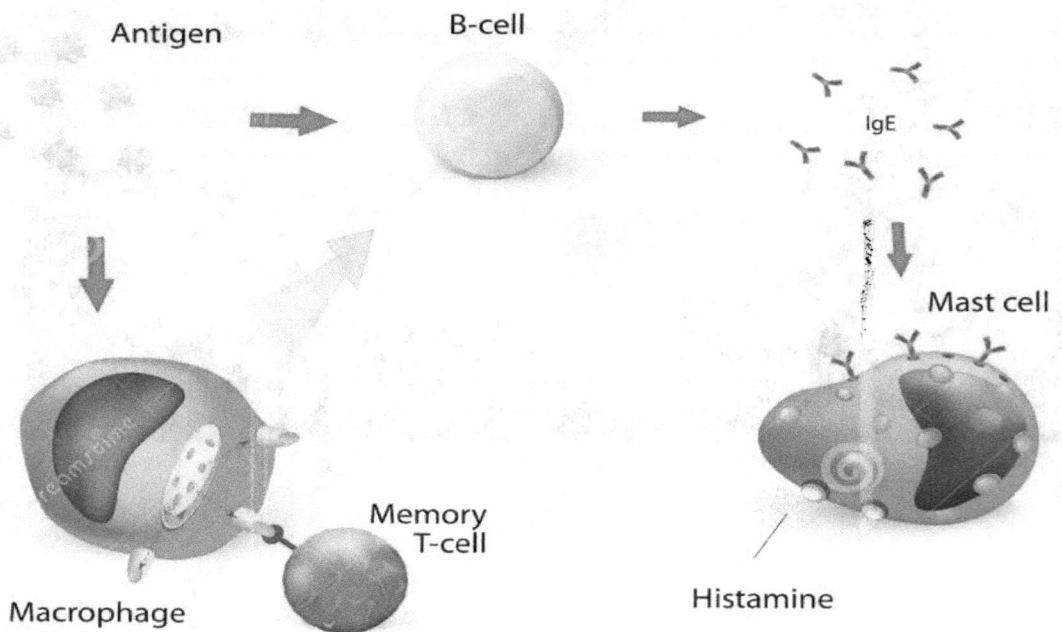

Antigen   B-cell

IgE

Mast cell

Memory
T-cell

Macrophage

Histamine

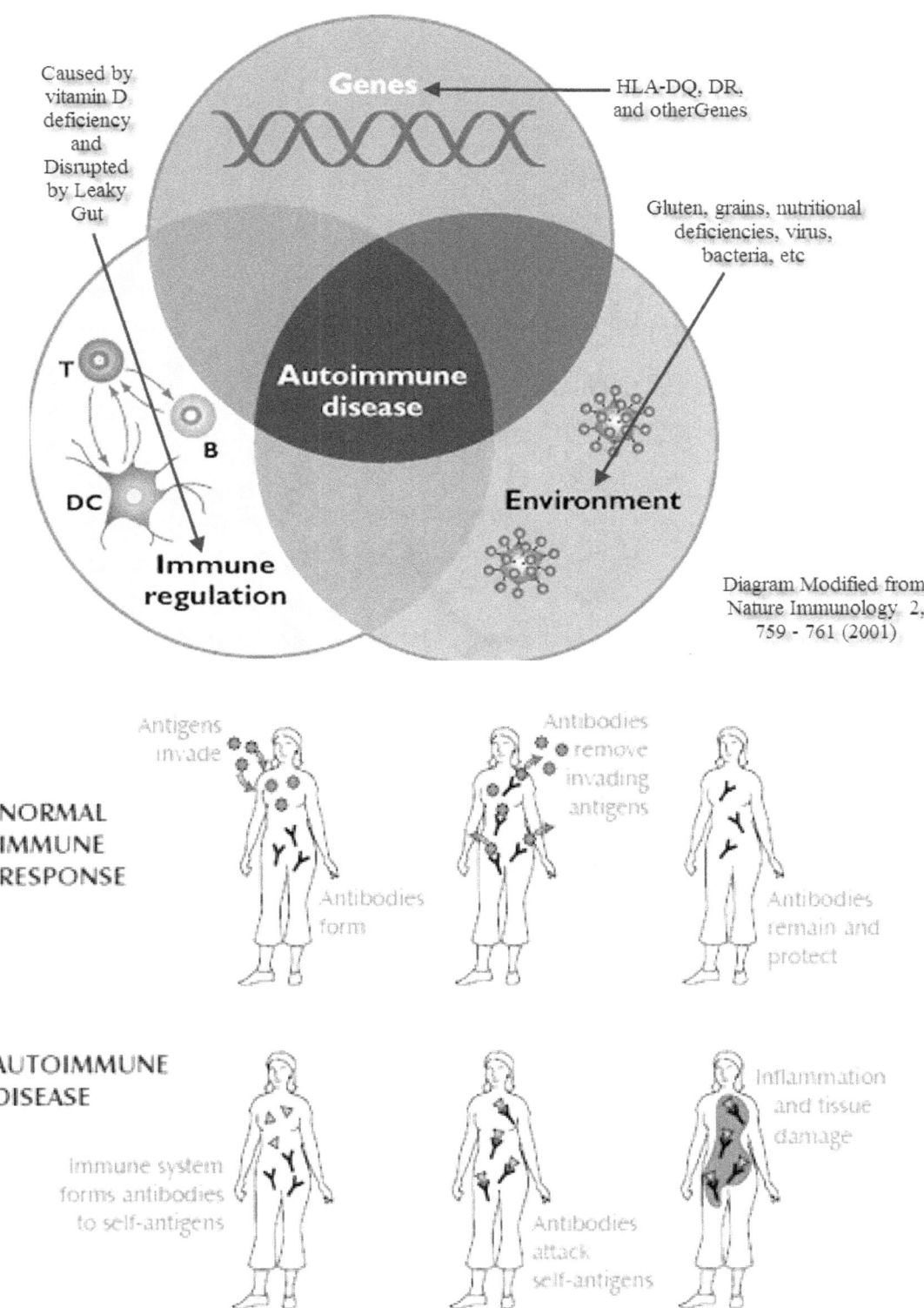

Genes

HLA-DQ, DR, and otherGenes

Caused by vitamin D deficiency and Disrupted by Leaky Gut

Gluten, grains, nutritional deficiencies, virus, bacteria, etc

T

B

DC

Autoimmune disease

Environment

Immune regulation

Diagram Modified from: Nature Immunology 2, 759 - 761 (2001)

NORMAL IMMUNE RESPONSE

Antigens invade

Antibodies form

Antibodies remove invading antigens

Antibodies remain and protect

AUTOIMMUNE DISEASE

immune system forms antibodies to self-antigens

Antibodies attack self-antigens

Inflammation and tissue damage

Gut Flora Controls Development of Immune Cells in Intestinal Lining and Treg Suppression Normally Prevents Autoimmunity

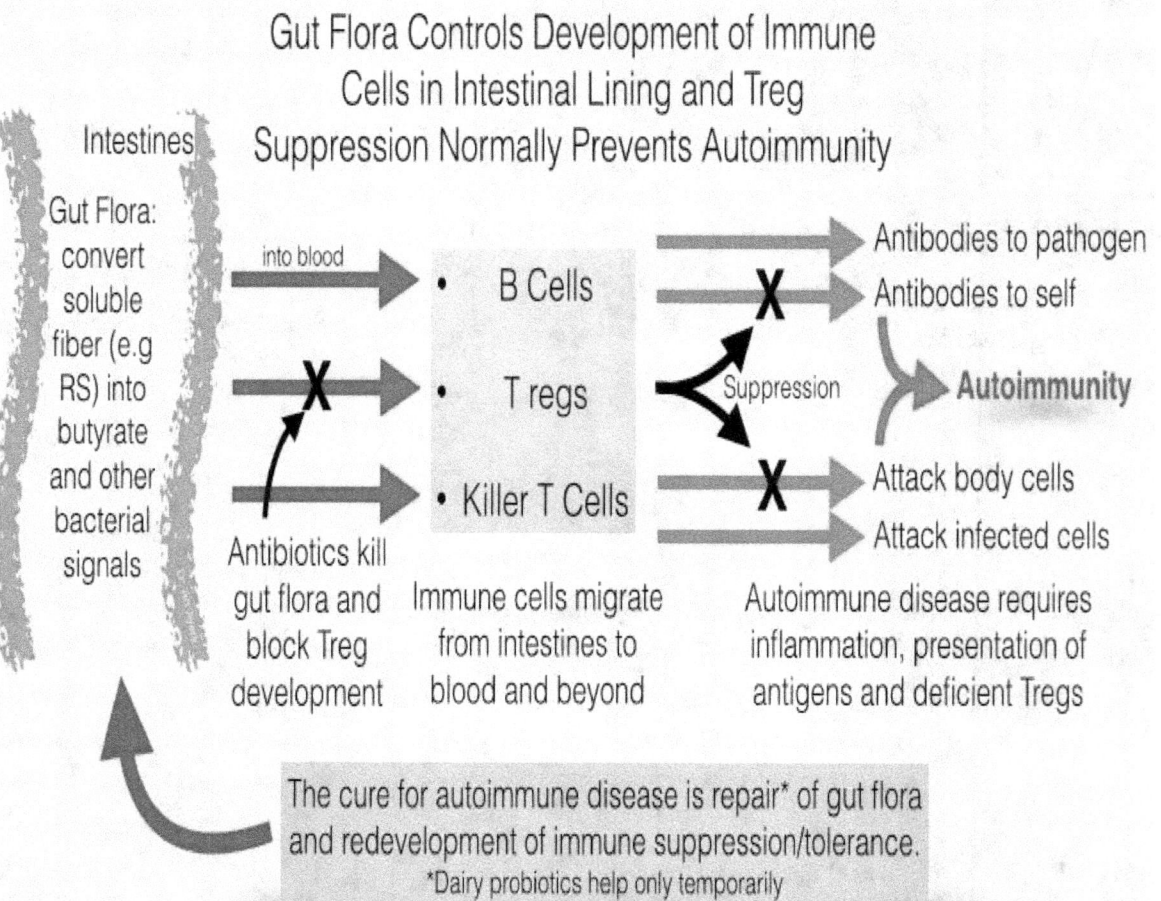

Intestines

Gut Flora: convert soluble fiber (e.g RS) into butyrate and other bacterial signals

into blood

• B Cells

• T regs

• Killer T Cells

Suppression

Antibodies to pathogen

Antibodies to self

Autoimmunity

Attack body cells

Attack infected cells

Antibiotics kill gut flora and block Treg development

Immune cells migrate from intestines to blood and beyond

Autoimmune disease requires inflammation, presentation of antigens and deficient Tregs

The cure for autoimmune disease is repair* of gut flora and redevelopment of immune suppression/tolerance.
*Dairy probiotics help only temporarily

Sugar is destroying your immune system. Can you see the problem.

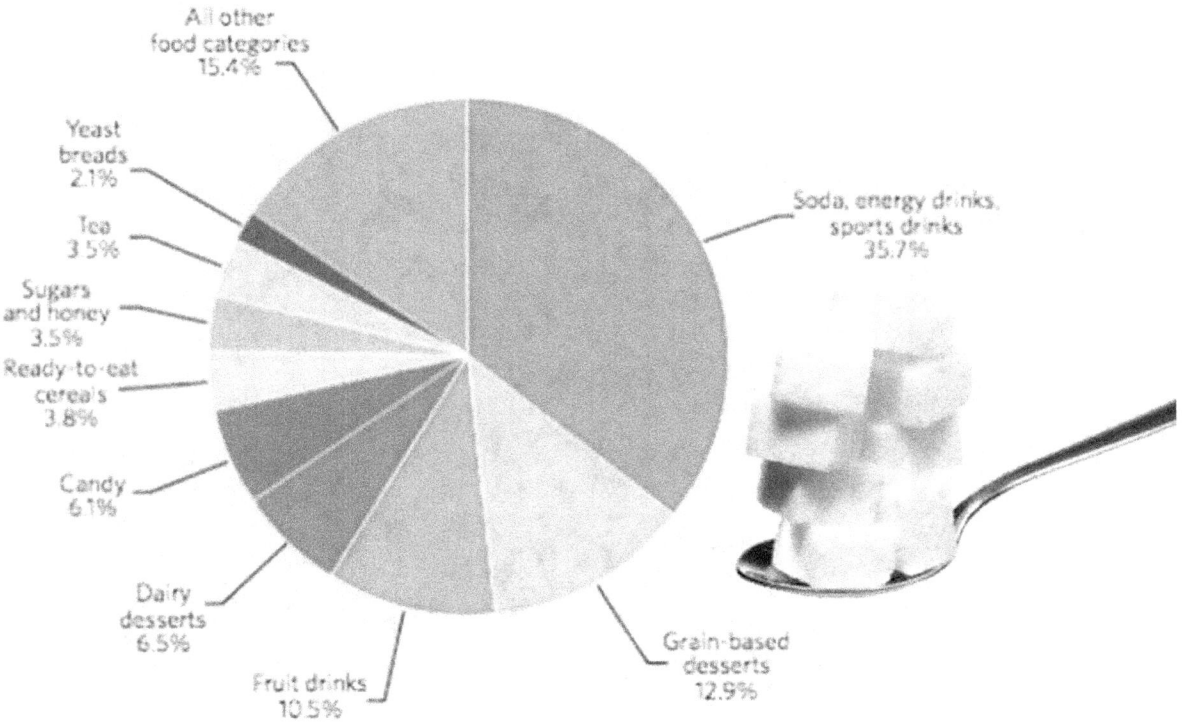

All other food categories 15.4%

Yeast breads 2.1%

Tea 3.5%

Sugars and honey 3.5%

Ready-to-eat cereals 3.8%

Candy 6.1%

Dairy desserts 6.5%

Fruit drinks 10.5%

Grain-based desserts 12.9%

Soda, energy drinks, sports drinks 35.7%

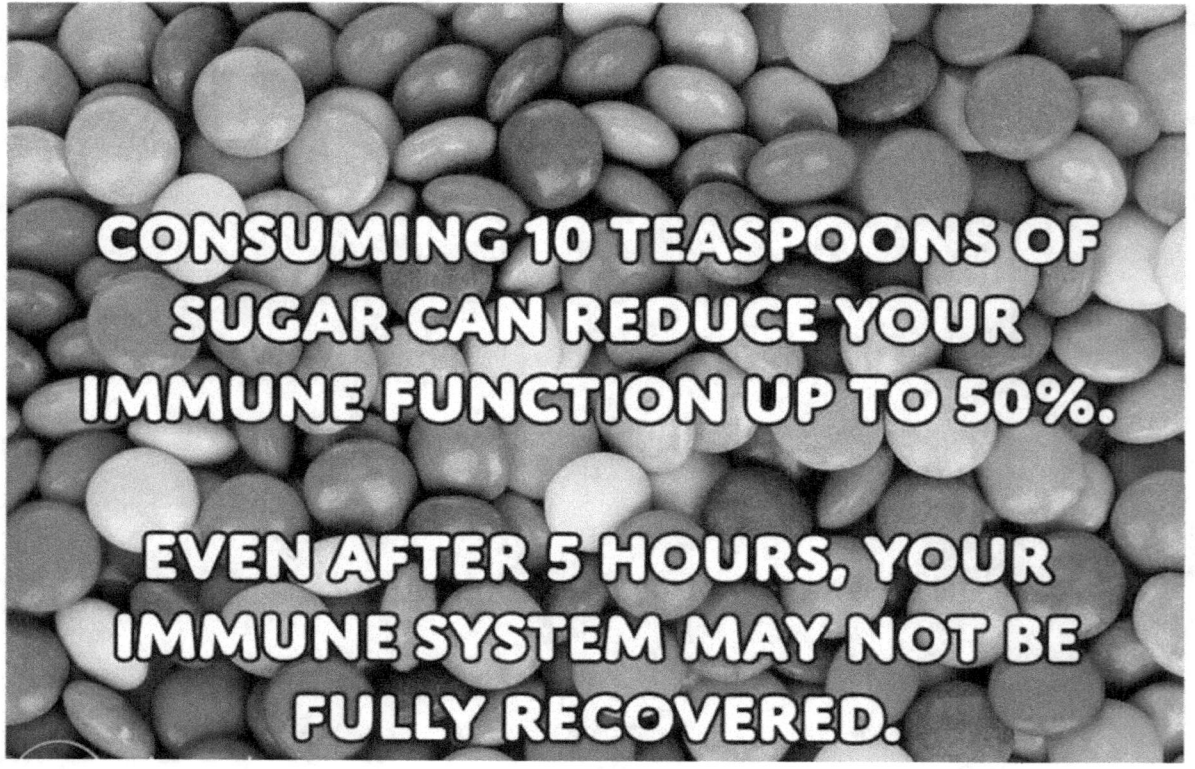

CONSUMING 10 TEASPOONS OF SUGAR CAN REDUCE YOUR IMMUNE FUNCTION UP TO 50%.

EVEN AFTER 5 HOURS, YOUR IMMUNE SYSTEM MAY NOT BE FULLY RECOVERED.

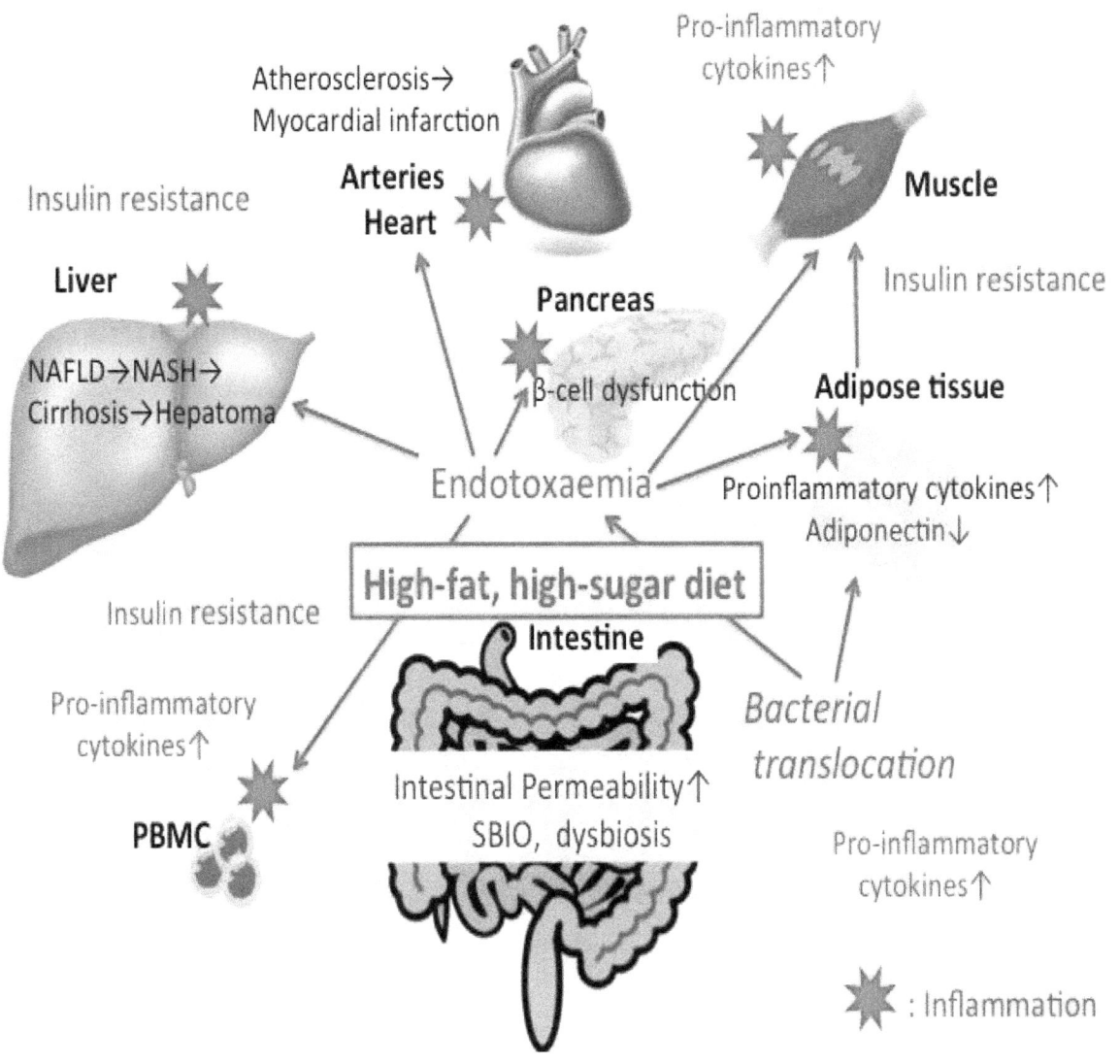

*****

Chapter 10 ... DEATH BY SUGAR

*****

By SUGAR I mean artificial, manufactured and/or process SUGAR. Glucose is the foundation of Sugar and Glucose is our #1 source for Life Energy. We NEED Sugar in the sense of GLUCOSE, but unfortunately many of us get lost in the commercial/advertising on TV and accept that as reality.

We fall for terms like sugar-free, or sugar substitutes or Low-sugar. Mis-leading terms because they don't disclose that they are referring to UNNATURAL Sugars and NOT from a Natural source like Sugar Cane, Honey, Molasses or Fruits.

So, with this chapter I want to show the affects of artificial, manufactured and/or processed (Unnatural) Sugar has on our Immune System.

Unnatural Sugar is scientifically and medically known to suppress the immune system, mess up your digestive system and cause a long list of side effects that are harsh enough to cause havoc all over your body.

Unnatural Sugar and junk foods can produce a burst of energy and feel comforting in the short term.

That's why we go for them when stressed, bored, sad, or short on time.

The pain-killing effect of sugar comes from the release of endorphins in your body when you eat the sweets.

Endorphins are a morphine-like chemical your body naturally circulates when you exercise, are excited, or eat sweet or spicy foods.

Despite how good you feel right after eating sweets, I'll bet you didn't know that sugar has a direct and dramatic effect on your immune system for hours after you eat it!

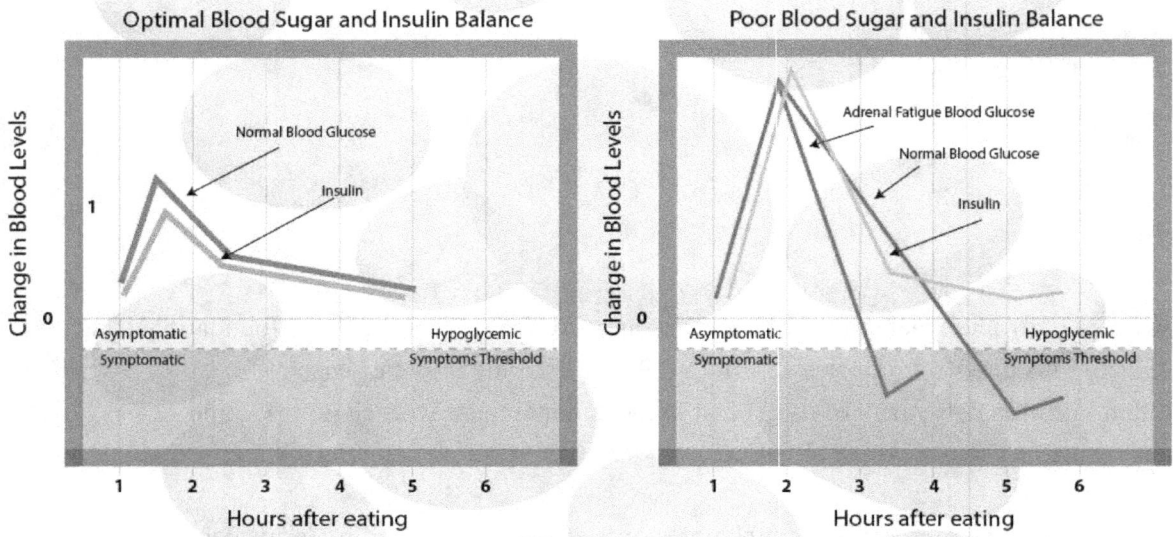

If you have an immune disorder sugar becomes even more of a problem.

According to a 1973 study done by Loma Linda University, when you eat 100 grams of sugar, about as much sugar as you find in a 1 liter bottle of soda, your white blood cells are 40 percent less effective at killing germs.

This can cripple your immune system for up to 5 hours after eating sugar!

Unnatural Sugar impacts your white blood cells by competing for space in those cells with Vitamin C. When Linus Pauling did research in the 1970s to find out how the body uses Vitamin C, he discovered that white blood cells need Vitamin C to destroy bacteria and viruses. Sugar and Vitamin C are similar in their chemical structure.

When you eat sugar, it directly competes for space in your immune cells with Vitamin C!

The more sugar in your system, the less Vitamin C can get into your white blood cells. Sugar DOES NOT help your immune system fight infection at all, resulting in a weakened defense from infections.

The tricky thing with sugar is that we are naturally set up to seek it out - in fact, human breast milk is sweet! In an orange or carrot, the sugar is packaged with nutrients, water, and fiber that help you digest it.

When you strip the vitamins and minerals from corn to make high fructose corn syrup, your body has to take nutrients from your bones, skin, and vital systems to break down the concentrated sweetener. Your kidneys will stimulate more urine production to water down the sugar, which is dehydrating and speeds up signs of aging and disease.

In the book "*Get The Sugar Out*" by Ann Louise Gittleman M.S. C.N.S Ms. Gittleman says, "**No matter what form it takes, sugar paralyzes the immune system in a variety of ways**:

- Sugar has been proven to destroy the germ-killing ability of white blood cells for up to five hours after ingestion.
- It reduces the production of antibodies, proteins that combine with and inactivate foreign invaders in the body.
- It interferes with the transport of vitamin C, one of the most important nutrients for all facets of immune function.
- It causes mineral imbalances and sometimes allergic reactions, both of which weaken the immune system.
- It neutralizes the action of essential fatty acids, thus making cells more permeable to invasion by allergens and microorganisms.

PAGE 148

Supreme Health & Fitness!   Health & Wellness Series Volume 1

A to Z Sugar Related Health Problems:

- Acne
- Addiction to drugs, caffeine & food
- Adrenal gland exhaustion
- Alcoholism
- Allergies
- Anxiety
- Appendicitis
- Arthritis
- Asthma
- Behavior problems
- Binge eating
- Bloating
- Bone loss
- Cancer (cancer cells feed on sugar)
- Candidiasis
- Cardiovascular disease
- Cataracts
- Colitis
- Constipation
- Depression
- Dermatitis
- Diabetes
- Difficulty concentrating
- Diverticulitis & diverticulosis
- Eczema
- Edema
- Emotional problems
- Endocrine gland dysfunction
- Fatigue
- Food cravings
- Gallstones

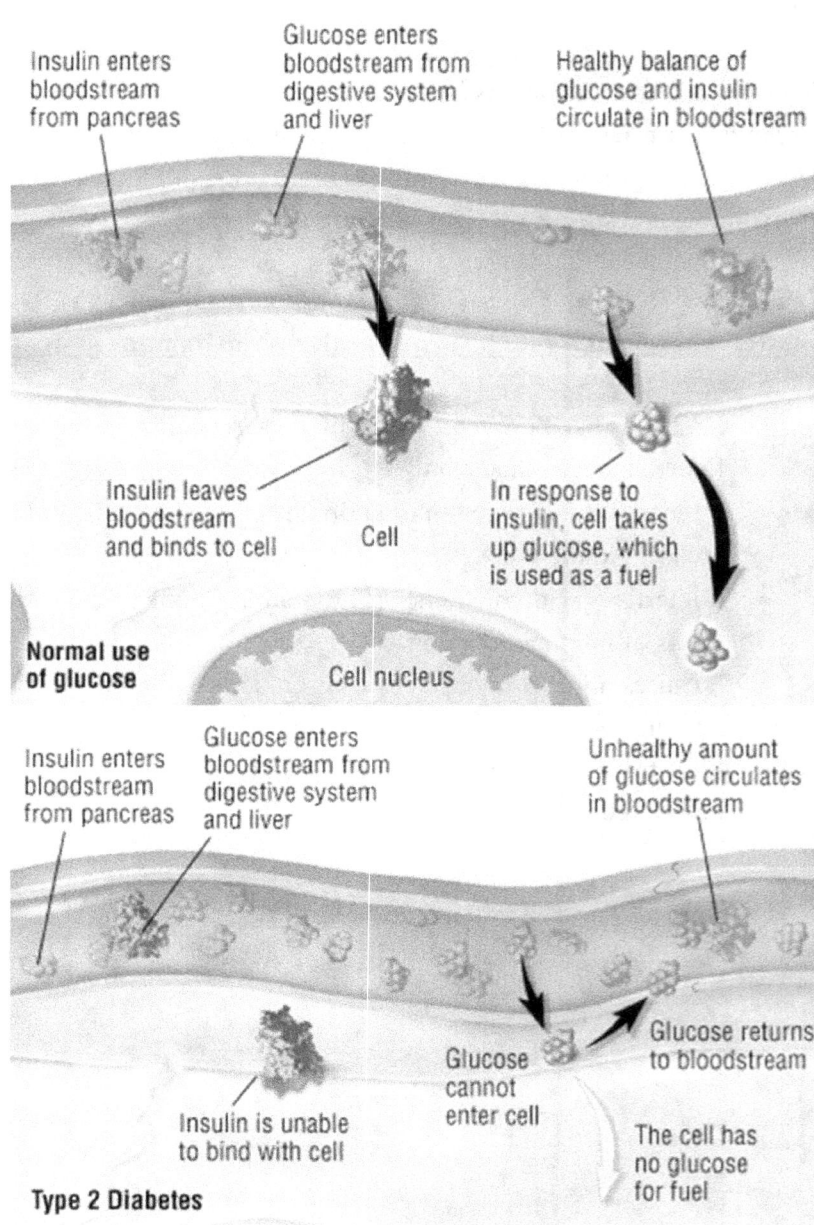

Insulin enters bloodstream from pancreas

Glucose enters bloodstream from digestive system and liver

Healthy balance of glucose and insulin circulate in bloodstream

Insulin leaves bloodstream and binds to cell

Cell

In response to insulin, cell takes up glucose, which is used as a fuel

Normal use of glucose

Cell nucleus

Insulin enters bloodstream from pancreas

Glucose enters bloodstream from digestive system and liver

Unhealthy amount of glucose circulates in bloodstream

Glucose cannot enter cell

Glucose returns to bloodstream

Insulin is unable to bind with cell

The cell has no glucose for fuel

Type 2 Diabetes

- Gout
- Heart Disease
- High blood cholesterol
- High estrogen levels
- High triglyceride levels
- Hormonal problems
- Hyperactivity
- High blood pressure
- Hypoglycemia
- Impaired digestion of all foods
- Indigestion
- Insomnia
- Kidney stones
- Liver dysfunction
- Liver enlargement & fatty liver syndrome
- Low HDL cholesterol
- Menstrual difficulties
- Mental illness
- Mood swings
- Muscle pain
- Nearsightedness
- Obesity
- Osteoporosis
- Parasitic infections
- Premature aging & wrinkles
- Premenstrual syndrome
- Psoriasis
- Rheumatism
- Shortened life span
- Tooth decay
- Ulcers
- Vaginal yeast infections

Sugar may not be the whole answer to why you are ill, but it could be an important part of the puzzle.

Sugar and Our Immune System

Your body has a very efficient system for protecting itself from outside "invaders" such as viruses, bacteria, fungi, etc. The single most important part of this system is the body's ability to identify and destroy any invaders that get inside.

There is a fact that you may not know about your body's immune system:

EATING ANY KIND OF SUGAR HAS THE POTENTIAL TO REDUCE YOUR BODY'S DEFENSES BY 75% OR MORE FOR FOUR TO SIX HOURS.

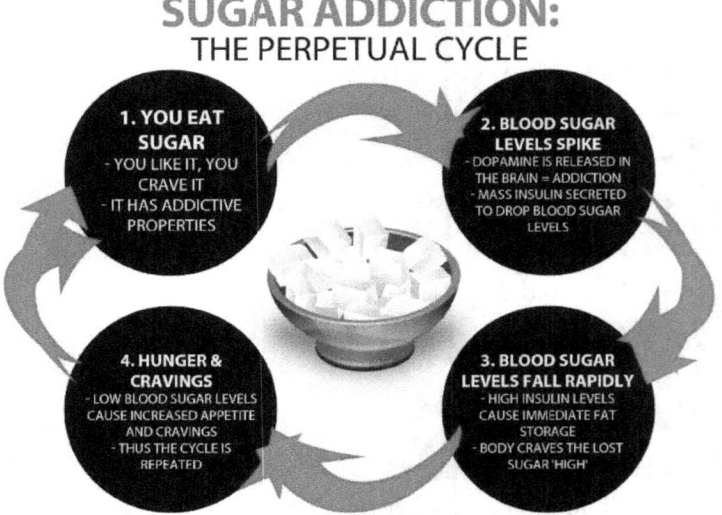

SUGAR ADDICTION:
THE PERPETUAL CYCLE

1. YOU EAT SUGAR
- YOU LIKE IT, YOU CRAVE IT
- IT HAS ADDICTIVE PROPERTIES

2. BLOOD SUGAR LEVELS SPIKE
- DOPAMINE IS RELEASED IN THE BRAIN = ADDICTION
- MASS INSULIN SECRETED TO DROP BLOOD SUGAR LEVELS

4. HUNGER & CRAVINGS
- LOW BLOOD SUGAR LEVELS CAUSE INCREASED APPETITE AND CRAVINGS
- THUS THE CYCLE IS REPEATED

3. BLOOD SUGAR LEVELS FALL RAPIDLY
- HIGH INSULIN LEVELS CAUSE IMMEDIATE FAT STORAGE
- BODY CRAVES THE LOST SUGAR 'HIGH'

This is not new data. In the 1970's Dr. Linus Pauling (one of the greatest researchers in the field of microbiology) discovered that vitamin C helps the body to combat the common cold. As part of the same research, Dr. Pauling found that sugar severely slows down this same process.

This is very important to know, as using this information can prevent illness and dramatically assist healing. Because the idea that sugar is "bad" for you is so controversial, I am going to give you a quick, simplified tour through your own immune system so you can see for yourself what Dr. Pauling discovered.

1. How Your Body Disposes Of Invaders: Bacteria, viruses, etc. are literally "swallowed" by a special type of cell called a "phagocyte." This is a cell, such as a white blood cell, that engulfs and absorbs waste material, harmful microorganisms, or other foreign bodies in the bloodstream and tissues.

2. Vitamin C: Dr. Pauling discovered that vitamin C is needed by white blood cells to engulf and absorb viruses and bacteria. In fact, a white blood cell has to contain 50 times the concentration of vitamin C as would normally be found in the blood around it. That's how Dr. Pauling came up with the "take vitamin C for a cold" theory. In order to continue to destroy bacteria and viruses, the white blood cells have to accumulate vitamin C all the time to keep up the 50-times concentration.

PAGE 151

Supreme Health & Fitness!   Health & Wellness Series Volume 1

So, vitamin C is being moved through the cell membranes into the white blood cells all over your body, all the time. That's why it's important to have plenty of vitamin C available to your body.

3. Sugar: Glucose (sugar in its simplest form, as found in the blood stream) and vitamin C have a similar chemical structure. So similar, in fact, that when a white blood cell tries to pull in more vitamin C from the blood around it, glucose can get substituted by mistake.

If the concentration of glucose in the blood goes beyond a certain concentration, the white blood cell's 50-times vitamin C concentration can start to drop because of the large amount of glucose it's pulling in as a substitute for vitamin C.

In fact, at a blood sugar level of 120, the white blood cell's ability to absorb and destroy viruses and bacteria is reduced by 75%. This blood sugar level would be easily obtained by any normal person eating some sugar (cake, cookies, candy, soda or even drinking fruit juice). Further, it can take four to six hours for the vitamin C concentration in the white blood cells to reach that optimum 50-times concentration again.

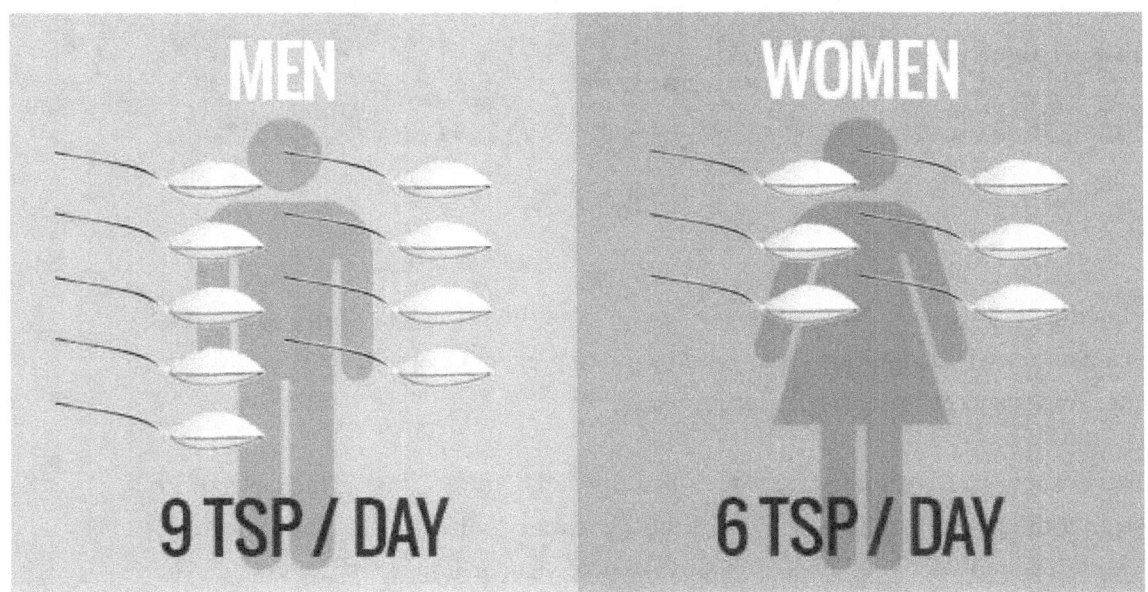

How much sugar is enough?

MEN — 9 TSP / DAY

WOMEN — 6 TSP / DAY

9 Ways Sugar Impacts Cancer

Are you eating too many carbs? Sweets and starches—even "healthy" whole—
grains—can lead to insulin resistance, which impacts cancer several ways.
Let us show you how to find the right amount of carbs for your body's metabolism.

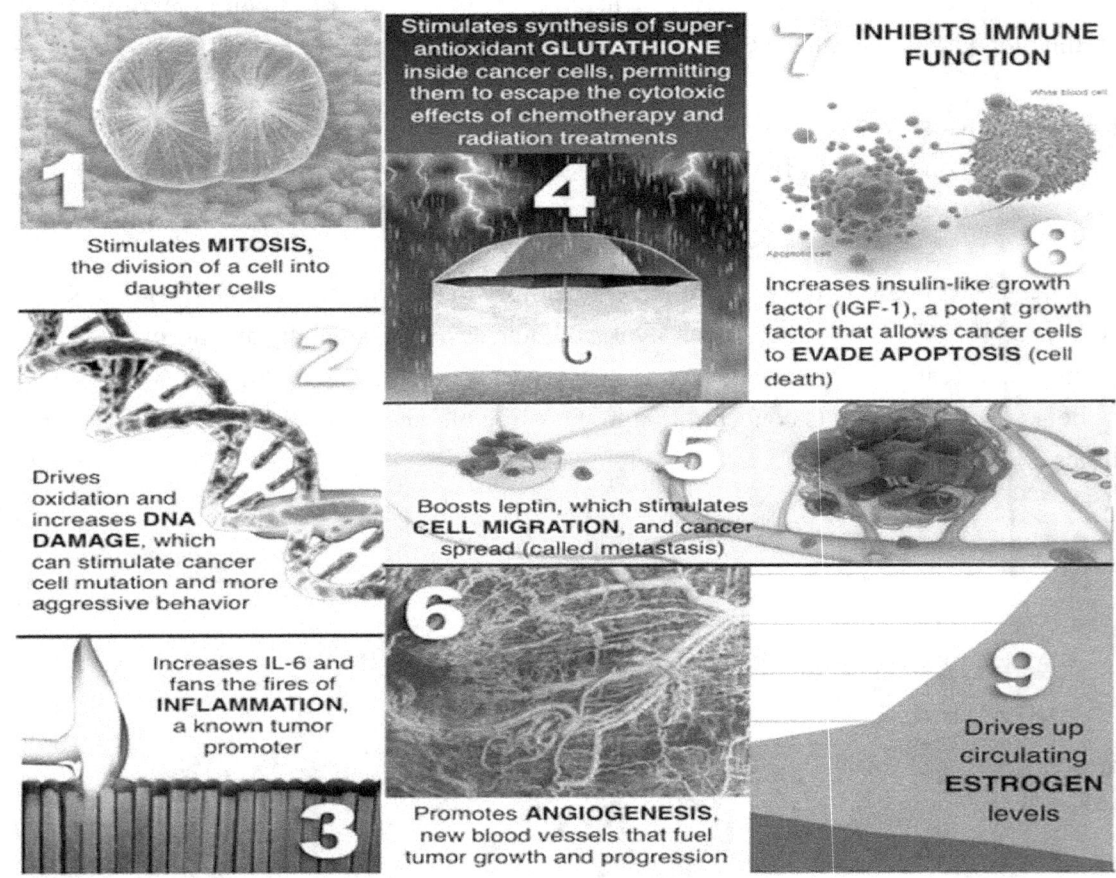

1 Stimulates **MITOSIS**, the division of a cell into daughter cells

2 Drives oxidation and increases **DNA DAMAGE**, which can stimulate cancer cell mutation and more aggressive behavior

3 Increases IL-6 and fans the fires of **INFLAMMATION**, a known tumor promoter

4 Stimulates synthesis of super-antioxidant **GLUTATHIONE** inside cancer cells, permitting them to escape the cytotoxic effects of chemotherapy and radiation treatments

5 Boosts leptin, which stimulates **CELL MIGRATION**, and cancer spread (called metastasis)

6 Promotes **ANGIOGENESIS**, new blood vessels that fuel tumor growth and progression

7 INHIBITS IMMUNE FUNCTION

8 Increases insulin-like growth factor (IGF-1), a potent growth factor that allows cancer cells to **EVADE APOPTOSIS** (cell death)

9 Drives up circulating **ESTROGEN** levels

Cancer Cells LOVE Sugar!

That is why refined carbohydrates like white sugar, white flour, high fructose corn syrup (HFCS) and soft drinks are extremely dangerous for anyone trying to prevent or reverse cancer. Sugar essentially feeds tumors and encourages cancer growth.

Cancer cells uptake sugar at 10-12 times the rate of healthy cells. In fact, that is the basis of PET (positron emission tomography) scans -- one of the most accurate tools for detecting cancer growth. PET scans use radioactively labeled glucose to detect sugar-hungry tumor cells. When patients drink the sugar water, it gets preferentially taken up into the cancer cells and they light up!

The 1931 Nobel laureate in medicine, German Otto Warburg, PhD, discovered that cancer cells have a fundamentally different energy metabolism compared to healthy cells. He found that malignant tumors exhibit increased glycolysis -- a process whereby glucose is used as a fuel by cancer -- as compared with normal cells.

Dr. Otto Warburg also found that cancers thrive in an acidic environment. Sugar is highly acidic. With a pH of about 6.4, it is 10 times more acidic than the ideal alkaline pH of blood at 7.4.

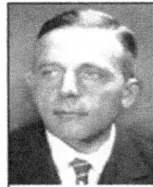

Dr. Otto Heinrich Warburg
1931 Nobel Prize Winner
The Root Cause of Cancer

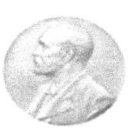

Dr. Otto Warburg discovered the root cause of cancer in 1923 and he received the Nobel Prize for doing so in 1931. Dr. Warburg was director of the Kaiser Wilhelm Institute (now Max Planck Institute) for cell physiology at Berlin. He investigated the metabolism of tumors and the respiration of cells, particularly cancer cells. Below are some direct quotes by Dr. Warburg during medical lectures where he was the keynote speaker:

"Cancerous tissues are acidic, whereas healthy tissues are alkaline. Water splits into H+ and OH- ions, if there is an excess of H+, it is acidic; if there is an excess of OH- ions, then it is alkaline."

In his work *The Metabolism of Tumours* he demonstrated that all forms of cancer are characterized by two basic conditions: acidosis and hypoxia (lack of oxygen). Lack of oxygen and acidosis are two sides of the same coin: where you have one, you have the other.

"All normal cells have an absolute requirement for oxygen, but cancer cells can live without oxygen - a rule without exception." – Dr. Otto Warburg

"Deprive a cell 35% of its oxygen for 48 hours and it may become cancerous." – Dr. Otto Warburg.

Dr. Warburg has made it clear that the prime cause of cancer is oxygen deficiency (brought about by Toxemia). Dr Warburg discovered that cancer cells are anaerobic (do not breathe oxygen) and cannot survive in the presence of high levels of oxygen.

He investigated the metabolism of tumors & the respiration of cells, particularly cancer cells.

All cancerous tissues are ACIDIC, whereas healthy tissues are ALKALINE.

All forms of cancer have two basic conditions, ACIDOSIS & HYPOXIA.

Deprive a cell of 35% of its oxygen for 48 hours & it may become cancerous.

CANCER *cannot survive* in the presence of OXYGEN!

In most people, when sugar in any form is consumed, the pancreas releases insulin. Breast tissue, for example, contains insulin receptors, and insulin is a powerful stimulant of cell growth.

One group of Australian researchers concluded that high levels of ***insulin*** and ***insulin-like growth factor*** (IGF) may actually be causative of cancers of the breast, prostate, endometrium and pancreas.

A broad study conducted in 21 countries in Europe, North America and Asia concluded that sugar intake is a strong risk factor contributing to higher breast cancer rates, particularly in older women. A four-year study at the National Institute of Public Health and Environmental Protection in the Netherlands compared 111 biliary tract cancer patients with 480 healthy controls. *Sugar intake was associated with more than double the cancer risk.*

Sugar ingestion seriously contributes to obesity, a known cause of cancer. Obesity also negatively affects survival. More than 100,000 cases of cancer each year are caused by excess body fat, according to the American Institute for Cancer Research. These include esophageal, pancreatic, kidney, gallbladder, breast and colorectal cancer.

How Sugar Feeds Cancer Growth

Could it be possible that sugar feeds cancer growth? Billions of dollars are funneled into cancer research every year… Yes it is in the **multiple BILLIONS!!!**

While we have made great technological advances in detection and treatment, it seems to be all on new versions of the same treatments.

With that being said, cancer remains the number 2 cause of all *preventable* deaths in the US today.

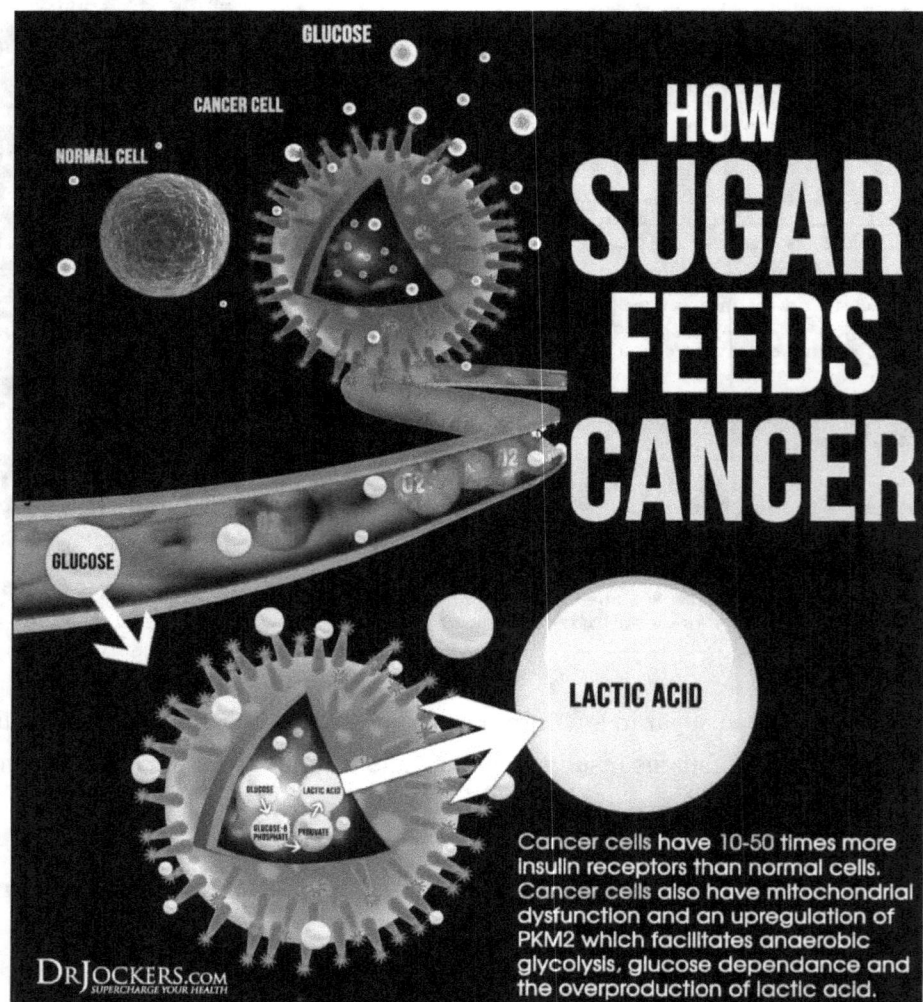

NORMAL CELL

CANCER CELL

GLUCOSE

GLUCOSE

LACTIC ACID

HOW SUGAR FEEDS CANCER

Cancer cells have 10-50 times more insulin receptors than normal cells. Cancer cells also have mitochondrial dysfunction and an upregulation of PKM2 which facilitates anaerobic glycolysis, glucose dependance and the overproduction of lactic acid.

DRJOCKERS.COM
SUPERCHARGE YOUR HEALTH

Take a look at almost any cancer treatment center in the US that uses the traditional treatment methods (chemotherapy, radiation, and surgery) and you'll notice something outright blasphemous.

To help keep weight on their patients, they offer snacks and meal replacements.

The problem? They are loaded with sugar and processed ingredients and… sugar feeds cancer.

Sugar suppresses a key immune response known as phagocytosis – the Pac-Man effect of the immune system. Consuming 10 teaspoons of sugar can cause about a 50% reduction in phagocytosis.

If you consider the sugar in your cereal, the syrup on your waffles and pancakes, the sugar added to your morning coffee or tea, the sugar in cold beverages like iced tea or lemonade, the HFCS in prepared foods, salad dressing and ketchup, and of course sugary snacks and desserts, you can see how easy it is to suppress your immune systems significantly.

Not only the amount of sugar, but also the frequency of ingesting sugar is relevant to immune function. In one study, research subjects were found to have nearly a 38% decrease in phagocytosis one hour after ingesting a moderate amount of sugar.

Two hours later, the immune system was suppressed 44%; immune function did not recover completely for a full five hours.

Sugar Substitutes

Please don't think I recommend artificial sugar substitutes!

Sweeteners containing aspartame, saccharin or sucralose have been shown to contribute to bladder cancer, lymphoma and leukemia, according to the National Institute of Environmental Health Sciences. A Good sugar substitutes are stevia (an all-natural herb from South America).

Artificial sweeteners	Sugar alcohols	Novel sweeteners	Natural sweeteners
Acesulfame potassium (Sunett, Sweet One)	Erythritol	Stevia extracts (Pure Via, Truvia)	Agave nectar
Aspartame (Equal, NutraSweet)	Hydrogenated starch hydrolysate	Tagatose (Naturlose)	Date sugar
Neotame	Isomalt	Trehalose	Fruit juice concentrate
Saccharin (SugarTwin, Sweet'N Low)	Lactitol		Honey
Sucralose (Splenda)	Maltitol		Maple syrup
	Mannitol		Molasses
	Sorbitol		
	Xylitol		
Advantame			

Even high-glycemic sweeteners like Sucanat, evaporated cane juice, molasses, honey and pure maple syrup are nutritionally superior to refined table sugar or HFCS, and you can avoid sugar spiking if you consume them in the presence of high fiber foods like ground flaxseeds.

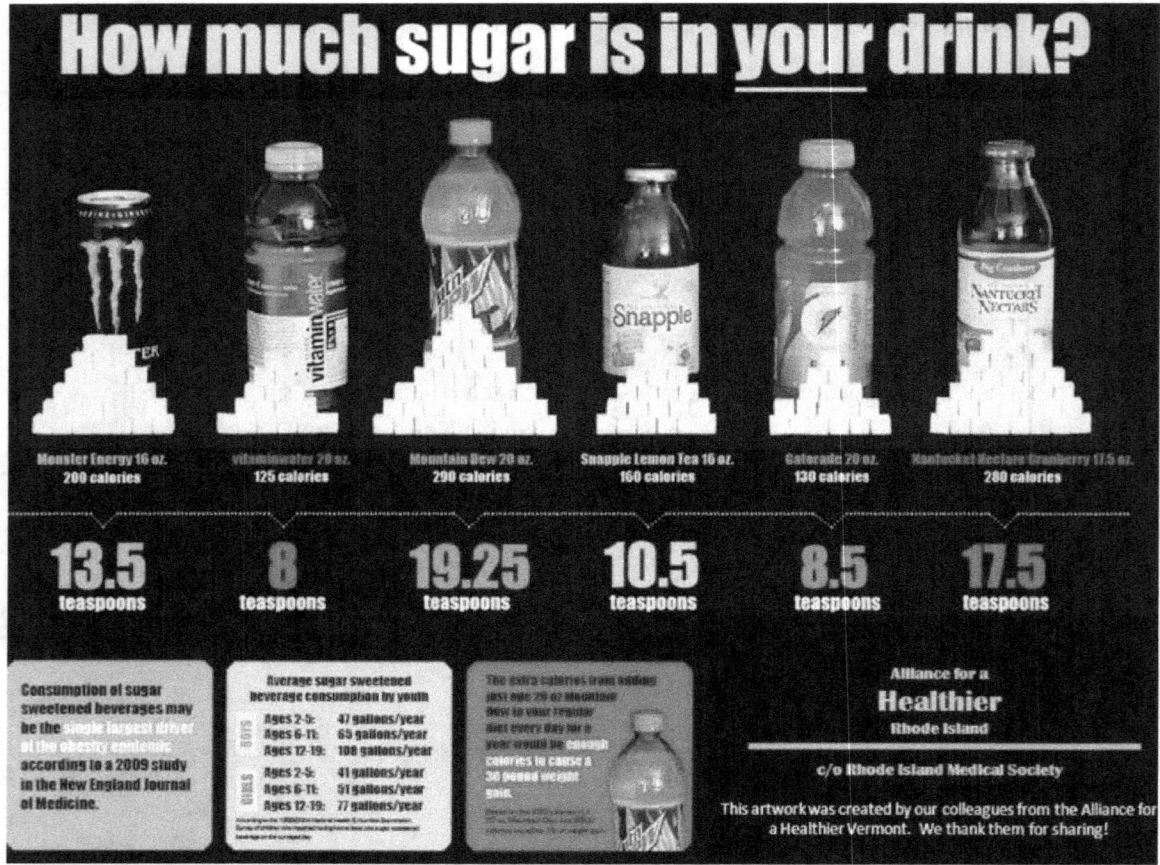

Conclusion

As you can see, it's not a great idea to eat any kind of sugar if you're sick, including the much-recommended orange juice (which may contain vitamin C, but this won't help if the white blood cells can't get past the sugar to use it!).

Further, if you were on a program of health improvement of any kind, sugar would be your number-1 enemy!

No matter if you're healing from an injury, either. White blood cells and other phagocytes remove dead tissue as well as other types of waste associated with injury healing.

A Balanced Immune System

Internal Threat	External Threat
Autoimmune problem (Hashimoto's Thyroiditis, Rheumatoid Arthritis, Lupus, Inflammatory bowel disease, Type 1 Diabetes)	**Allergic Reaction** (food sensitivities, allergies, eczema, asthma, sinusitis)

Immune Over-reaction

Balanced Immune System = Optimal Effectiveness

Immune Under-reaction

Cancer (Hepatitis, HIV, Shingles, TB)	**Infection** (Bacteria, Mold/Fungus, Parasites, Viruses)

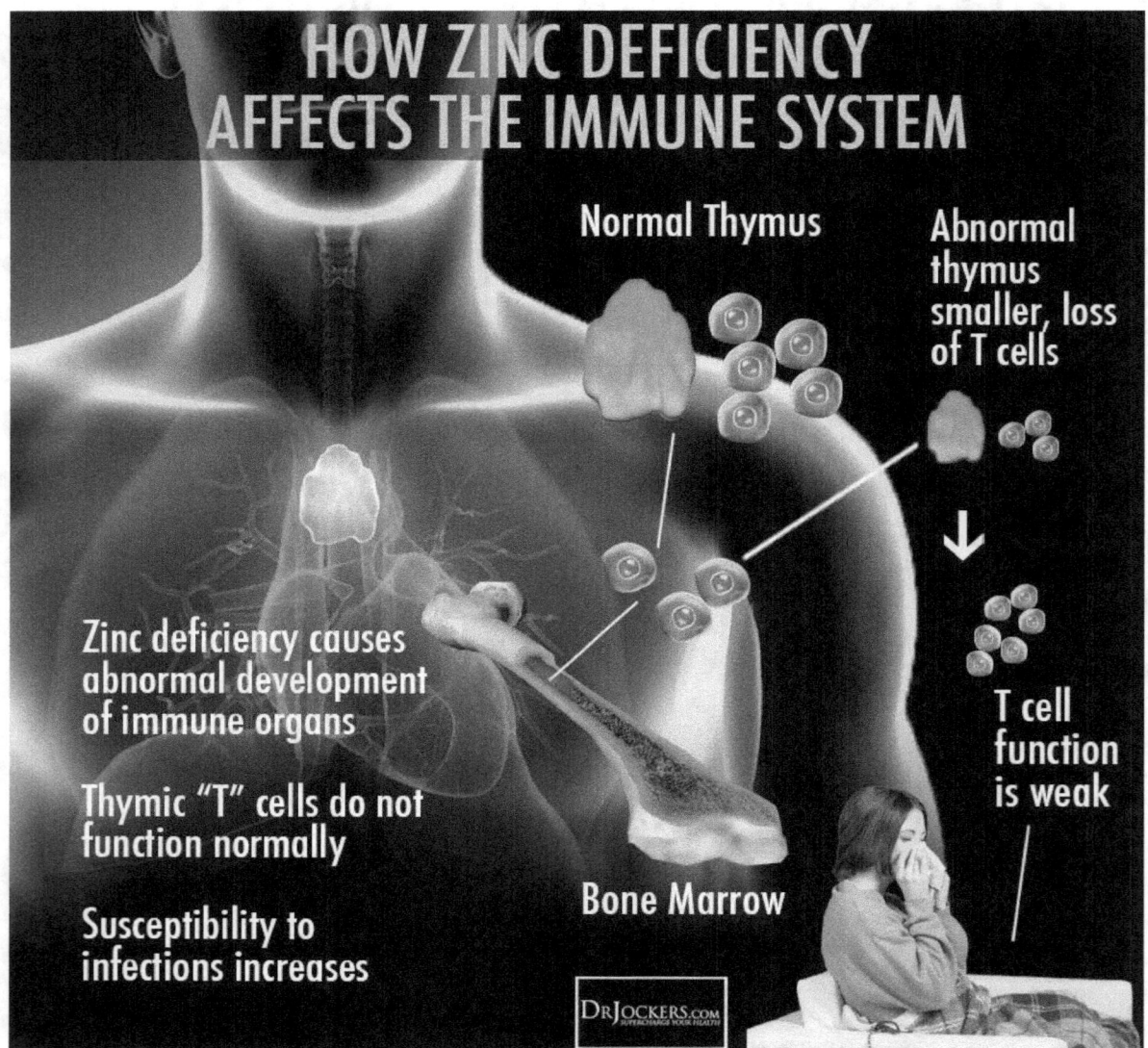

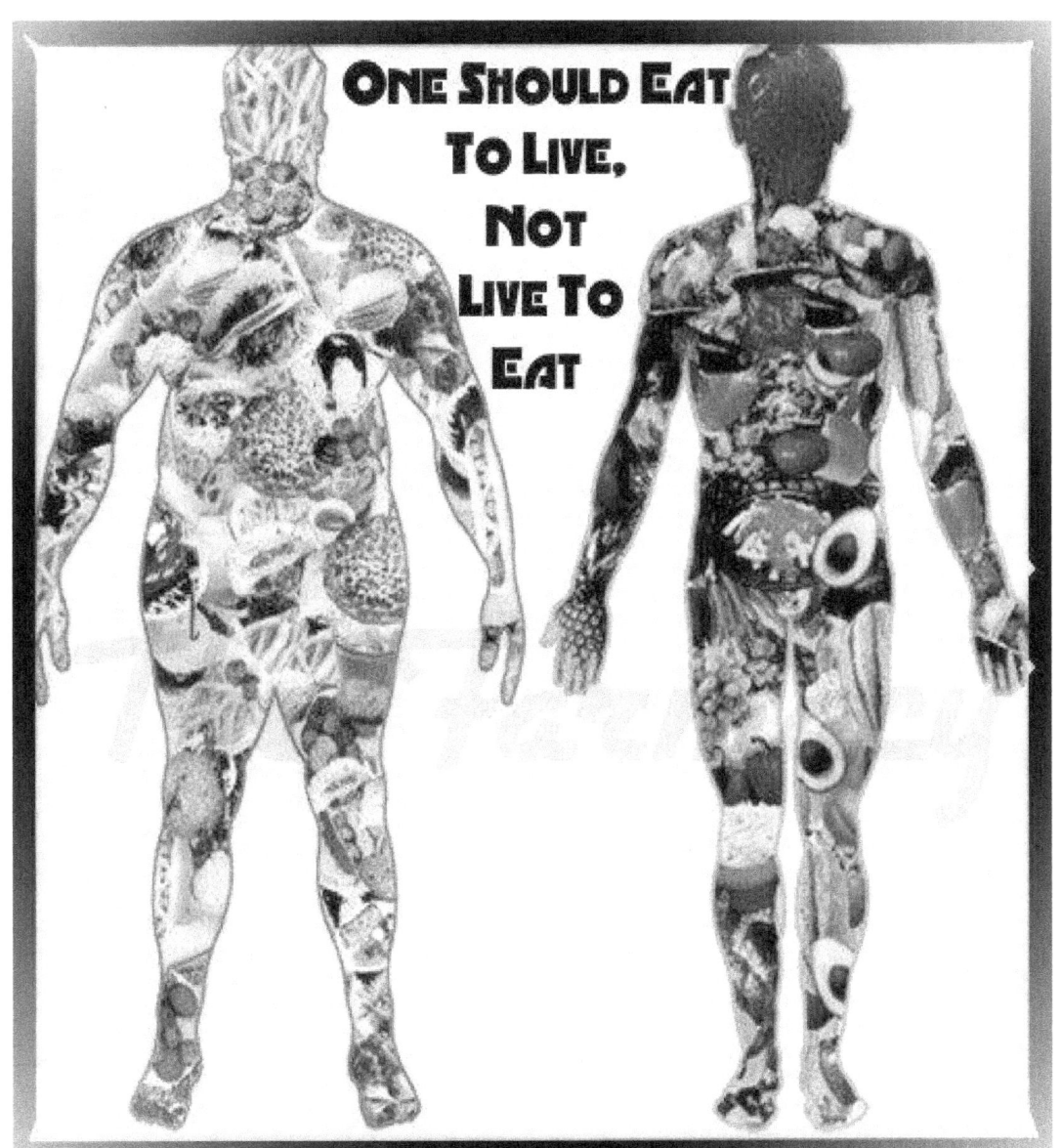

*****

Chapter 11 … Fasting – God's Prescription for Health

*****

Fasting Boosts Immune Properties

Fasting for as little as three days can regenerate the entire immune system, even in the elderly, scientists have found in a breakthrough described as "remarkable".

Although fasting diets have been criticized by nutritionists for being unhealthy, new research suggests starving the body kick-starts stem cells into producing new white blood cells, which fight off infection.

Scientists at the University of Southern California say the discovery could be particularly beneficial for people suffering from damaged immune systems, such as cancer patients on chemotherapy

The researchers say fasting "flips a regenerative switch" which prompts stem cells to create brand new white blood cells, essentially regenerating the entire immune system.

"It gives the 'OK' for stem cells to go ahead and begin proliferating and rebuild the entire system," said Prof Valter Longo, Professor of Gerontology and the Biological Sciences at the University of California.

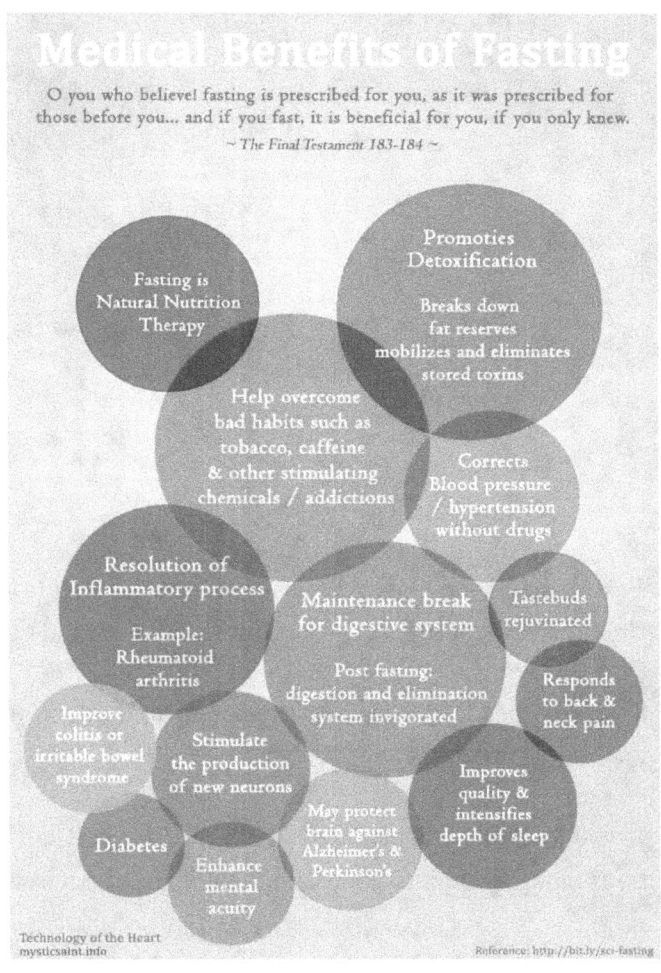

Medical Benefits of Fasting

O you who believe! fasting is prescribed for you, as it was prescribed for those before you... and if you fast, it is beneficial for you, if you only knew.
~ The Final Testament 183-184 ~

Fasting is Natural Nutrition Therapy

Promoties Detoxification
Breaks down fat reserves mobilizes and eliminates stored toxins

Help overcome bad habits such as tobacco, caffeine & other stimulating chemicals / addictions

Corrects Blood pressure / hypertension without drugs

Resolution of Inflammatory process
Example: Rheumatoid arthritis

Maintenance break for digestive system

Tastebuds rejuvinated

Post fasting: digestion and elimination system invigorated

Responds to back & neck pain

Improve colitis or irritable bowel syndrome

Stimulate the production of new neurons

Improves quality & intensifies depth of sleep

Diabetes

May protect brain against Alzheimer's & Perkinson's

Enhance mental acuity

Technology of the Heart
mysticsaint.info

Reference: http://bit.ly/sci-fasting

"And the good news is that the body got rid of the parts of the system that might be damaged or old, the inefficient parts, during the fasting.

Prolonged fasting forces the body to use stores of glucose and fat but also breaks down a significant portion of white blood cells.

During each cycle of fasting, this depletion of white blood cells induces changes that trigger stem cell-based regeneration of new immune system cells.

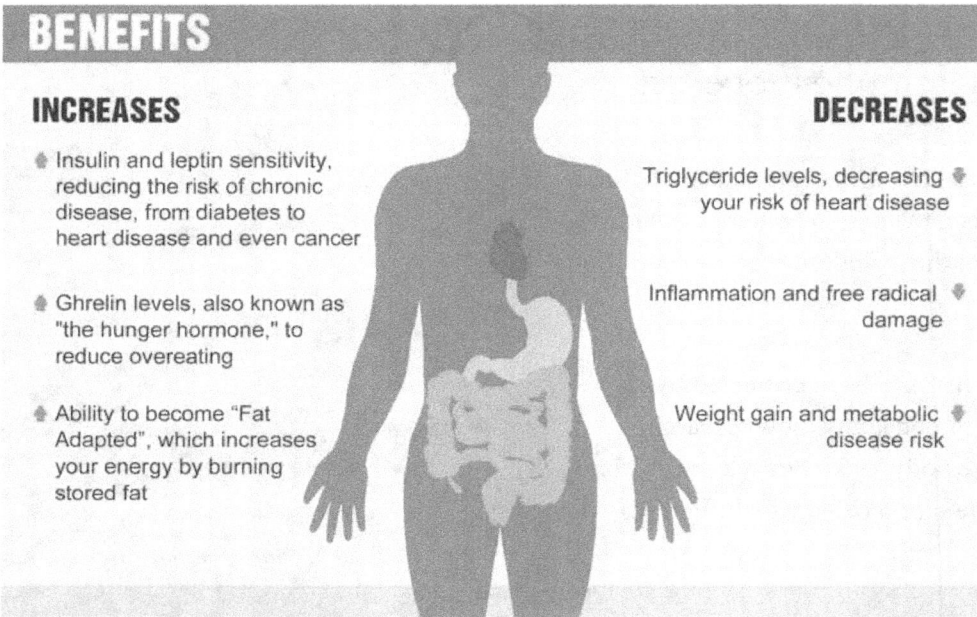

BENEFITS

INCREASES

☀ Insulin and leptin sensitivity, reducing the risk of chronic disease, from diabetes to heart disease and even cancer

☀ Ghrelin levels, also known as "the hunger hormone," to reduce overeating

☀ Ability to become "Fat Adapted", which increases your energy by burning stored fat

DECREASES

Triglyceride levels, decreasing ☀ your risk of heart disease

Inflammation and free radical ☀ damage

Weight gain and metabolic ☀ disease risk

Fasting helps the body recover from small ailments and areas of weakness since the body has time to fix them before the next onslaught of food comes in.

The body needs all its power to transform the food into nourishment while removing the toxins and disposing of the waste.

If you look at a waste management facility, you can see the work involved in turning your household waste into something that is more environmentally friendly and less toxic.

Your body has an even more difficult job with the foods and drinks you consume. Not only does it have to filter out all the toxins that are inherent in them, but the food itself must be broken down to a level that the cells can utilize it.

There is no machinery in the world that is as complex as the human body.

This process is so efficient that it may take anywhere from a few minutes to a few days to break down the foods so the body can use it properly and whisk away the waste and the toxins.

This daily ritual of eating, drinking and pooping is what makes the body stay healthy, yet, it is a rigorous undertaking. When a person chooses to fast, perhaps on juices only for a period of time, it's as if they are giving their digestive system a little vacation.

The nutrition from the juices will adequately sustain their energy levels, as well as continue to assist the creation of new, healthy cells and dispose of the cellular waste—all without taxing the digestive system.

This allows the NK (natural killer) cells the luxury to begin to work on areas of the body that have been neglected due to constant food manufacturing processes each day, all day long. In trials humans were asked to regularly fast for between two and four days over a six-month period.

Scientists found that prolonged fasting also reduced the enzyme PKA, which is linked to aging and a hormone which increases cancer risk and tumor growth.

"We could not predict that prolonged fasting would have such a remarkable effect in promoting stem cell-based regeneration of the hematopoietic system," added Dr. Longo.

"When you starve, the system tries to save energy, and one of the things it can do to save energy is to recycle a lot of the immune cells that are not needed, especially those that may be damaged," Dr. Longo said.

"What we started noticing in both our human work and animal work is that the white blood cell count goes down with prolonged fasting. Then when you re-feed, the blood cells come back. So we started thinking, well, where does it come from?"

Fasting for 72 hours also protected cancer patients against the toxic impact of chemotherapy.

"While chemotherapy saves lives, it causes significant collateral damage to the immune system. The results of this study suggest that fasting may mitigate some of the harmful effects of chemotherapy," said co-author Tanya Dorff, assistant professor of clinical medicine at the USC Norris Comprehensive Cancer Center and Hospital.

By fasting, though, cancer sufferers can basically force their bodies to reboot their immune system. It will help them to increase the production of the white blood cells that have been destroyed in the cancer treatment and will make it possible for their body to protect itself even after it is flooded with chemotherapy drugs and radiation.

The Effects of Fasting on our Immune system doesn't stop there!

Fasting Activates Your Body's 'survival' Mode, Boosting Your Immune System

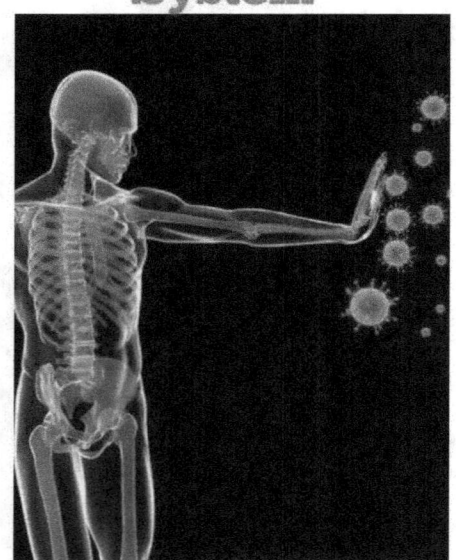

When you fast, your body basically has to scramble to find nutrients and energy, so it burns up a lot of what your body has stored in case of emergencies.

This means that a lot of the inefficient or damaged parts of the body are eliminated during the fasting, basically resetting your overall health at the same time.

Fasting forces the body to store sugars, fats, and ketones, and to break down a significant amount of white blood cells. Ketones are produced when the body turns fat into energy or fuel and are a major player in weight loss.

Intermittent fasting allows the body to use fat as its primary source of energy, which is why many athletes use it to hit lower body-fat percentages for competitions.

It can help speed up the metabolism and improve bowel movements by giving your digestive system a rest. Periods without food boost the metabolism to burn through calories more efficiently — in a way reminding the body how healthy digestion is done.

Think of fasting as a reset button for the body. It creates a healthy environment for the body to release regulated hormones in order to experience what true hunger feels like. People who eat every three to four hours don't get to experience the body's ability to signal true, natural hunger.

PAGE 165

Supreme Health & Fitness!   Health & Wellness Series Volume 1

When the body is temporarily freed from digestion for 12 to 24 hours, it's also able to focus its regenerative abilities on other systems, such as the skin. Fasting is known to help the body remove toxins and regulate filtering organs such as the liver and kidney.

With each fast the white blood cell depletion triggered new cells in the immune system. When the enzyme PKA was reduced along with the cells in the fasting process, that's when Long and his team realized there was a switch being flicked on. The switch made it possible to create new cells and also lowered the levels of IGF-1, a hormone that's linked to aging, tumor growth, and cancer risk.

"PKA is the key gene that needs to shut down in order for these stem cells to switch into regenerative mode," Longo said. "It gives the 'OK' for stem cells to go ahead and begin proliferating and rebuild the entire system. And the good news is that the body got rid of the parts of the system that might be damaged or old, the inefficient parts, during the fasting. Now, if you start with a system heavily damaged by chemotherapy or aging, fasting cycles can generate, literally, a new immune system."

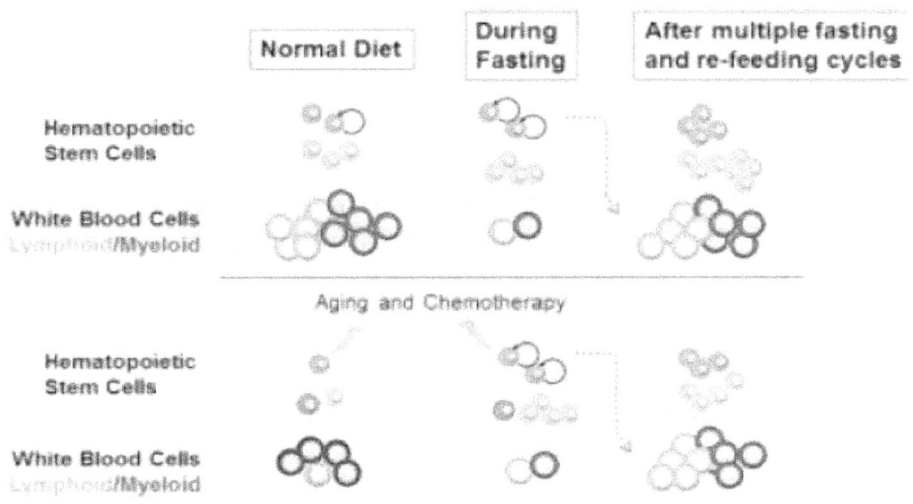

The fasting cycle of two or three days can actually help to restore a system that was severely damaged or decimated. White blood cells are broken down during the fast, which in turn forces the stem cells in your body to produce more.

These new white blood cells are not just brand new, but they're healthier and more effective than the previous cells—meaning they're more effective at combatting disease and illness.

PAGE 166

Supreme Health & Fitness!　　　　　　　　　Health & Wellness Series Volume 1

To sum it up, fasting reboots your immune system, regenerates white blood cells, and replenishes any blood cells that have been lost!

Pretty awesome reason to fast, right?!

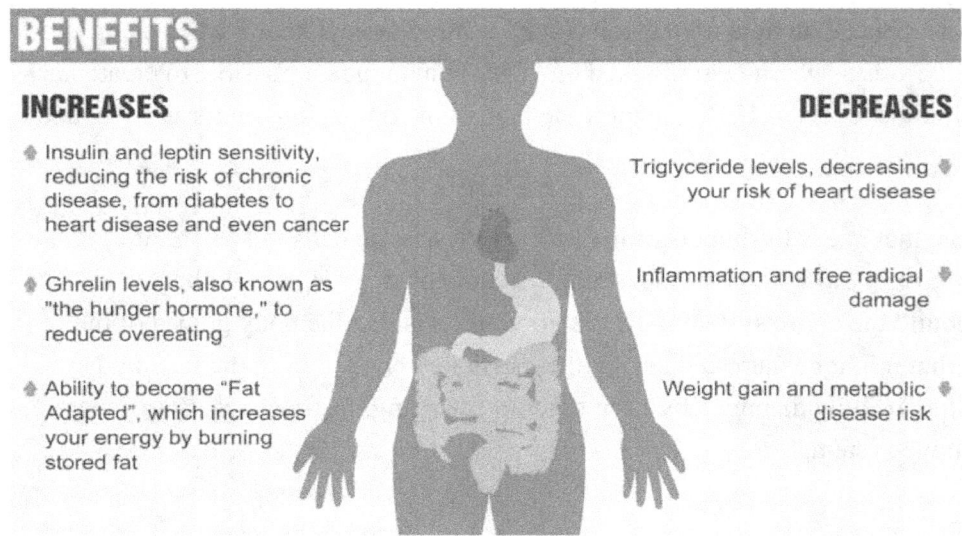

How to Fast Safely

If you want to benefit from the effect of fasting on immune system, it's important that you go about it the right way. Fasting is a Prescribed Action from The CREATOR for us to gain Control and Balance of Self.

If you do it right, you should be able to make it through the 48 to 72 hours of fasting without too much suffering.

It's important to prepare yourself for your 2 or 3-day fast BEFORE you start fasting. In the week leading up to the fast, slowly wean yourself off coffee, sugar, alcohol, and any other stimulants. Cut back on meat, fish, and dairy until you are accustomed to just eating fruits and veggies for a few days. Focus on soups, as they are water-heavy and will acclimate your body to getting more liquid. Eat some veggies, seeds, but focus on fruits.

For the 3 days before your fast, have nothing but liquids and easily digestible fruits and veggies. This will be easier on your digestive system and will help acclimate you to the fast.

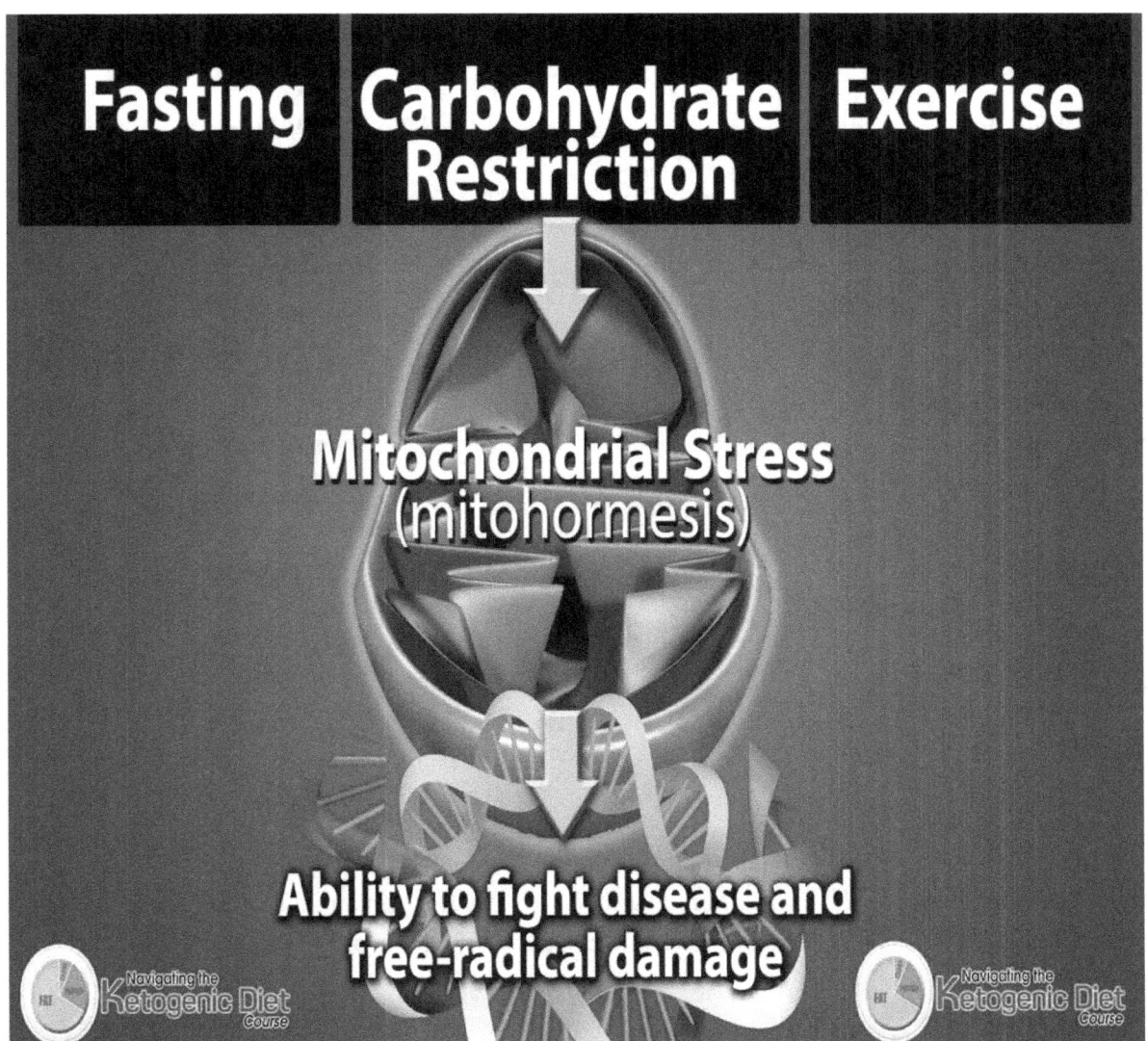

PAGE 168

Supreme Health & Fitness!   Health & Wellness Series Volume 1

The Process of Detoxification and Elimination

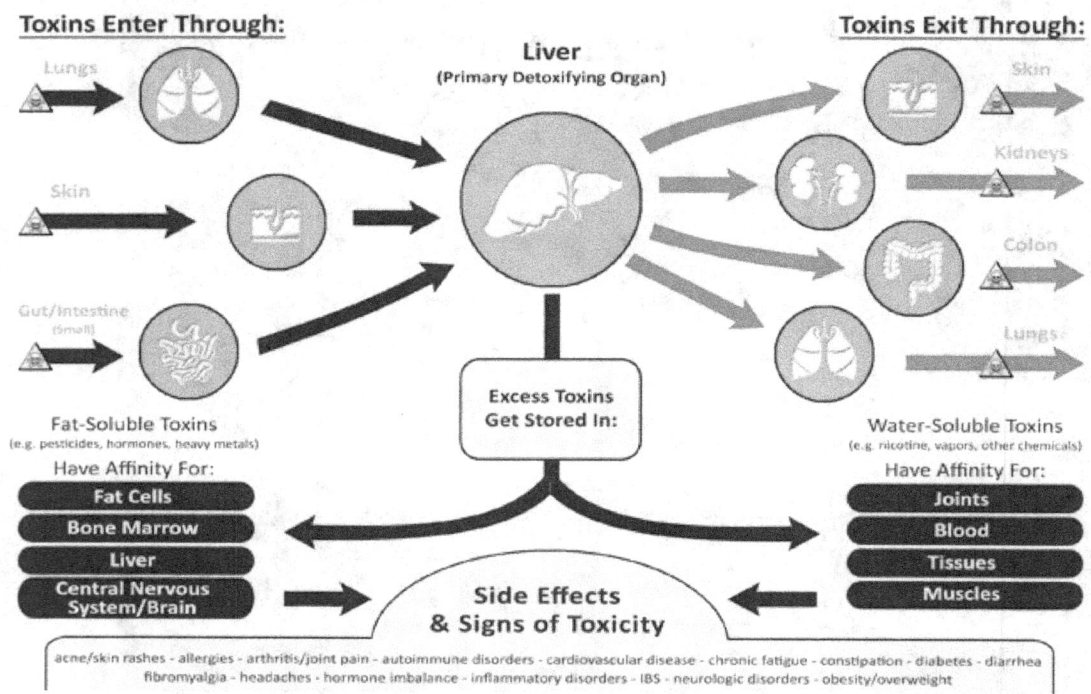

Toxins Enter Through:

Lungs

Skin

Gut/Intestine (Small)

Fat-Soluble Toxins
(e.g. pesticides, hormones, heavy metals)

Have Affinity For:
- Fat Cells
- Bone Marrow
- Liver
- Central Nervous System/Brain

Liver
(Primary Detoxifying Organ)

Excess Toxins Get Stored In:

Toxins Exit Through:

Skin

Kidneys

Colon

Lungs

Water-Soluble Toxins
(e.g. nicotine, vapors, other chemicals)

Have Affinity For:
- Joints
- Blood
- Tissues
- Muscles

Side Effects & Signs of Toxicity

acne/skin rashes · allergies · arthritis/joint pain · autoimmune disorders · cardiovascular disease · chronic fatigue · constipation · diabetes · diarrhea
fibromyalgia · headaches · hormone imbalance · inflammatory disorders · IBS · neurologic disorders · obesity/overweight

Unfortunately, in the world we live in it is hard for our body to keep up with amount of toxins we are exposed to on a daily basis. We also need to make sure that the exit pathways are functioning properly as well.

It seems pretty simple you just need to make sure more toxins are going out through your colon, kidneys, lungs and skin than are coming in through your digestive system, lungs and skin. If you don't whatever toxins don't get eliminated end up getting stored in other parts of your body. One of the major 'storage' locations for toxins is fat cells, this is why normally when people do a detox or cleanse they also lose weight.

Cleansing or doing a detox is has recently become a trendy thing to do. The only problem with a quick magic cure all detox is they don't support all the areas that are needed to have a healthy and complete detox.

So, the toxins don't get eliminated like planned and you may not notice any benefit or difference at all.

Detoxification Pathways

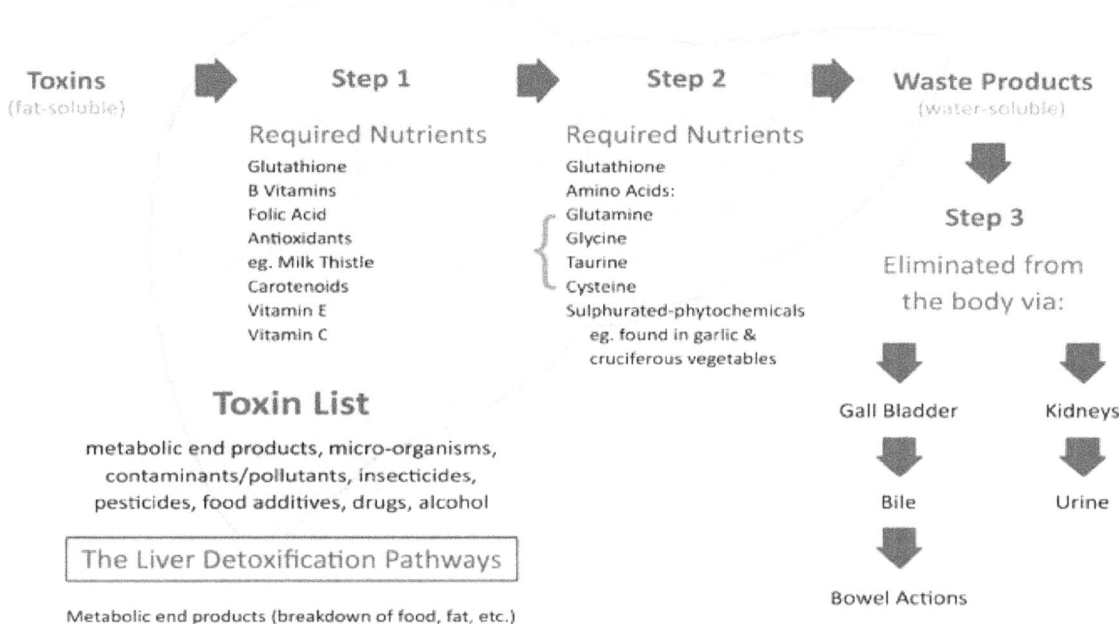

Toxins (fat-soluble)

Step 1

Required Nutrients
Glutathione
B Vitamins
Folic Acid
Antioxidants
eg. Milk Thistle
Carotenoids
Vitamin E
Vitamin C

Step 2

Required Nutrients
Glutathione
Amino Acids:
Glutamine
Glycine
Taurine
Cysteine
Sulphurated-phytochemicals
eg. found in garlic &
cruciferous vegetables

Waste Products (water-soluble)

Step 3

Eliminated from
the body via:

Gall Bladder — Bile — Bowel Actions

Kidneys — Urine

Toxin List

metabolic end products, micro-organisms,
contaminants/pollutants, insecticides,
pesticides, food additives, drugs, alcohol

The Liver Detoxification Pathways

Metabolic end products (breakdown of food, fat, etc.)

8 Keys to a Proper Comprehensive Detox:

1. Nutrients to promote detox pathways

As you can see in the image above Step 1 and Step 2 of the detoxification pathway have a list of nutrients that are needed to make each step work. If there isn't an adequate amount of these nutrients the toxin will not proceed through the detox pathway or even get eliminated. The major required nutrient for both step 1 and 2 is glutathione. A proper detox supplement must have the needed nutrients to make the pathway flow but especially must have extra support for step 2 because without step 2 your liver will not be able to detox.

2. Limit new toxins coming in

This seems like a pretty obvious. If our systems are overloaded then for us to start removing the burden we must stop adding to it. A vital part of this is the foods that are allowed during the detox program. The preferred diet would be centered on organic foods.

PAGE 170

Supreme Health & Fitness!   Health & Wellness Series Volume 1

An often over-looked source of toxins is the actual detox supplements themselves. If what you are taking is bringing in more toxins you will not be able to detox properly. Only use supplements from companies that are 3rd party tested for purity and harmful contaminants.

3. Healthy elimination via digestive and urinary systems

If you are not able to perform step 3 of detoxification which is elimination the toxins will end up being reabsorbed and redistributed back to your cells. While doing a detox program you must be having at least 1 bowel movement per day (more is not a bad thing) and urinating frequently. Making sure your liver, digestive system and urinary system is ready for an upgraded detox is essential to having a successful detox.

4. Protein (hypoallergenic)

A healthy protein source is needed to rebuild and restore function to the cells and tissues that were damaged by the toxins. Giving your body all the building blocks (amino acids, vitamins, minerals, and other nutrients) is how you get healthier. If you are not rebuilding your cells stronger than you are becoming weaker overall. Especially during a detox it is best to use protein sources that don't promote inflammation, which would be counterproductive. Usually a pea, rice or potato protein is the best fit.

5. Safely Stimulate All steps in the detoxification process.

The products used to stimulate detoxification must be used safely and be in the right dosages. Ensuring that all steps are properly supported is necessary. If the whole pathway isn't supported the toxins won't be eliminated and could potentially even make your health worse.

6. Digestive Enzymes

While taking the shake or any type of liquid nutrition taking digestive enzymes is a good idea. When you are drinking the shake the liquid passes through the stomach and intestines at a faster rate which lowers the amount of nutrients that are absorbed. Digestive enzymes help speed up the digestive process and provide a greater rate of absorption and also decrease in inflammation and any gas and bloating that may occur.

PAGE 171

Supreme Health & Fitness!   Health & Wellness Series Volume 1

7. Diet rich in nutrients without causes of inflammation

A clean and healthy diet is a must for a comprehensive detoxification program. Combining the points from limiting toxins coming in and providing the building blocks mentioned with proteins. To rebuild and strengthen your cells and tissues you must give them building blocks to do so. You wouldn't remodel your house by tearing it down and rebuilding it with lower quality products.

8. Probiotics

A healthy microbe balance is needed for a healthy digestive system and a healthy detox. There are around 100 trillion bacteria in our digestive systems and must be in balance. Probiotics work to promote that delicate balance. Probiotics alone have been shown to remove toxins (such as BPA) and prevents toxin recycling.

PAGE 172

Supreme Health & Fitness!   Health & Wellness Series Volume 1

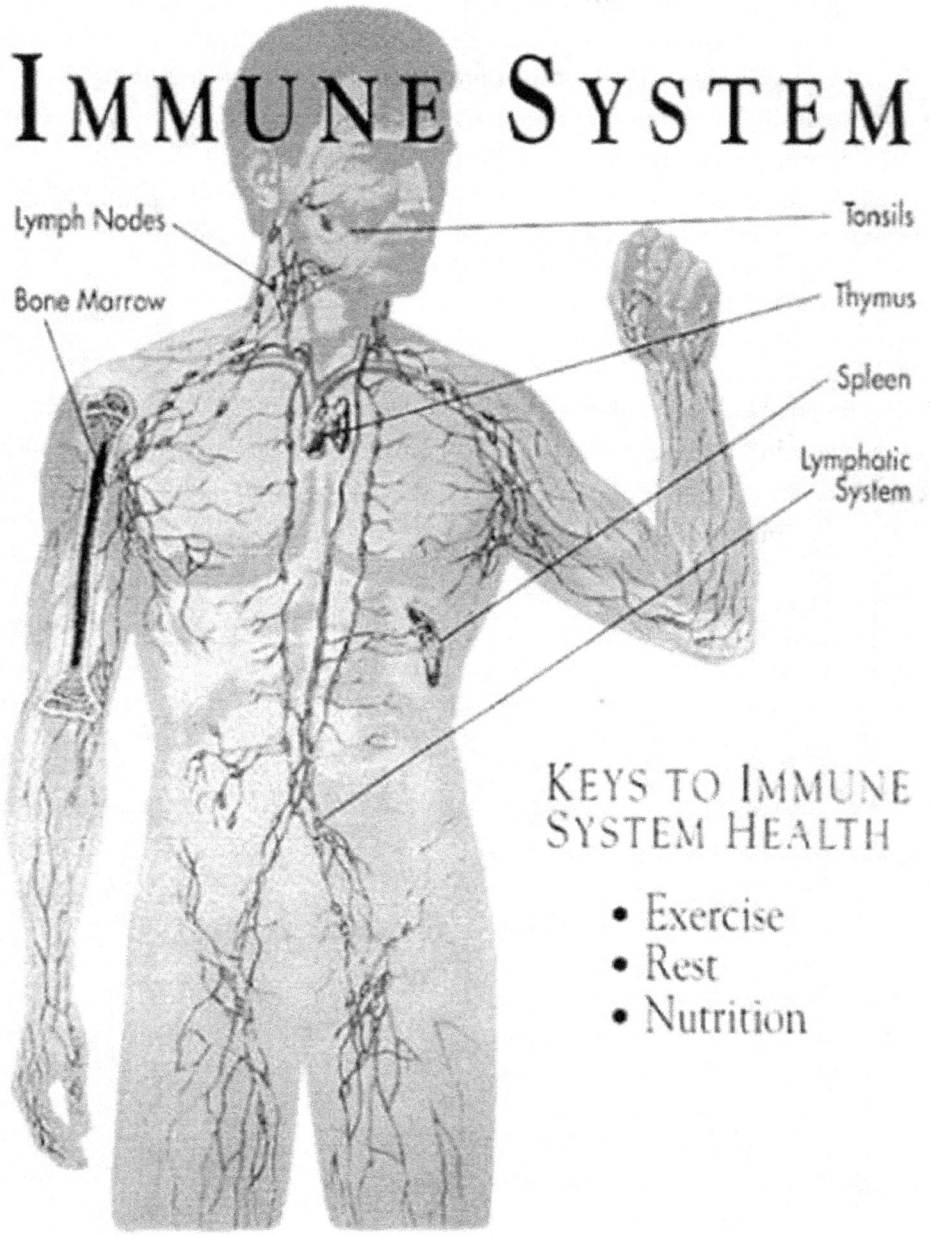

IMMUNE SYSTEM

Lymph Nodes

Bone Marrow

Tonsils

Thymus

Spleen

Lymphatic System

KEYS TO IMMUNE SYSTEM HEALTH

- Exercise
- Rest
- Nutrition

Are you living to eat?

-or-

Eating to live?

*****

Chapter 12 ... Eating 2 LIVE – Glucose & Navy Beans!

*****

Carbohydrates are our Primary Source of Life Energy. The element or 'food' that our Cells need to grow and develop manifests in the form of GLUCOSE (a Carbohydrate). Whole Wheat is one of our BEST forms of Naturally occurring Carbohydrates.

Sugar is what our bodies use for fuel, which is why we crave a sugary drink/food when we are low on Energy and Why we get that Boost after we consume it.

NOTICE that there aren't any Animal meats listed as a source of Life Energy!

Sources of sugar

Sugar Components	Food Sources
Glucose	Fruits, vegetables, table sugar, honey, milk products, cereals
Fructose	Fruits, vegetables, honey
Galactose	Milk products
Sucrose	Fruits, vegetables, table sugar, honey
Lactose	Milk products
Maltose	Malt products, some cereals

Glucose – Life Energy for Cells

Glucose is the human body's key source of energy as it provides energy to all the cells in our body.

Glucose also is critical in the production of proteins, lipid metabolism and is a precursor for vitamin C production.

Glucose is the sole source of fuel to create energy for all brain and red blood cells. The availability of glucose influences many psychological processes.

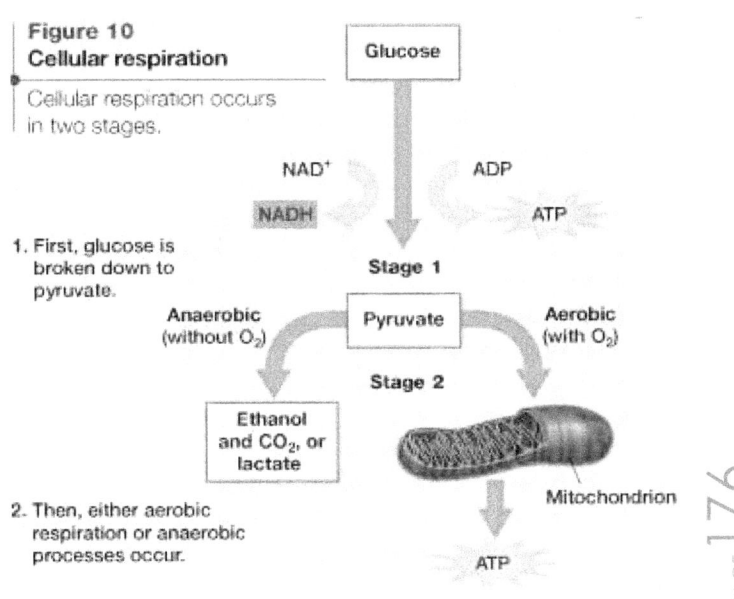

Figure 10
Cellular respiration

Cellular respiration occurs in two stages.

1. First, glucose is broken down to pyruvate.

2. Then, either aerobic respiration or anaerobic processes occur.

Glucose → Stage 1 → Pyruvate

NAD+ → NADH
ADP → ATP

Anaerobic (without O₂) → Ethanol and CO₂, or lactate

Aerobic (with O₂) → Mitochondrion → ATP

Stage 2

PAGE 176

Supreme Health & Fitness!   Health & Wellness Series Volume 1

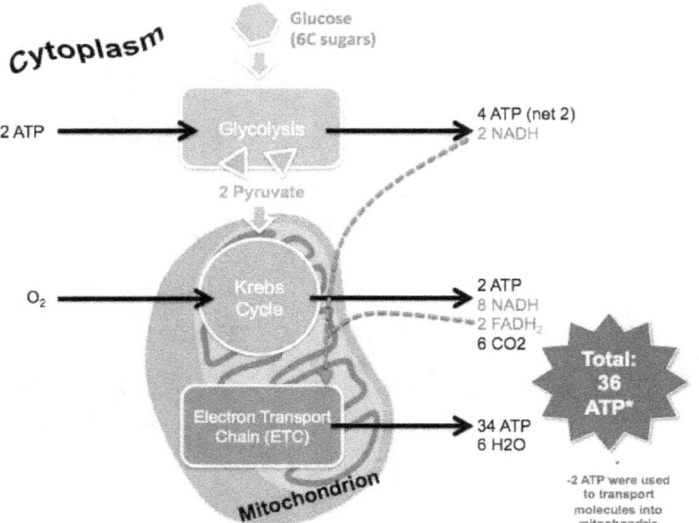

Cytoplasm

Glucose
(6C sugars)

2 ATP → Glycolysis → 4 ATP (net 2)
2 NADH

2 Pyruvate

O₂ → Krebs Cycle → 2 ATP
8 NADH
2 FADH₂
6 CO2

Electron Transport Chain (ETC) → 34 ATP
6 H2O

Mitochondrion

Total:
36
ATP*

-2 ATP were used
to transport
molecules into
mitochondria

When glucose levels are low, psychological processes requiring mental effort l(self-control, critical thinking and decision-making) become impaired.

The human body converts carbohydrates, particularly glucose, into glycogen for storage, mainly in liver and muscle cells for daily use and in adipose cells and tissues as body fat for long term energy use.

Nature is amazing!

Plants obtain energy from the sun by capturing the sun's photons during the photosynthesis process creating glucose and oxygen. Glucose is present in many fruits and vegetables.

Glucose is mostly found in food as a building block in more complex carbohydrates. Complex carbohydrates are composed of thousands of glucose units linked together in chains. Our digestive system breaks down complex carbohydrates into many molecules of glucose for use by our cells to create energy.

The majority of our carbohydrates intake should come from complex carbohydrates (starches) and naturally occurring sugars, rather than processed or refined sugars, which do not have the vitamins, minerals, and fiber found in complex and natural carbohydrates.

Refined sugars like high-fructose corn syrup are often called "empty calories" because they have little to no nutritional value.

High-fructose corn syrup is not to be confused with corn syrup, which has a high glucose content. Diets containing foods with high-fructose corn syrup contribute to the development of Type 2 Diabetes.

(a) Phase 1: Preparation and cleavage. The six-carbon glucose molecule is phosphorylated twice by ATP and split to form two molecules of glyceraldehyde-3-phosphate. This requires an input of two ATP per glucose.

(b) Phase 2: Oxidation and ATP generation. The two molecules of glyceraldehyde-3-phosphate are oxidized to 3-phosphoglycerate. Some of the energy from this oxidation is conserved as two ATP and two NADH molecules are produced.

(c) Phase 3: Pyruvate formation and ATP generation. The two 3-phosphoglycerate molecules are converted to pyruvate, with accompanying synthesis of two more ATP molecules.

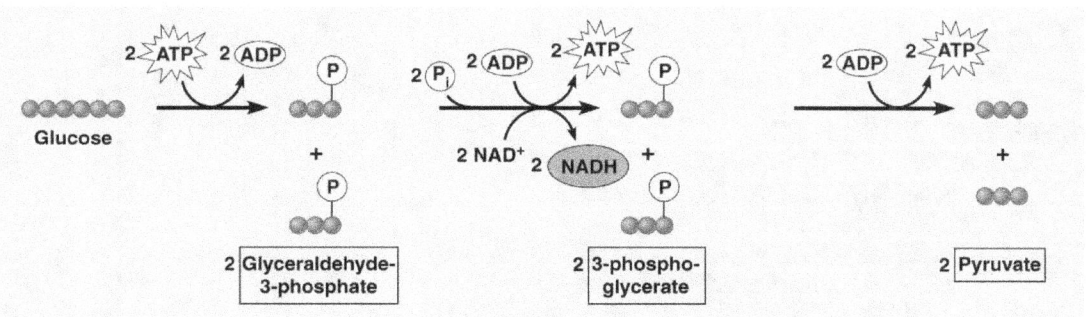

Food, Glucose and the Body

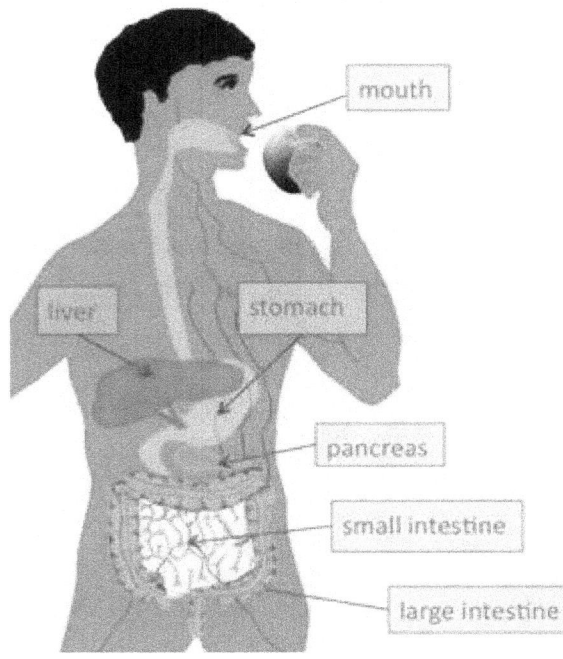

- Glucose comes from food that contains carbohydrate (eg, starch, sugar, rice, pasta, bread, cakes, etc.)

- The mouth, the stomach and the small intestine digest (break down) food to glucose

- Glucose enters the blood stream from the small intestine

- The blood then carries glucose to muscles and the brain

Natural Food Sources of Glucose:

- **Fruit and Vegetables**

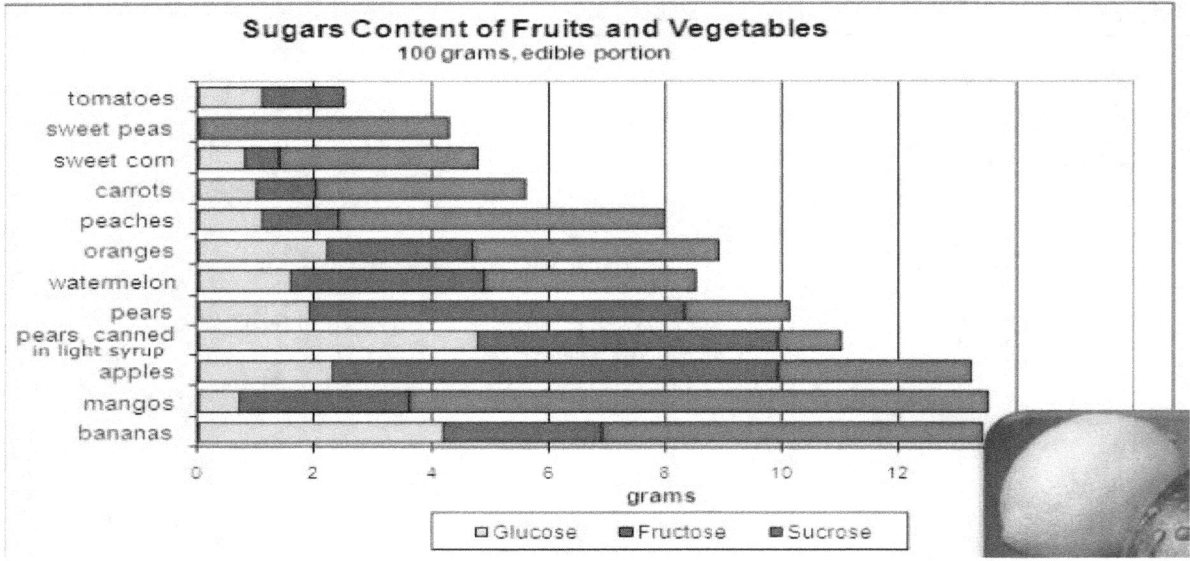

Sugars Content of Fruits and Vegetables
100 grams, edible portion

Categories (top to bottom): tomatoes, sweet peas, sweet corn, carrots, peaches, oranges, watermelon, pears, pears canned in light syrup, apples, mangos, bananas

x-axis: grams (0, 2, 4, 6, 8, 10, 12)

Legend: □ Glucose   ■ Fructose   ■ Sucrose

1. Whole Grains and Whole Grain Cereals made without high-fructose corn syrup are also nutritious sources of complex carbohydrates. See Health Benefits of Whole Grains - Nutrient Comparison between Whole Grains and Refined Flour Products

2. Legumes which includes beans, lentils and peas are high sources of complex carbohydrates and also contain protein.

3. Vegetables contain glucose often in the form of starch. Starch is the energy storage molecule of plants. It is formed by long chains of a glucose molecules linked together. Vegetable high in starch include, corn, squash and zucchini.

Low starch vegetables include asparagus, eggplant, mushrooms, brussels sprouts, cabbage, cauliflower, celery, cucumbers, okra, green beans, red and green peppers, onions, and tomatoes, and are all packed with nutrition.

4. Grapes are an especially rich source of glucose.

5. Honey contains about 38% glucose.

PAGE 179

Supreme Health & Fitness!   Health & Wellness Series Volume 1

6. Dairy products including milk, yogurt and cottage cheese all contain lactose. Lactose is composed of one glucose molecule joins a galactose molecule, which is digested into glucose. Raw Milk is your best natural food source for glucose - Read why here!

***Complex carbs keep us satisfied for longer time than foods containing simple sugars/high-fructose corn syrup. Consumption of complex carbohydrates requires less food intake and this results in less caloric intake. That is why complex carbs are suggested in weight maintenance diets.*

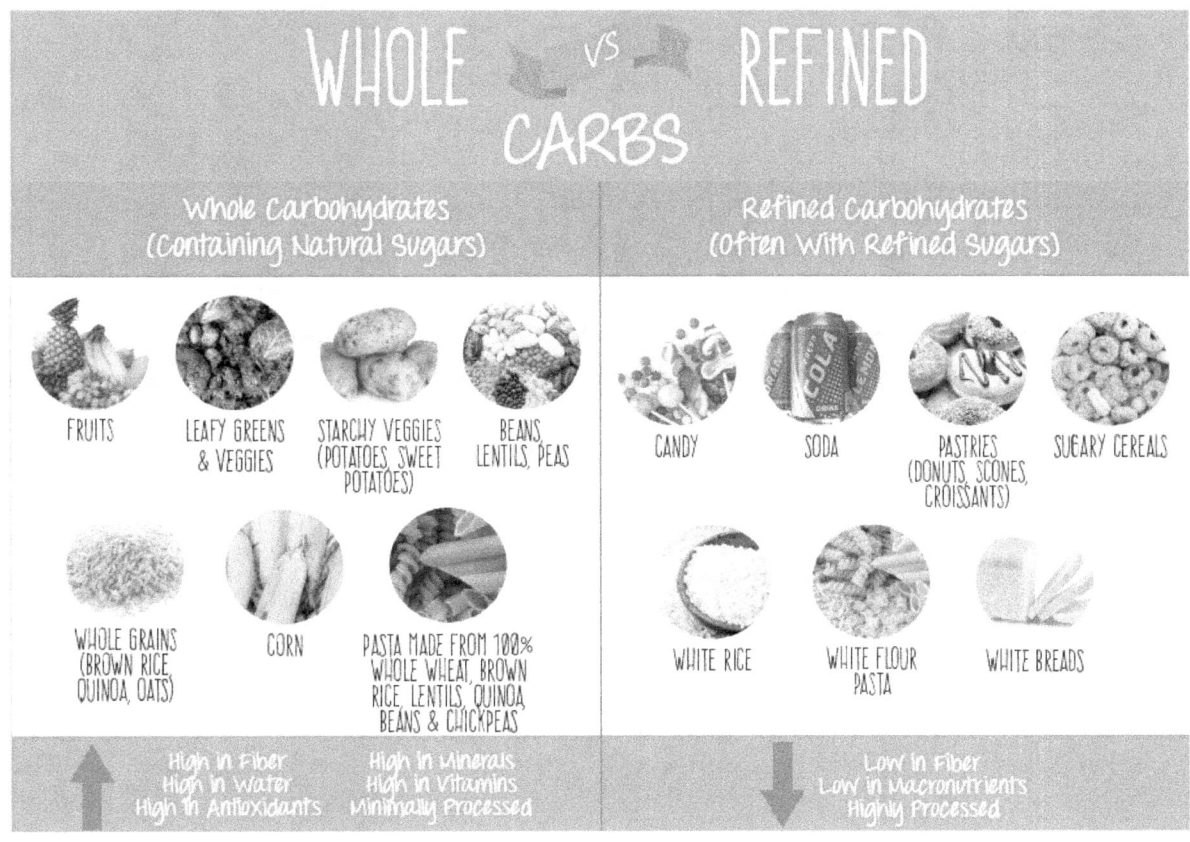

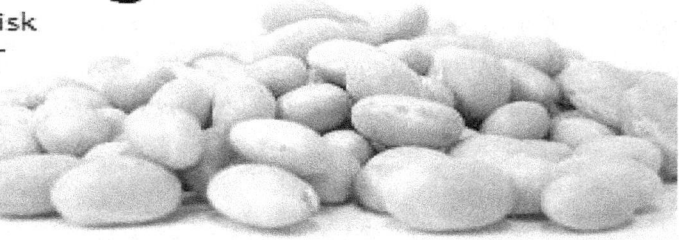

10 Health Benefits of...
Navy Beans

1. Lower Heart-Attack Risk
2. Stabilises Blood-Sugar
3. Good Folate Source
4. Full of Fibre
5. Full of Iron
6. Protein Rich
7. Anti-Oxidant
8. Energy Booster
9. Immune Booster
10. Improve Memory

EatHealthyLiveFit.com

The Awesome Pulse of the Earth - Navy Bean

The Navy Bean is one of the most Complete Sources of Energy in 1 Element. These natural foods have a lot of the stuff that you need to function well, without a lot of the unwanted elements that are often found in processed foods, such as sugar, fat and sodium.

Due to their high nutritive value and protein content, they have become staple foods in many different cultures, and can be stored for long periods of time or canned without losing their nutritional value, unlike many other vegetables or legumes.

While it may seem like all beans are created equal, that isn't exactly true, and navy beans do possess certain unique chemical components, such as phosphatidylserine. Now, without further ado, let's take a more in-depth look at the many health benefits of navy beans.

Health Benefits of Navy Beans

**Memory and Cognition**: Folate is a key nutrient for many different reasons within the body, including the prevention of neural tube defects and anemia, but it also affects the nervous system in a meaningful way. A deficiency of folate has been directly linked to an increase in homocysteine levels, which can often lead to neurodegenerative diseases like Alzheimer's and Parkinson's disease.

PAGE 181

Supreme Health & Fitness!   Health & Wellness Series Volume 1

Furthermore, one of the B vitamins found in navy beans, thiamin, can help to increase certain neurotransmitters we need for memory and cognition, so these little legumes can also keep our memory sharp as we age.

Growth and Repair: One of the most notable and important aspects of navy beans are their high content of protein. Proteins are the building blocks of all life, and we need a steady stream for the growth of new cells, tissues, muscles, bones, blood vessels and every other part of our body. Protein is essential for normal development, but also in the function of repairing damaged areas of the body and speeding the healing process.

Navy beans are an excellent source of protein, with more than 15 grams of protein in a single cup!

Circulatory System: Keeping the blood flowing normally in our body is obviously important for the oxygenation of our organ systems and normal overall function. Iron is a key component of red blood cells, and without proper iron intake, your circulation suffers, making you susceptible to anemia, weakness, bone mineral loss, fatigue and poor circulation. Copper is also very important in this regard, as it is necessary for the synthesis of hemoglobin.

In other words, without copper, iron is practically useless in the body. Navy beans, fortunately, contain high levels of both.

Antioxidant Activity: Manganese isn't a mineral you often hear about, but it is a key cofactor in many antioxidant enzymes that can prevent the spread and impact of free radicals. This can help to lower your risk of cancer and chronic illness. Secondly, copper plays an important role as an enzyme cofactor as well, and can help to stimulate blood flow, joint mobility and overall flexibility by cutting back on oxidative stress in those areas.

Calorie Counting: A serving of about 180 grams of navy beans contains around 250 calories. That's more calories per gram than a lot of green vegetables and fresh produce. This calorie count even approaches the caloric value of some processed foods. Looking at the nutrients that navy beans contain, however, can show you how using these beans in moderation can be part of a good, wholesome meal.

For example, a bean salad may use only half of this serving size, and can contain other ingredients for a better overall nutritional value.

Navy beans are an excellent source of cholesterol-lowering fiber, as are most other beans. In addition to lowering cholesterol, navy beans' high fiber content prevents blood sugar levels from rising too rapidly after a meal, making these beans an especially good choice for individuals with diabetes, insulin resistance or hypoglycemia. But this is far from all navy beans have to offer.

Navy beans are a very good source of folate and manganese and a good source of protein and vitamin B1 as well as the minerals phosphorus, copper, magnesium and iron.

Navy Beans, cooked 1.00 cup 182.00 grams				Calories: 255 GI: low
Nutrient	Amount	DRI/DV (%)	Nutrient Density	World's Healthiest Foods Rating
fiber	19.11 g	76	5.4	excellent
folate	254.80 mcg	64	4.5	very good
manganese	0.96 mg	48	3.4	very good
copper	0.38 mg	42	3.0	good
phosphorus	262.08 mg	37	2.6	good
vitamin B1	0.43 mg	36	2.5	good
protein	14.98 g	30	2.1	good
magnesium	96.46 mg	24	1.7	good
iron	4.30 mg	24	1.7	good

World's Healthiest Foods Rating	Rule
excellent	DRI/DV>=75% OR Density>=7.6 AND DRI/DV>=10%
very good	DRI/DV>=50% OR Density>=3.4 AND DRI/DV>=5%
good	DRI/DV>=25% OR Density>=1.5 AND DRI/DV>=2.5%

Navy beans are a good supply of magnesium puts yet another plus in the column of its beneficial cardiovascular effects.

Magnesium is Nature's own calcium channel blocker. When there is enough magnesium around, veins and arteries breathe a sigh of relief and relax, which lessens resistance and improves the flow of blood, oxygen and nutrients throughout the body. Studies show that a deficiency of magnesium is not only associated with heart attack but that immediately following a heart attack, lack of sufficient magnesium promotes free radical injury to the heart.

Potassium, an important electrolyte involved in nerve transmission and the contraction of all muscles including the heart, is another mineral that is essential for maintaining normal blood pressure and heart function. Navy beans are ready to promote your cardiovascular health by being a good source of this mineral, too.

A one cup serving of navy beans provides over 700 mg of potassium, making these beans an especially good choice to protect against high blood pressure and atherosclerosis.

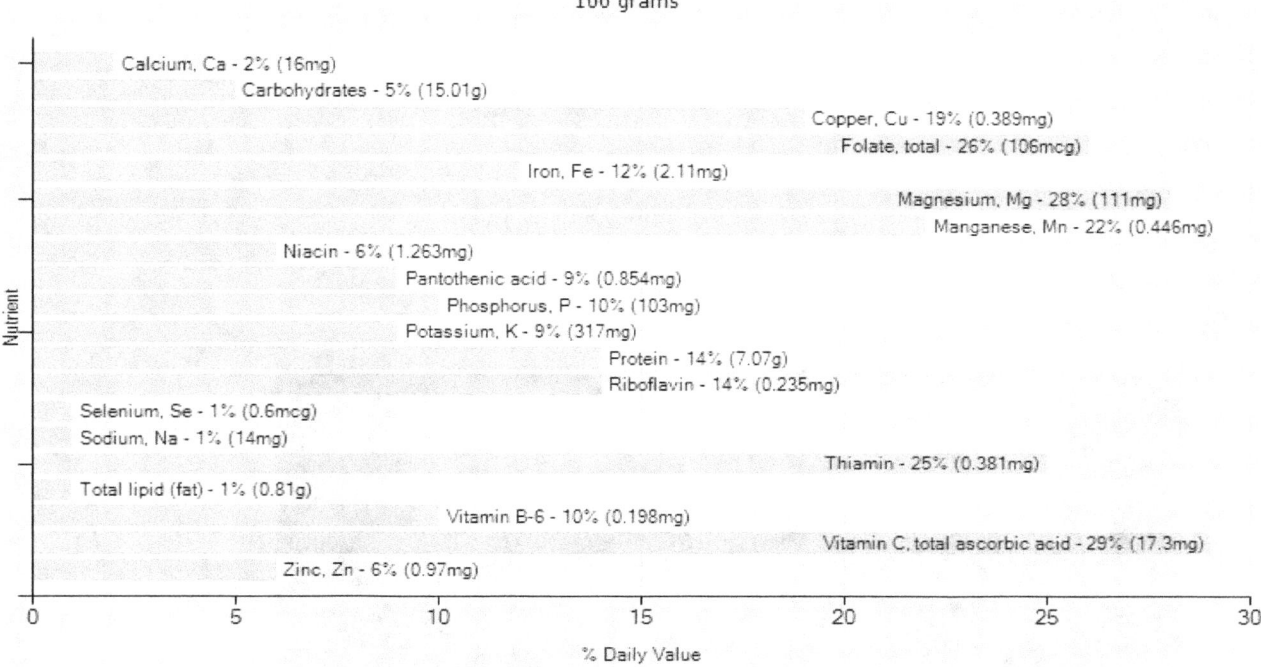

Beans, navy, mature seeds, sprouted, cooked, boiled, drained, without salt
100 grams

Calcium, Ca - 2% (16mg)
Carbohydrates - 5% (15.01g)
Copper, Cu - 19% (0.389mg)
Folate, total - 26% (106mcg)
Iron, Fe - 12% (2.11mg)
Magnesium, Mg - 28% (111mg)
Manganese, Mn - 22% (0.446mg)
Niacin - 6% (1.263mg)
Pantothenic acid - 9% (0.854mg)
Phosphorus, P - 10% (103mg)
Potassium, K - 9% (317mg)
Protein - 14% (7.07g)
Riboflavin - 14% (0.235mg)
Selenium, Se - 1% (0.6mcg)
Sodium, Na - 1% (14mg)
Thiamin - 25% (0.381mg)
Total lipid (fat) - 1% (0.81g)
Vitamin B-6 - 10% (0.198mg)
Vitamin C, total ascorbic acid - 29% (17.3mg)
Zinc, Zn - 6% (0.97mg)

% Daily Value

Navy Beans Give You Energy to Stabilize Blood Sugar

In addition to its beneficial effects on the digestive system and the heart, the dietary fiber found in navy beans helps stabilize blood sugar levels. If you have insulin resistance, hypoglycemia or diabetes, navy beans can really help you balance blood sugar levels while providing steady, slow-burning energy.

Studies of high fiber diets and blood sugar levels have shown the dramatic benefits provided by these high fiber foods.

Researchers compared two groups of people with type 2 diabetes who were fed different amounts of high fiber foods. One group ate the standard American Diabetic diet, which contained 24 grams of fiber/day, while the other group ate a diet containing 50 grams of fiber/day.

Those who ate the diet higher in fiber had lower levels of both plasma glucose (blood sugar) and insulin (the hormone that helps blood sugar get into cells).

The high fiber group also reduced their total cholesterol by nearly 7%, their triglyceride levels by 10.2% and their VLDL (Very Low Density Lipoprotein—the most dangerous form of cholesterol) levels by 12.5%.

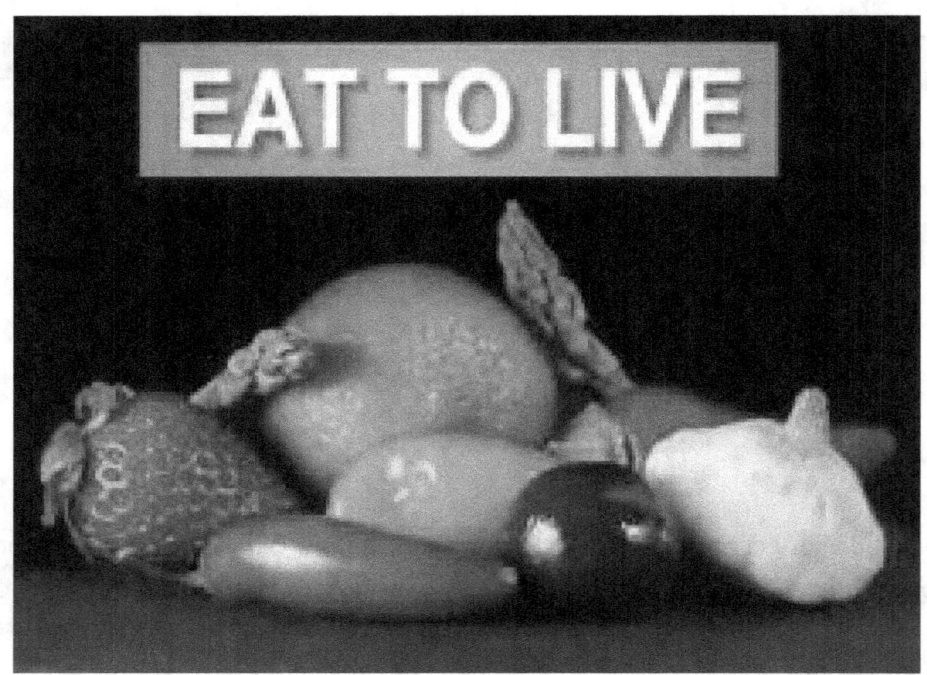

*****

Eating 2 LIVE ... Skin

*****

Eating more fresh fruits and vegetables is a great way to get immune boosting benefits from Vitamin C and other phytonutrients found in fresh raw foods. The colors of produce give you a clue for how they help the immune system.

Choose orange fruits and vegetables like carrots to get more beta carotene, the precursor your body turns into Vitamin A. This nutrient helps your immune system by supporting healthy lungs and lymph.

Dark greens like spinach contain beta carotene and Vitamin E that help your body fend off cold and flu infections.

Fresh red and pink produce like tomatoes, strawberries and pink grapefruit are especially high in Vitamin C.

Caring for your skin can be a challenge. There are various products sold that claim to grant you a perfectly smooth and blemish-free face, but the fact is that problems will always arise if you are not eating healthy.

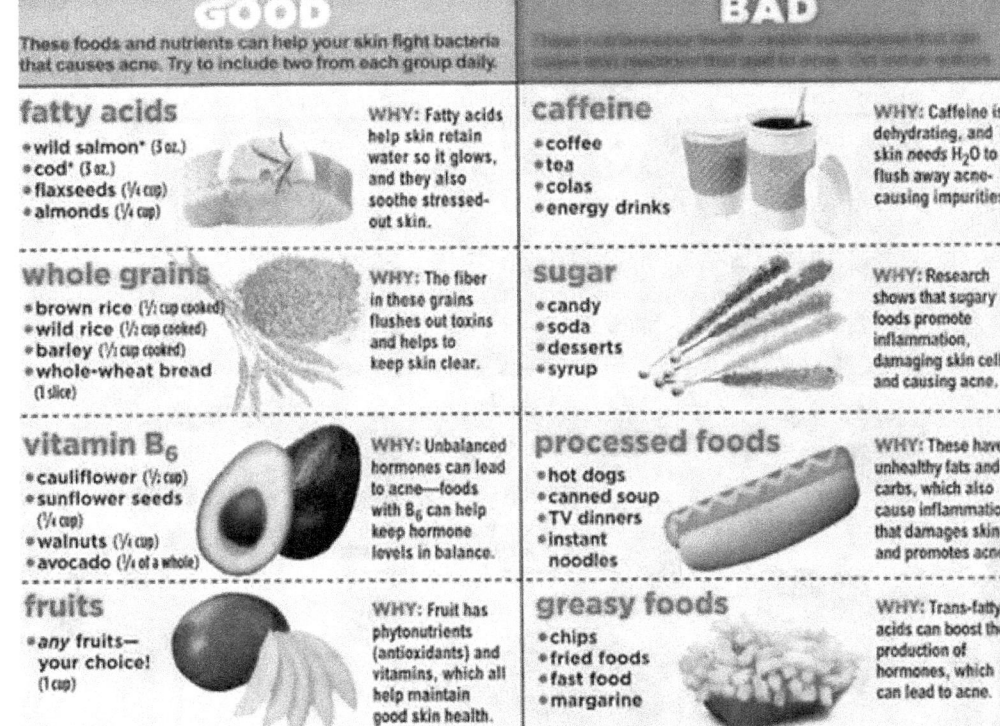

GOOD

These foods and nutrients can help your skin fight bacteria that causes acne. Try to include two from each group daily.

fatty acids
- wild salmon* (3 oz.)
- cod* (3 oz.)
- flaxseeds (¼ cup)
- almonds (¼ cup)

WHY: Fatty acids help skin retain water so it glows, and they also soothe stressed-out skin.

whole grains
- brown rice (½ cup cooked)
- wild rice (½ cup cooked)
- barley (½ cup cooked)
- whole-wheat bread (1 slice)

WHY: The fiber in these grains flushes out toxins and helps to keep skin clear.

vitamin B₆
- cauliflower (½ cup)
- sunflower seeds (¼ cup)
- walnuts (¼ cup)
- avocado (⅓ of a whole)

WHY: Unbalanced hormones can lead to acne—foods with B₆ can help keep hormone levels in balance.

fruits
- any fruits—your choice! (1 cup)

WHY: Fruit has phytonutrients (antioxidants) and vitamins, which all help maintain good skin health.

BAD

caffeine
- coffee
- tea
- colas
- energy drinks

WHY: Caffeine is dehydrating, and skin needs H₂0 to flush away acne-causing impurities.

sugar
- candy
- soda
- desserts
- syrup

WHY: Research shows that sugary foods promote inflammation, damaging skin cells and causing acne.

processed foods
- hot dogs
- canned soup
- TV dinners
- instant noodles

WHY: These have unhealthy fats and carbs, which also cause inflammation that damages skin and promotes acne.

greasy foods
- chips
- fried foods
- fast food
- margarine

WHY: Trans-fatty acids can boost the production of hormones, which can lead to acne.

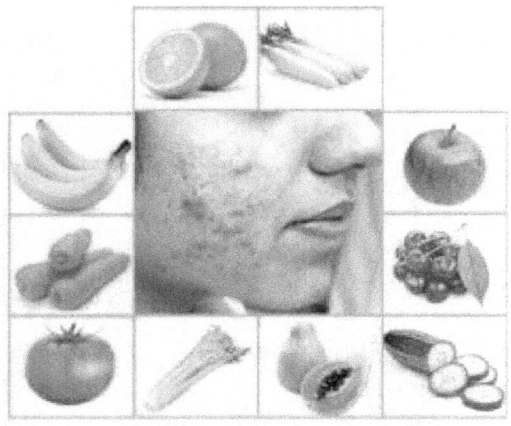

Best foods for acne

By simply cutting certain foods out of your diet, you will get clearer skin in no time, without having to purchase expensive creams and soaps.

Processed foods such as packaged cookies, tv dinners, candy bars, and crackers, are known for causing acne. On top of keeping your body from running efficiently, too much of these foods can also cause your blood sugar to shoot up. This will then cause more oily skin, which eventually leads to more acne.

These food-like items are not natural, and all of their good nutrients are sucked out during the manufacturing process. These food-like items aren't okay for a snack at anytime and should not be eaten on a regular basis.

Dull, congested skin that appears to have aged prematurely is a common problem for many people.

While microdermabrasion, laser treatments and face lifts can help to make you look younger, there are some natural ways to alter your skin's overall look simply by adding certain foods to your diet on a regular basis.

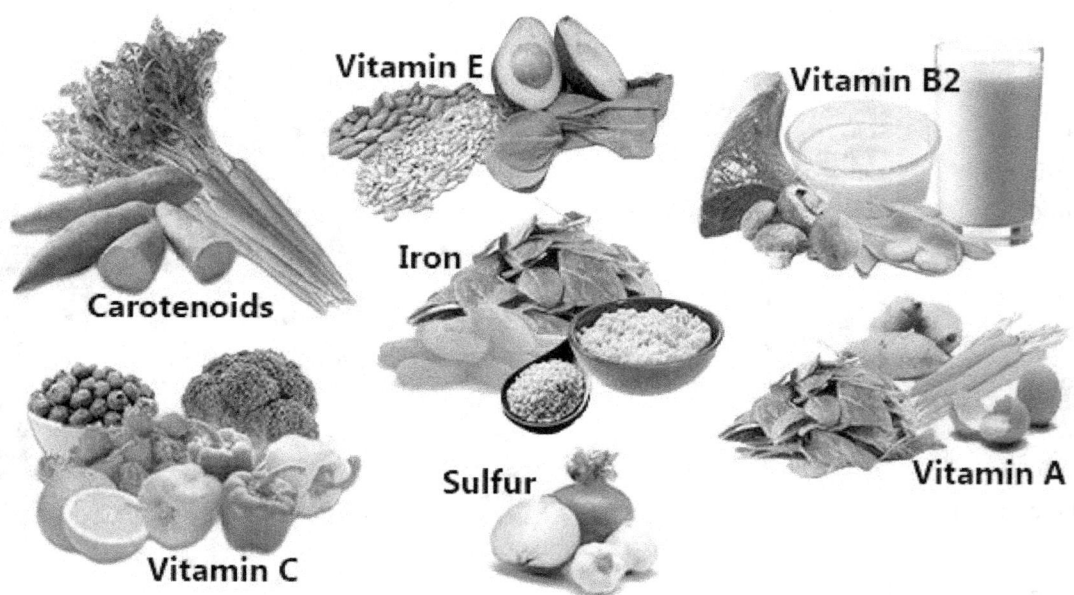

PAGE 187

Supreme Health & Fitness!   Health & Wellness Series Volume 1

4 Steps to Improving Skin Health:

Step 1: Eat more vitamin E rich foods like raw sunflower seeds, olives, papaya and boiled greens like Swiss chard, spinach and mustard greens. According to World'sHealthiestFoods.com, foods high in vitamin E help keep the skin looking healthy because they protect the skin from harmful UV light.

Step 2: Consume foods that contain high amounts of omega-3 fatty acids like salmon, tuna, halibut, flaxseeds, walnuts and raw tofu. Omega-3 fatty acids can help to reduce skin inflammation and keep cell membranes healthy. Foods rich in omega-3 fatty acids have also been shown to help those with sun sensitivity and psoriasis, according to the University of Maryland Medical Center.

Step 3: Add regular servings of berries like blackberries, blueberries, raspberries, cranberries and strawberries to your diet. Berries can help your skin look smoother, firmer and more supple because they help to produce collagen, and they are extremely high in the antioxidants which can help to get rid of free radicals that damage the skin and lead to premature aging, according to Healthy-Skincare.com.

Step 4: Eat vitamin A-rich foods like sweet potatoes, carrots, spinach, broccoli, apricots, asparagus, green beans, yellow corn, peas, eggs and beef liver regularly to keep your skin looking radiant and smooth. If you can't add more vitamin A to your diet, the Women's Health website recommends beta carotene supplements instead.

Tips: Eliminate caffeine from coffee and tea, or at least reduce the amount you consume. Caffeine dehydrates the skin, which can lead to fine lines and wrinkles, according to the Best Natural Cures Health Guide, who recommends replacing caffeinated beverages with water, natural fruit juice or coconut milk for optimum skin health. Eating properly is important to your skin, and so is a proper skin care regimen. If you are unclear about products you should or should not be using for your skin type, ask your doctor or dermatologist.

Warnings: Avoid too much synthetic vitamin A. Vitamin A, unlike many vitamins, is not water soluble, and it will not be flushed from your system properly.

PAGE 188

Supreme Health & Fitness!   Health & Wellness Series Volume 1

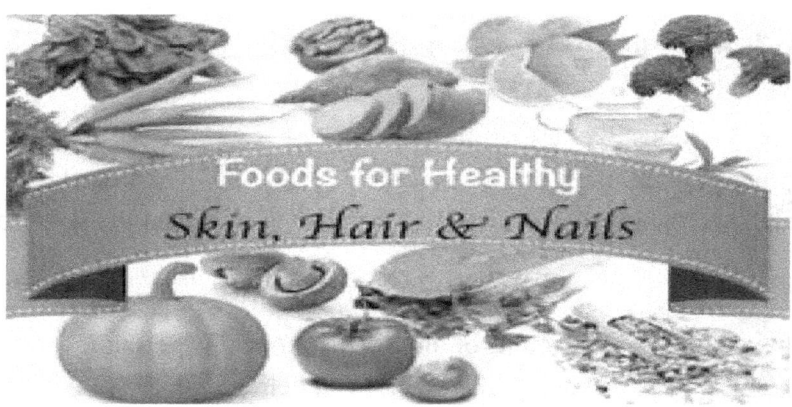

Foods for Healthy
Skin, Hair & Nails

Watermelon: Watermelon falls into the sun protector/cancer fighter categories when it comes to skincare. While protecting you from cancer doesn't necessarily help with maintaining a healthy glow, it's definitely something you should be looking for when choosing foods for your diet. This mouth-watering fruit will help clear your blemishes, smooth your skin and improve your skin's elasticity – all important elements of a healthy, fresh looking face.

Blueberries: Blueberries fall into the tightener/re-newer category when it comes to skincare. This healthy and delicious antioxidant-rich fruit is high in fiber, vitamin A and vitamin C and low in saturated fat, cholesterol and sodium. In addition, these tasty berries will help clear acne and blotchy spots on your skin, leaving you with a healthier, happier glow.

Berries: All berries (particularly raspberries, blackberries and strawberries) are great in achieving a healthy glow. Like oranges and grapefruits, these fruits are high in vitamin C – a strong antioxidant which keeps the collagen in your skin healthy. They're also high in anthocyanins and quercetin, which will help reduce inflammation and keep your skin looking evenly toned and radiant.

Kiwi: Kiwis fall into the category of firming when it comes to skincare. This sour fruit will help prevent wrinkles while keeping your bones and teeth healthy as well. The antioxidants found in this delicious fruit will also help protect you from cancer – a definite bonus when it comes to a healthy diet.

Avocados: Avocados are great for preventing blemishes and enhancing the quality of your skin. This popular fruit is high in vitamins A, D and E. These vitamins help prevent the signs of aging.

PAGE 189

Supreme Health & Fitness!   Health & Wellness Series Volume 1

Avocados are also high in minerals like copper and iron. These minerals help the skin fight the signs of aging by defending against free radicals.

Furthermore, this delicious fruit will help promote skin elasticity and pigment – leaving your skin (and hair) looking healthy refreshed all day long.

Oranges: Oranges (and grapefruits, for that matter) are considered very effective wrinkle preventers by nutritionists all over the world. This delicious fruit is known for its toning properties. It's also a great source of vitamin C (as most of you already know) which helps improve the texture and color of your skin. To finish things off, this citrus fruit helps restore collagen, leaving your skin firm and equipped to fight the signs of early aging.

Spinach: Leafy green vegetables, particularly spinach, are rich in nutrients and antioxidants. This particular vegetable is packed with lutein which helps to keep your eyes sparkling white. This healthy vegetable is also a great source of vitamin B, C and E as well as potassium, iron, calcium, magnesium and omega-3 fatty acids. Swapping your normal lettuce for spinach will work wonders for your skin.

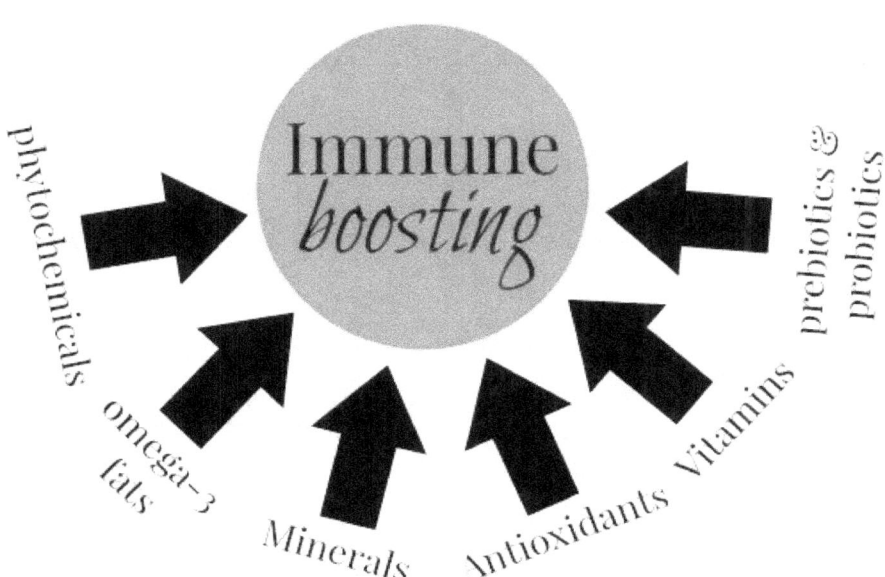

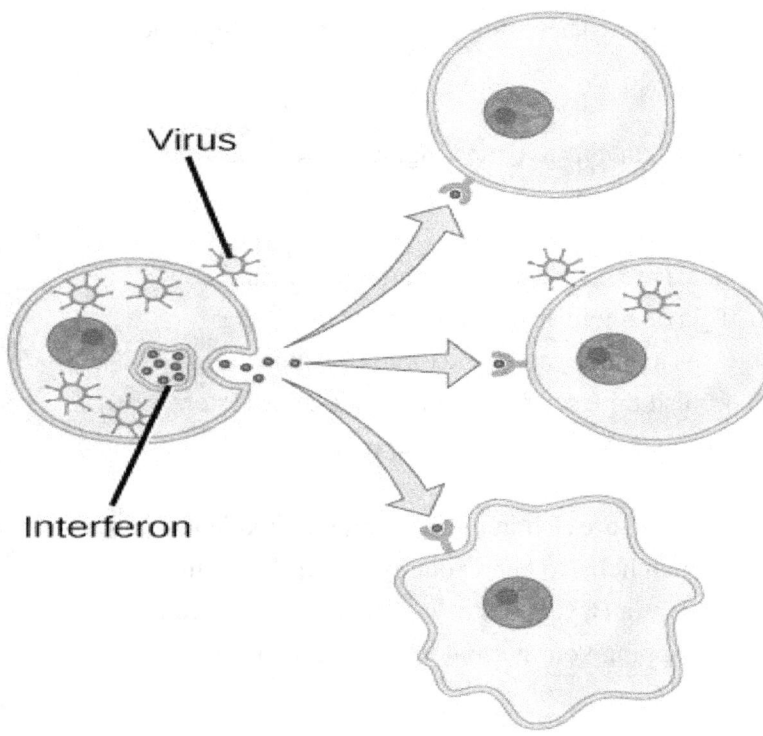

Signals neighboring
uninfected cells to
destroy RNA and
reduce protein
synthesis.

Signals neighboring
infected to cells to
undergo apoptosis.

Activates
immune cells.

ANTIVIRAL ACTION OF INTERFERON (INF)

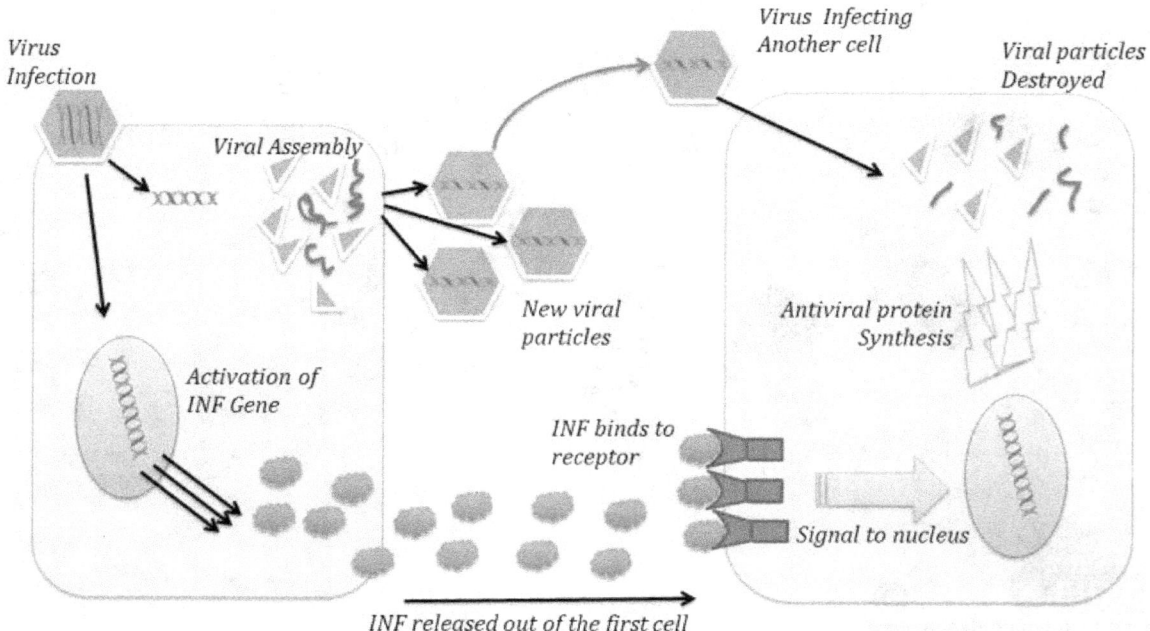

*****

Eating 2 LIVE ... Interferons

*****

Interferon is a Natural substance produced by our body's **white cells** to fight **infections, cancer, allergies** and **toxic** chemical poisoning. It can be made artificially and injected for some cancers and viral infections like HIV and hepatitis C, however there are side effects.

Interferons were discovered in 1957 by British bacteriologist Alick Isaacs and Swiss microbiologist Jean Lindenmann.

Licorice

- Strengthens the immune system by increasing interferon production
- Exhibits anti-inflammatory and anti-arthritic properties
- More than 10 anti-inflammatory favonoids isolated from licorice
- Chemical components help reduce swelling

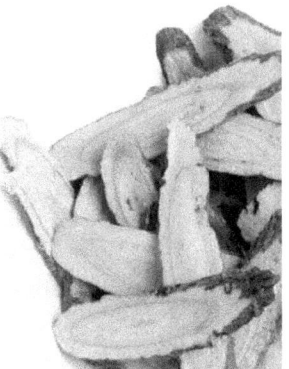

Interferon, any of several related proteins that are produced by the body's cells as a defensive response to viruses. They are important modulators of the immune response.

Interferon was named for its ability to interfere with viral proliferation. The various forms of interferon are the bodies most rapidly produced and important defense against viruses. Interferons can also combat bacterial and parasitic infections, inhibit cell division, and promote or impede the differentiation of cells. They are produced by all vertebrate animals and possibly by some invertebrates as well.

Interferons are categorized as cytokines, small proteins that are involved in intercellular signaling. Interferon is secreted by cells in response to stimulation by a virus or other foreign substance, but it does not directly inhibit the virus's multiplication. Rather, it stimulates the infected cells and those nearby to produce proteins that prevent the virus from replicating within them. Further production of the virus is thereby inhibited and the infection is stemmed.

Astragalus stimulates the body's production of interferon – our body's early warning system.

Interferons also have immunoregulatory functions—they inhibit B-lymphocyte (B-cell) activation, enhance T-lymphocyte (T-cell) activity, and increase the cellular-destruction capability of natural killer cells.

Three Types of Interferons

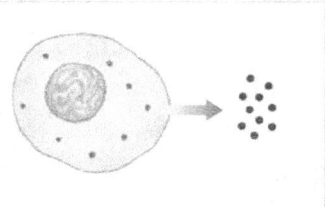

① Alpha (α)-interferons are produced by cells infected with viruses. They attract and stimulate NK cells and enhance resistance to viral infection.

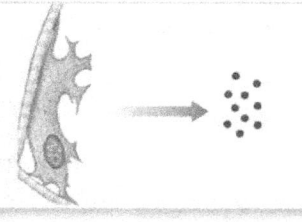

② Beta (β)-interferons, secreted by fibroblasts, slow inflammation in a damaged area.

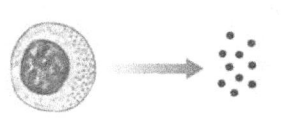

③ Gamma (γ)-interferons, secreted by T cells and NK cells, stimulate macrophage activity.

There are 3 forms of Interferon - **Alpha** (α), **Beta** (β), and **Gamma** (γ)—have been recognized. These interferons have been classified into 2 types: **type I** includes the **alpha** and **beta** forms, and **type II** consists of the **gamma** form.

This division is based on the type of cell that produces the interferon and the functional characteristics of the protein.

Type I interferons can be produced by almost any cell upon stimulation by a virus; their primary function is to induce viral resistance in cells. Type II interferon is secreted only by natural killer cells and T lymphocytes; its main purpose is to signal the immune system to respond to infectious agents or cancerous growth.

Research conducted in the 1970s revealed that these substances could not only prevent viral infection but also suppress the growth of cancers in some laboratory animals.

The many natural substances that activate the body's own production of interferon:

- Astragalus: a Chinese herb that enhances the antibody reaction to foreign invaders of all types including cancer.
- Boneset: a native American Indian herb with antiseptic, anti-viral properties used for the treatment of colds and flus, coughs, fevers, indigestion and pain.
- Chlorophyll: a plant pigment which can be found in a long list of green leafy vegetables and algae like spirulina, chlorella and barley green.
- Echinacea: the most popular herb in North America used as a treatment for toothaches, bites or stings and all types of infections.

- Ginkgo: a potent central nervous system antioxidant for the treatment of circulation disorders, memory problems, high blood pressure, depression, tinnitus and immune system disorders.
- Licorice: an anti-inflammatory and anti-allergic herb used to boost energy, treat respiratory tract infections as well as female disorders, ulcers, adrenal insufficiency and congestion.
- Melatonin: a hormone produced by the pineal gland with strong antioxidant and immune system boosting properties.
- Milk Thistle (Silymarin): a herb most commonly recommended as a liver cleanser and complementary medical treatment for hepatitis.
- Medicinal Mushrooms: Reishi, Maitake, Shiitake, Kombucha and others stimulate many aspects of the immune system including the production of interferon.
- Siberian Ginseng: stimulates T-cell and B-cell activity, energy, libido, body fat burning and many stress-related conditions.
- Vitamin C and bioflavonoids, especially proanthocyanidins (pycnogenols) like grape seed extract, pine bark extract and bilberry, quercetin, hesperidin and catechin are powerful antioxidants.

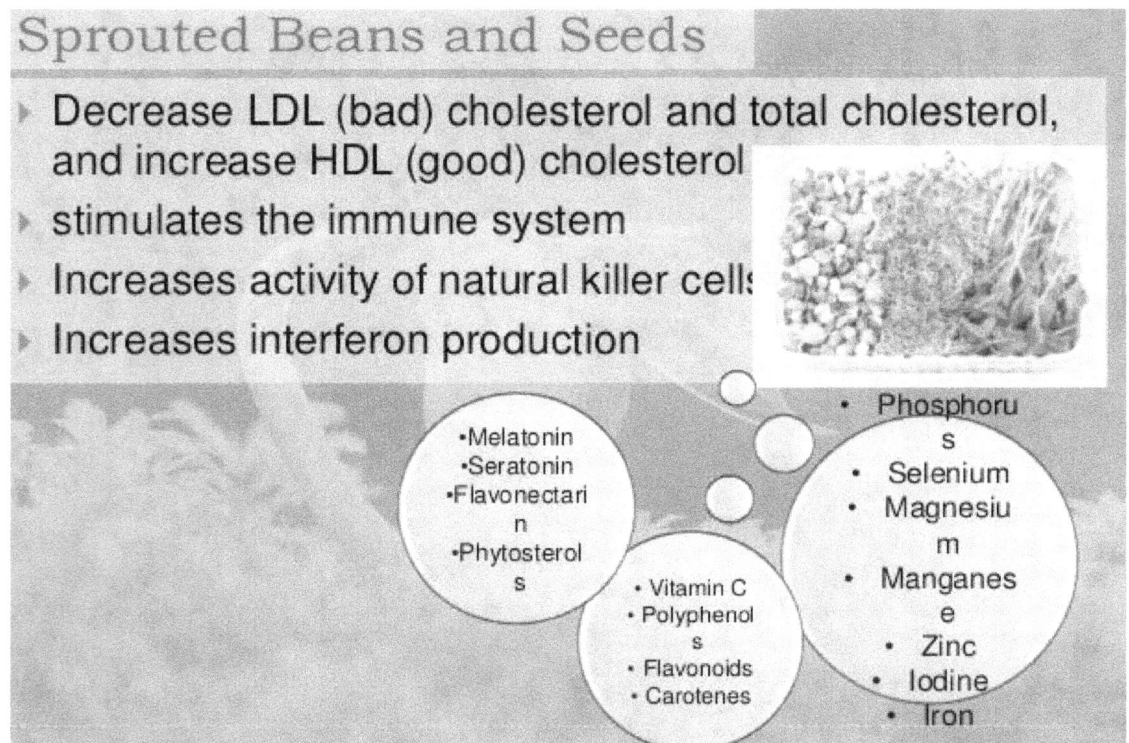

Sprouted Beans and Seeds

▸ Decrease LDL (bad) cholesterol and total cholesterol, and increase HDL (good) cholesterol
▸ stimulates the immune system
▸ Increases activity of natural killer cells
▸ Increases interferon production

- Melatonin
- Seratonin
- Flavonectarin
- Phytosterols

- Vitamin C
- Polyphenols
- Flavonoids
- Carotenes

- Phosphorus
- Selenium
- Magnesium
- Manganese
- Zinc
- Iodine
- Iron

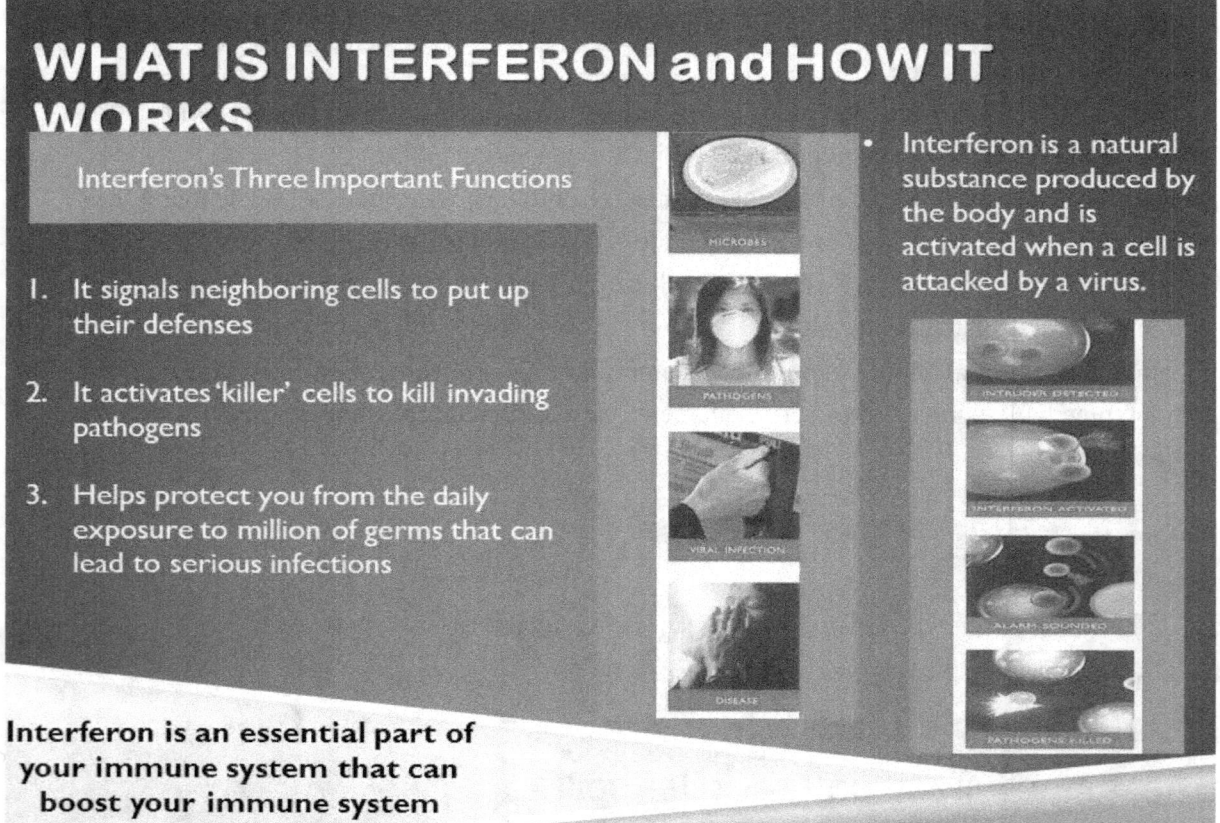

WHAT IS INTERFERON and HOW IT WORKS

Interferon's Three Important Functions

1. It signals neighboring cells to put up their defenses

2. It activates 'killer' cells to kill invading pathogens

3. Helps protect you from the daily exposure to million of germs that can lead to serious infections

- Interferon is a natural substance produced by the body and is activated when a cell is attacked by a virus.

MICROBES

PATHOGENS

VIRAL INFECTION

DISEASE

INTRUDER DETECTED

INTERFERON ACTIVATED

ALARM SOUNDED

PATHOGENS KILLED

Interferon is an essential part of your immune system that can boost your immune system

*****

Eating 2 LIVE … White Blood Cells

*****

Low white blood cell counts are indicative of a suppressed immune system and can have many causes. Emotional state and stress, an unhealthy diet and lifestyle, and nutritional intake can all cause lower immune system response and low white blood cell counts. Low immunity can also be caused by a number of health conditions, by surgical or medical treatments and by the natural aging process. Whatever the cause, low immunity and low white blood cell counts prevent the body from being able to have an optimum response to infections and illness. Here are some things which can help prevent low immunity and keep white blood cell counts high:

White blood cells

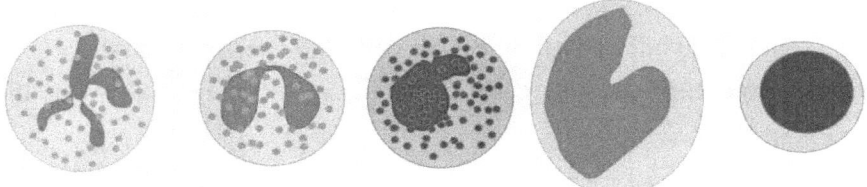

neutrophil   eosinophil   basophil   monocyte   lymphocyte

- Avoid sugar and keep sweet stuff to a minimum. Sugar prevents white blood cells from being their strongest

- Eliminate unhealthy fats. Polyunsaturated fats in vegetable oils such as corn, safflower, and sunflower oil are deterrents to a healthy immune system.

- If you are overweight, lose a few pounds. Being overweight is very detrimental to your immune system and studies have shown that overweight people are less able to fight off infection.

- Drink plenty of water to boost the immune system as well as flush out toxins

- Exercise is a proven immune system booster. Exercise is best in moderation, however, since too much exercise may wear the body down and create immune system problems.

- Avoid stress and try to relax. Stress is rightly called the silent killer and too much stress invariably leads to a lowered immune system.

Many food items help boost immune function and white blood cell counts. For example:

Navy beans, Carrots and other red, yellow, orange, and dark-green leafy vegetables contain beta carotene which helps protect the immune system, especially the thymus gland. Beta carotene and other carotenes also strengthen white blood cell production, and foods rich in beta-carotene help the body better fight off infection.

Yogurt can be very beneficial for the immune system. It helps the body produce antibodies and strengthens white blood cells.

Vitamin A is an antioxidant that helps your body fight cancer cells and is essential in the formation of white blood cells. Vitamin A also increases the ability of antibodies to respond to invaders.

People who eat more garlic have more natural killer white blood cells.

Other helpful foods include dark grapes and guava.

** Supplements can play a big role in boosting immune function and white blood cell counts. Some examples:

- Oleander extract in herbal supplement form. One herbal oleander based supplement was 100% effective in a clinical trial of raising white blood cell counts in HIV/AIDS patients with extremely compromised immune systems.

- Astragalus root helps stimulate white blood cells and protects against invading organisms. It also enhances production of the important natural compound interferon to fight against viruses.

- Zinc is necessary for white blood cell function and it acts as a catalyst in the immune system's killer response to foreign bodies.

- Vitamin C is an immune enhancer that helps white blood cells perform at their peak and quickens the immune system response.

- The trace mineral selenium is vital to the development and movement of white blood cells.

- Both Siberian ginseng (eleuthero) and Asian ginseng provide support for the immune system.

- Echinacea helps stimulate the immune system in a variety of ways, including increased white blood cell production.

- Green Tea also stimulates production of white blood cells.

Some other potent immune boosters are pau d arco, suma, medicinal mushrooms, beta glucans and aloe vera.

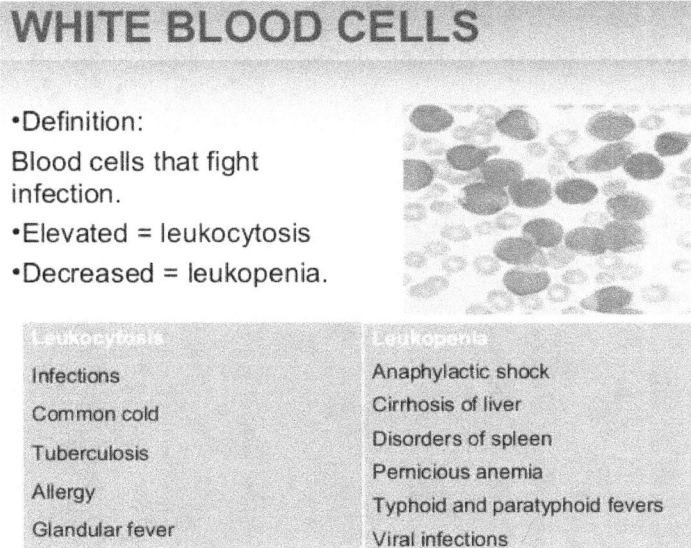

WHITE BLOOD CELLS

•Definition:
Blood cells that fight infection.
•Elevated = leukocytosis
•Decreased = leukopenia.

Leukocytosis	Leukopenia
Infections	Anaphylactic shock
Common cold	Cirrhosis of liver
Tuberculosis	Disorders of spleen
Allergy	Pernicious anemia
Glandular fever	Typhoid and paratyphoid fevers
	Viral infections

PAGE 198

Supreme Health & Fitness!   Health & Wellness Series Volume 1

The Effect of Diet

Diet and nutrition can affect white blood cell count. Individuals with a low count are advised to eat foods that help boost the immune system. These include live yogurt, fruit, garlic, spinach and other vegetables, and foods rich in zinc such as shiitake mushrooms. Caution should also be taken about foods that carry a risk of infection, such as raw milk and cheese.

If you have low WBC (leukopenia), it is very important to practice good hygiene, hand-washing, and food safety practices. Neutrophils are the cells that fight bacterial infection. Neutropenia, which simply means low levels of neutrophils, occurs when Absolute neutrophil count (ANC) falls below 1500. When this happens, a person is more susceptible to infections.

If your ANC is low, you can minimize your risk of infection by using an anti-bacterial soap and warm water, and scrubbing your hands for 15-30 seconds several times per day, and every time before you prepare food.

If you have neutropenia, you should avoid raw meat, eggs and fish, moldy or expired food, unwashed or moldy fruit and vegetables, and unpasteurized beverages, including fruit and vegetable juice, beer, milk, as well as unpasteurized honey. You do not need to avoid fresh fruit and vegetables, because this practice has not been shown to reduce the number of major infections. However, you should wash these foods thoroughly before you eat them. The American Cancer Society's recommendations for foods to avoid for neutropenia can be found here.

Good quality protein is important for cancer patients to include in their diet, because our bodies need the building blocks (amino acids) from the protein we eat to make the new WBCs.

FOODS THAT BOOST
YOUR IMMUNE SYSTEM NATURALLY!

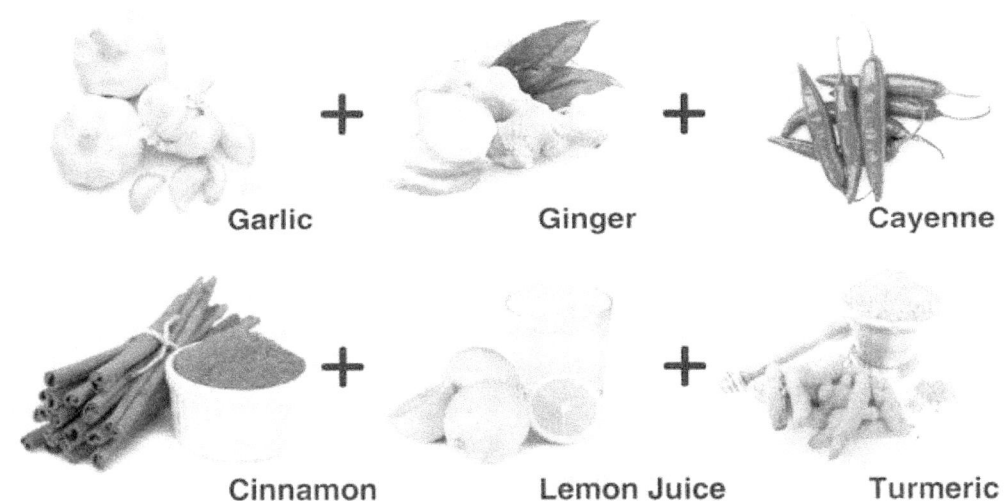

Garlic + Ginger + Cayenne

Cinnamon + Lemon Juice + Turmeric

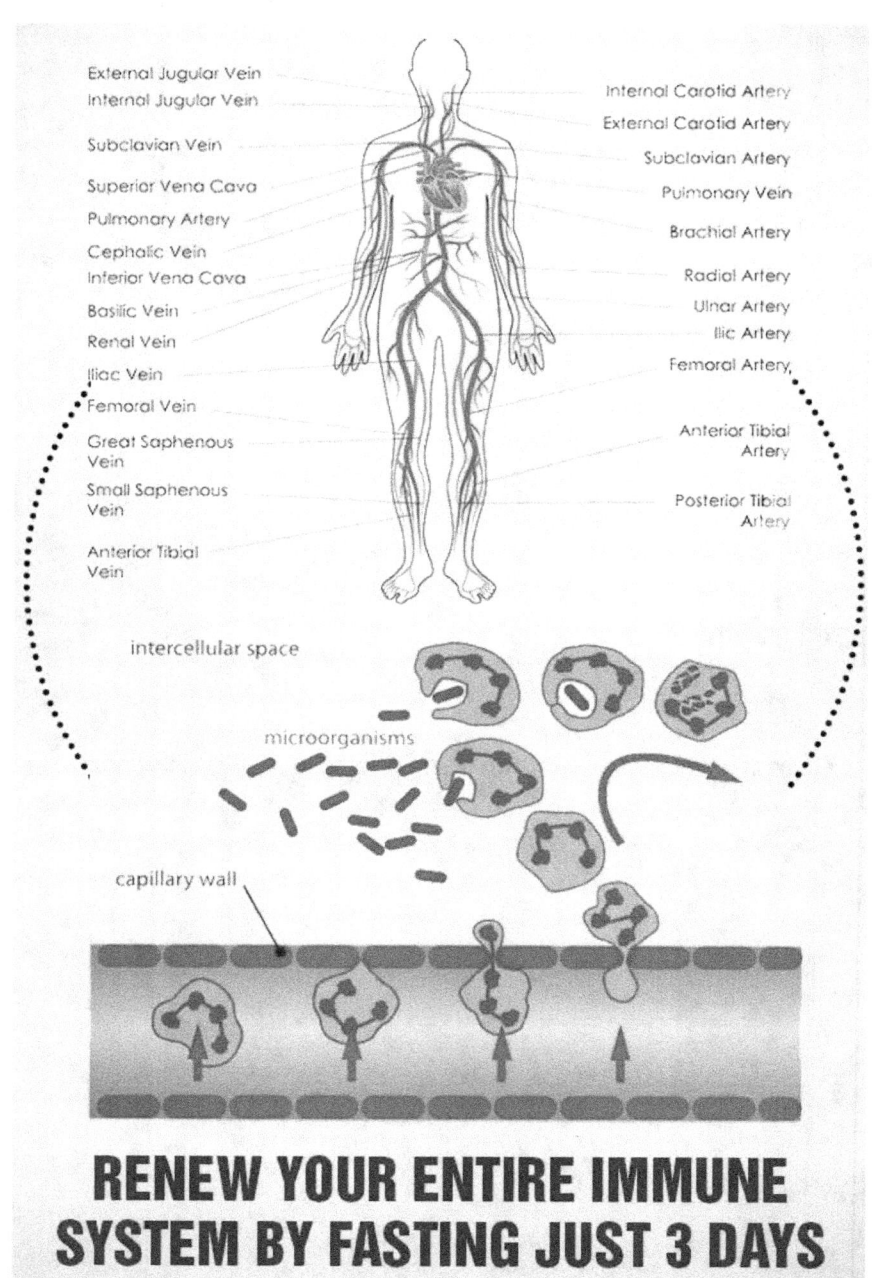

External Jugular Vein
Internal Jugular Vein

Subclavian Vein

Superior Vena Cava
Pulmonary Artery
Cephalic Vein
Inferior Vena Cava
Basilic Vein
Renal Vein
Iliac Vein
Femoral Vein
Great Saphenous Vein
Small Saphenous Vein

Anterior Tibial Vein

Internal Carotid Artery
External Carotid Artery
Subclavian Artery
Pulmonary Vein
Brachial Artery
Radial Artery
Ulnar Artery
Ilic Artery
Femoral Artery,

Anterior Tibial Artery

Posterior Tibial Artery

intercellular space

microorganisms

capillary wall

RENEW YOUR ENTIRE IMMUNE SYSTEM BY FASTING JUST 3 DAYS

IMMUNE SYSTEM

The immune system protects the body against disease or other potentially damaging foreign bodies. When functioning properly, the immune system identifies and attacks a variety of threats, including viruses, bacteria and parasites, while distinguishing them from the body's own healthy tissue.

LYMPHATIC SYSTEM
consists of bone marrow, spleen, thymus and lymph nodes.

Lymph nodes:
Produce and store cells that fight infection and disease.

Bone marrow:
Produces white blood cells, or leukocytes.

Thymus:
This organ is where T-cells mature. T-cells help destroy infected or cancerous cells.

Spleen:
The largest lymphatic organ in the body contains white blood cells that fight infection or disease.

LYMPHOCYTES AND LEUKOCYTES

These small white blood cells play a large role in defending the body against disease.

Leukocytes are white blood cells that identify and eliminate pathogens.

The two types of lymphocytes are B-cells, which make antibodies that attack bacteria and toxins, and T-cells, which help destroy infected or cancerous cells.

Pathogen

Red blood cell

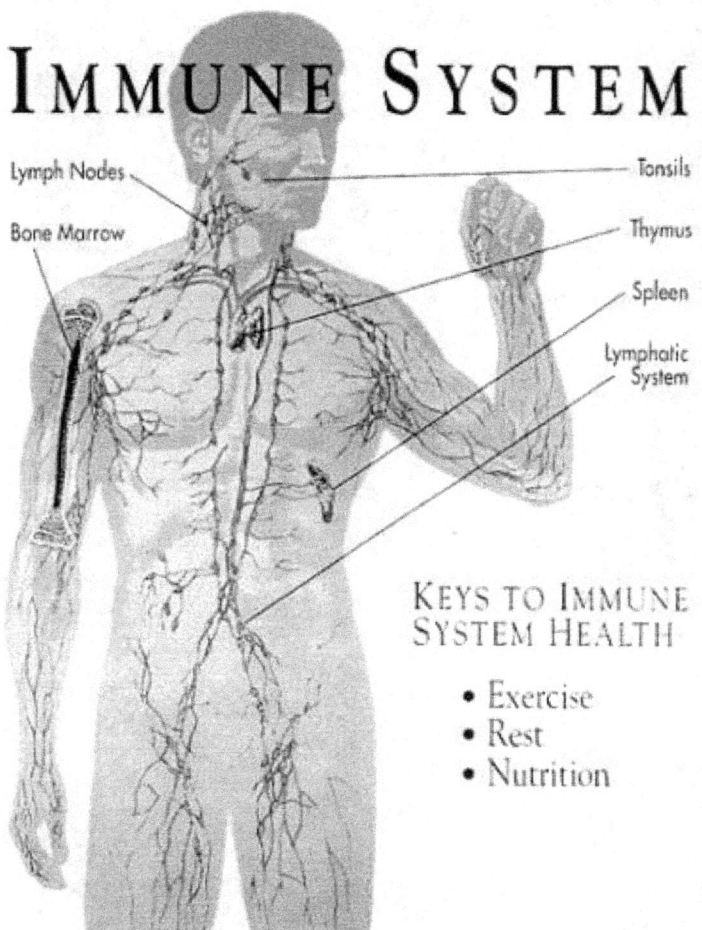

IMMUNE SYSTEM

Lymph Nodes

Bone Marrow

Tonsils

Thymus

Spleen

Lymphatic System

KEYS TO IMMUNE SYSTEM HEALTH

- Exercise
- Rest
- Nutrition

*****

Chapter 13 … SLEEP

*****

Sleep — the irresistible tempter to whom we inevitably succumb. Sleep—sweet, renewing, mysterious sleep. While sleeping, you may feel "dead to the world," but you are not. Even when you are deeply asleep, your perceptual window is open a crack.

The State of Sleep is very important to our Immune System as well as our overall health and well-being. Our Bodies do not begin the Healing process until we are SLEEP … So, no matter what condition we are in, we Need Sleep to Heal, increase our Health and manifest our Power!

You move around on your bed, but you manage not to fall out. The occasional roar of passing vehicles may leave your deep sleep undisturbed, but a cry from a baby's nursery quickly interrupts it. So, does the sound of your name. EEG recordings confirm that the brain's auditory cortex responds to sound stimuli even during sleep (Kutas, 1990).

And when you are asleep, as when you are awake, you process most information outside your conscious awareness.

"I love to sleep. Do you? Isn't it great? It really is the best of both worlds. You get to be alive and unconscious." *Comedian Rita Rudner, 1993*

Many of sleep's mysteries are now being solved as some people sleep, attached to recording devices, while others observe.

By recording brain waves and muscle movements, and by observing and occasionally waking sleepers, researchers are glimpsing things that a thousand years of common sense never told us.

Biological Rhythms and Sleep

Like the ocean, life has its rhythmic tides. Over varying time periods, our bodies fluctuate, and with them, our minds. Let's look more closely at two of those biological rhythms—our 24-hour biological clock and our 90-minute sleep cycle.

Circadian Rhythm

How do our biological rhythms influence our daily functioning?

The rhythm of the day parallels the rhythm of life—from our waking at a new day's birth to our nightly return to what Shakespeare called "death's counterfeit."

Our bodies roughly synchronize with the 24-hour cycle of day and night by an internal biological clock called the **circadian rhythm** (from the Latin *circa*, "about," and *diem*, "day"). As morning approaches, body temperature rises, then peaks during the day, dips for a time in early afternoon (when many people take siestas), and begins to drop again in the evening.

Thinking is sharpest and memory most accurate when we are at our daily peak in circadian arousal. Try pulling an all-nighter or working an occasional night shift. You'll feel groggiest in the middle of the night but may gain new energy when your normal wake-up time arrives.

Circadian [ser-KAY-dee-an] Rhythm the biological clock; regular bodily rhythms (for example, of temperature and wakefulness) that occur on a 24-hour cycle.

Age and experience can alter our circadian rhythm. Most 20-year-olds are evening-energized "owls," with performance improving across the day (May & Hasher, 1998). Most older adults are morning-loving "larks," with performance declining as the day wears on.

By mid-evening, when the night has hardly begun for many young adults, retirement homes are typically quiet. After about age 20 (slightly earlier for women), we begin to shift from being owls to being larks (Roenneberg et al., 2004).

Women become more morning oriented as they have children and also as they transition to menopause (Leonhard & Randler, 2009; Randler & Bausback, 2010). Morning types tend to do better in school, to take more initiative, and to be less vulnerable to depression (Randler, 2008, 2009; Randler & Frech, 2009).

Sleep Stages

Sooner or later, sleep overtakes us and consciousness fades as different parts of our brain's cortex stop communicating (Massimini et al., 2005). But rather than emitting a constant dial tone, the sleeping brain has its own biological rhythm.

What is the biological rhythm of our sleeping and dreaming stages?

Sleep researchers measure brain-wave activity, eye movements, and muscle tension by electrodes that pick up weak electrical signals from the brain, eyes, and facial muscles.

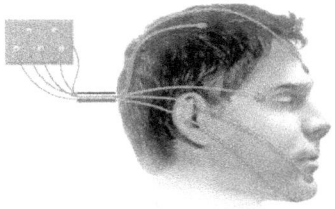

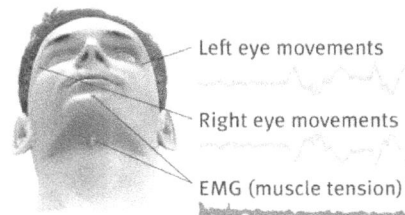

Left eye movements

Right eye movements

EMG (muscle tension)

About every 90 minutes, you cycle through four distinct sleep stages. This simple fact apparently was

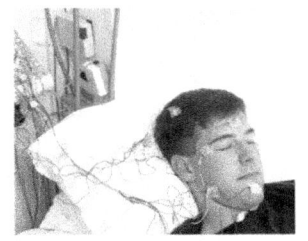

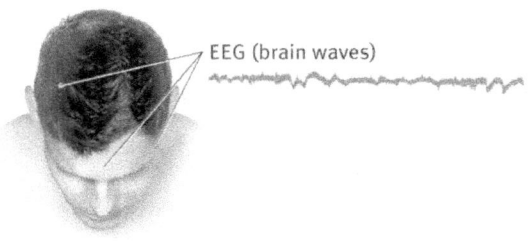

EEG (brain waves)

unknown until 8-year-old Armond Aserinsky went to bed one night in 1952. His father, Eugene, a University of Chicago graduate student, needed to test an electroencephalograph he had repaired that day (Aserinsky, 1988; Seligman & Yellen, 1987).

Placing electrodes near Armond's eyes to record the rolling eye movements then believed to occur during sleep, Aserinsky watched the machine go wild, tracing deep zigzags on the graph paper.

Could the machine still be broken? As the night proceeded and the activity recurred, Aserinsky realized that the periods of fast, jerky eye movements were accompanied by energetic brain activity. Awakened during one such episode, Armond reported having a dream. Aserinsky had discovered what we now know as **REM sleep** (*r*apid *e*ye *m*ovement sleep).

REM sleep rapid eye movement sleep; a recurring sleep stage during which vivid dreams commonly occur. Also known as *paradoxical sleep*, because the muscles are relaxed (except for minor twitches) but other body systems are active.

Similar procedures used with thousands of volunteers showed the cycles were a normal part of sleep (Kleitman, 1960).

To appreciate these studies, imagine yourself as a participant. As the hour grows late, you feel sleepy and yawn in response to reduced brain metabolism. (Yawning, which can be socially contagious, stretches your neck muscles and increases your heart rate, which increases your alertness [Moorcroft, 2003].)

When you are ready for bed, a researcher comes in and tapes electrodes to your scalp (to detect your brain waves), on your chin (to detect muscle tension), and just outside the corners of your eyes (to detect eye movements). Other devices will record your heart rate, respiration rate, and genital arousal.

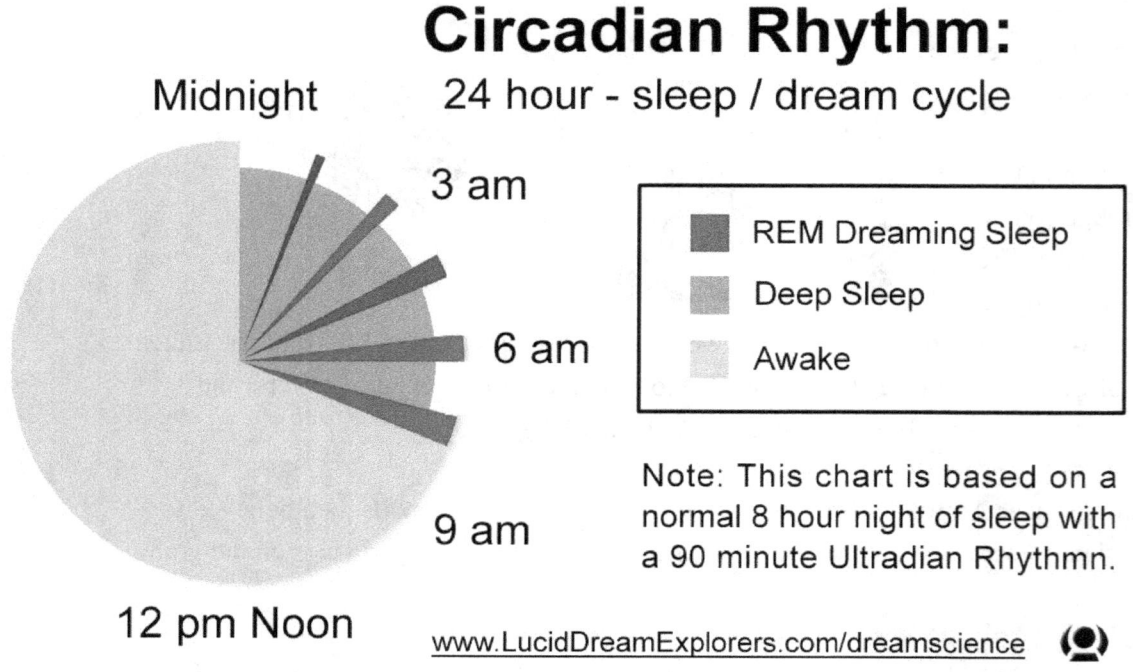

Circadian Rhythm:
24 hour - sleep / dream cycle

Midnight

3 am

6 am

9 am

12 pm Noon

REM Dreaming Sleep
Deep Sleep
Awake

Note: This chart is based on a normal 8 hour night of sleep with a 90 minute Ultradian Rhythmn.

www.LucidDreamExplorers.com/dreamscience

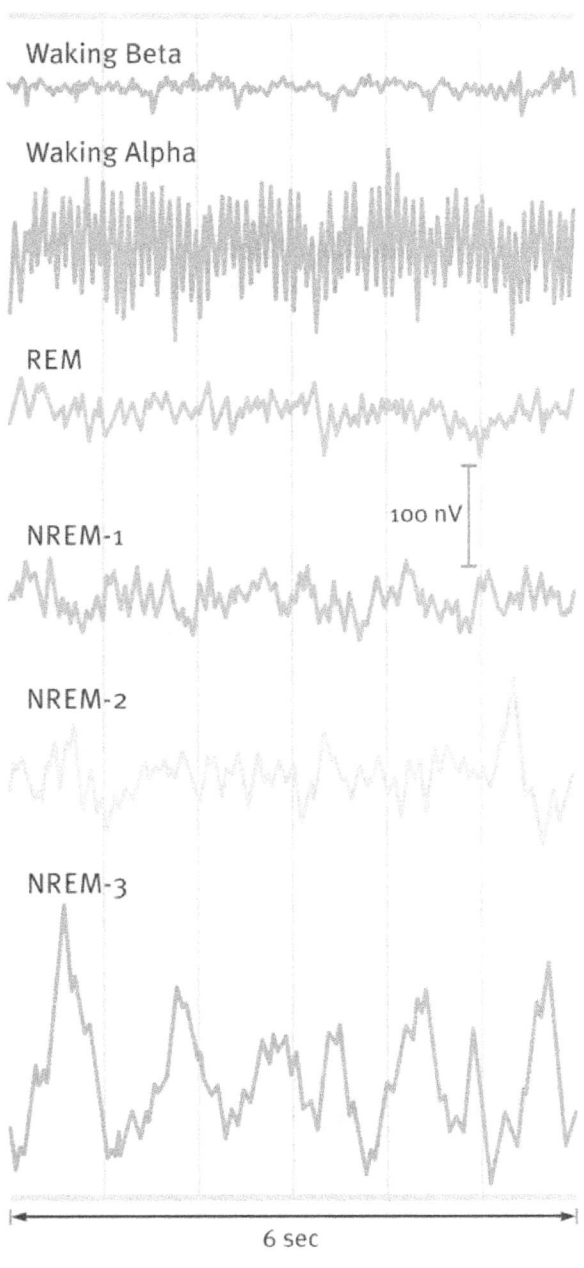

Waking Beta

Waking Alpha

REM

100 nV

NREM-1

NREM-2

NREM-3

6 sec

Dement, 1999.)

When you are in bed with your eyes closed, the researcher in the next room sees on the EEG the relatively slow **alpha waves** of your awake but relaxed state. As you adapt to all this equipment, you grow tired and, in an unremembered moment, slip into **sleep**.

The transition is marked by the slowed breathing and the irregular brain waves of non-REM stage 1 sleep. Using the new American Academy of Sleep Medicine classification of sleep stages, this is called NREM-1 sleep (Silber et al., 2008).

Alpha waves The relatively slow brain waves of a relaxed, awake state.

The beta waves of an alert, waking state and the regular alpha waves of an awake, relaxed state differ from the slower, larger delta waves of deep NREM-3 sleep.

Although the rapid REM sleep waves resemble the near-waking NREM-1 sleep waves, the body is more aroused during REM sleep than during NREM sleep.

Rebecca Spencer, University of Massachusetts assisted with this illustration.

Sleep Periodic, natural loss of consciousness—as distinct from unconsciousness resulting from a coma, general anesthesia, or hibernation. (Adapted from Dement, 1999.)

We seem unaware of the moment we fall into sleep, but someone watching our brain waves could tell. (From Dement, 1999.)

Sleep

1 second

In one of his 15,000 research participants, William Dement (1999) observed the moment the brain's perceptual window to the outside world slammed shut. Dement asked this sleep-deprived young man, lying on his back with eyelids taped open, to press a button every time a strobe light flashed in his eyes (about every 6 seconds). After a few minutes the young man missed one. Asked why, he said, "Because there was no flash." But there was a flash. He missed it because (as his brain activity revealed) he had fallen asleep for 2 seconds, missing not only the flash 6 inches from his nose but also the awareness of the abrupt moment of entry into sleep.

During this brief NREM-1 sleep you may experience fantastic images resembling **hallucinations**—sensory experiences that occur without a sensory stimulus. You may have a sensation of falling (at which moment your body may suddenly jerk) or of floating weightlessly. These *hypnagogic* sensations may later be incorporated into your memories.

People who claim to have been abducted by aliens—often shortly after getting into bed—commonly recall being floated off (or pinned down on) their beds (Clancy, 2005).

Hallucinations False sensory experiences, such as seeing something in the absence of an external visual stimulus.

To catch your own hypnagogic experiences, you might use your alarm's snooze function.

You then relax more deeply and begin about 20 minutes of NREM-2 sleep, with its periodic *sleep spindles*—bursts of rapid, rhythmic brain-wave activity (see Figure 3.7). Although you could still be awakened without too much difficulty, you are now clearly asleep.

Then you transition to the deep sleep of NREM-3. During this slow-wave sleep, which lasts for about 30 minutes, your brain emits large, slow **delta waves** and you are hard to awaken. (It is at the end of the deep, slow-wave NREM-3 sleep that children may wet the bed.)

Delta waves The large, slow brain waves associated with deep sleep.

REM Sleep

About an hour after you first fall asleep, a strange thing happens. Rather than continuing in deep slumber, you ascend from your initial sleep dive. Returning through NREM-2 (where you spend about half your night), you enter the most intriguing sleep phase—REM sleep. For about 10 minutes, your brain waves become rapid and saw-toothed, more like those of the nearly awake NREM-1 sleep.

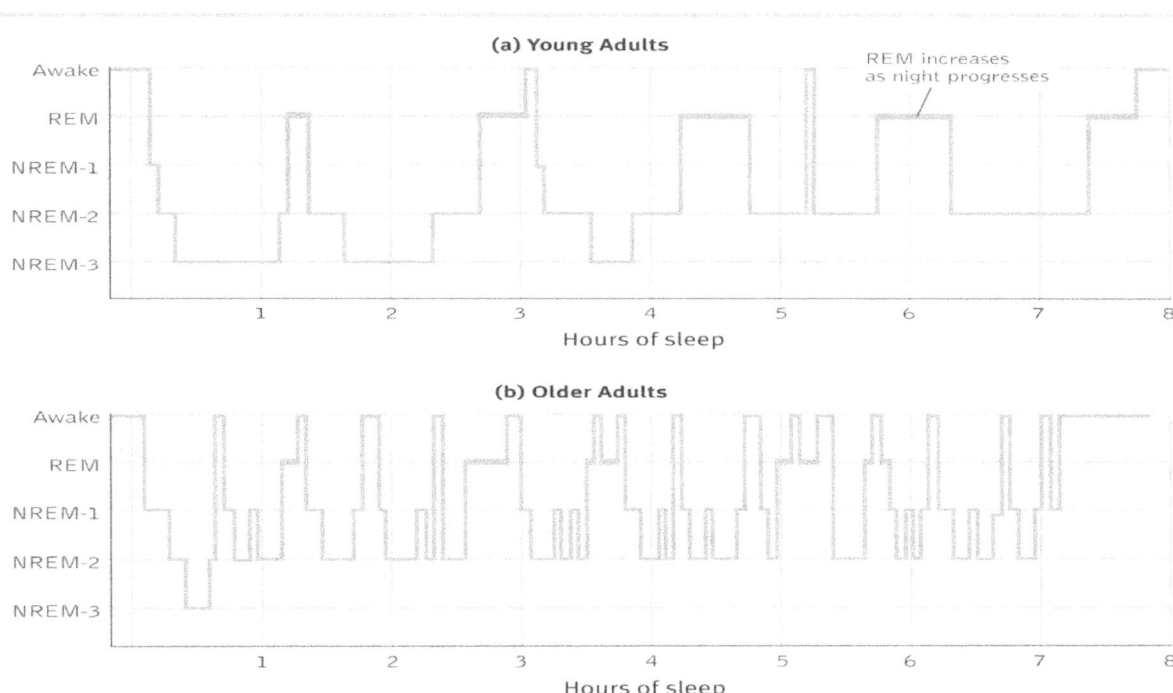

But unlike NREM-1, during REM sleep your heart rate rises, your breathing becomes rapid and irregular, and every half-minute or so your eyes dart around in momentary bursts of activity behind closed lids. These eye movements announce the beginning of a dream—often emotional, usually story-like, and richly hallucinatory.

Because anyone watching a sleeper's eyes can notice these REM bursts, it is amazing that science was ignorant of REM sleep until 1952.

People rarely snore during dreams. When REM starts, snoring stops.

People pass through a multistage sleep cycle several times each night, with the periods of deep sleep diminishing and REM sleep periods increasing in duration.

As people age, sleep becomes more fragile, with awakenings common among older adults (Kamel et al., 2006; Neubauer, 1999).

Except during very scary dreams, your genitals become aroused during REM sleep. You have an erection or increased vaginal lubrication and clitoral engorgement, regardless of whether the dream's content is sexual (Karacan et al., 1966).

Men's common "morning erection" stems from the night's last REM period, often just before waking. In young men, sleep-related erections outlast REM periods, lasting 30 to 45 minutes on average (Karacan et al., 1983; Schiavi & Schreiner-Engel, 1988). A typical 25-year-old man therefore has an erection during nearly half his night's sleep, a 65-year-old man for one-quarter. Many men troubled by *erectile disorder* (impotence) have sleep-related erections, suggesting the problem is not between their legs.

Horses, which spend 92 percent of each day standing and can sleep standing, must lie down for REM sleep (Morrison, 2003).

Your brain's motor cortex is active during REM sleep, but your brainstem blocks its messages. This leaves your muscles relaxed, so much so that, except for an occasional finger, toe, or facial twitch, you are essentially paralyzed.

Moreover, you cannot easily be awakened. REM sleep is thus sometimes called *paradoxical* sleep: The body is internally aroused, with waking-like brain activity, yet asleep and externally calm.

The sleep cycle repeats itself about every 90 minutes for younger adults (somewhat more frequently for older adults). As the night wears on, deep NREM-3 sleep grows shorter and disappears. The REM and NREM-2 sleep periods get longer.

By morning, we have spent 20 to 25 percent of an average night's sleep—some 100 minutes—in REM sleep. Thirty-seven percent of people report rarely or never having dreams "that you can remember the next morning" (Moore, 2004). Yet even they will, more than 80 percent of the time, recall a dream after being awakened during REM sleep.

We spend about 600 hours a year experiencing some 1500 dreams, or more than 100,000 dreams over a typical lifetime—dreams swallowed by the night but not acted out, thanks to REM's protective paralysis.

What Affects Our Sleep Patterns?

How do biology and environment interact in our sleep patterns?

The idea that "everyone needs 8 hours of sleep" is untrue. Newborns sleep nearly two-thirds of their day, most adults no more than one-third. Still, there is more to our sleep differences than age. Some of us thrive with fewer than 6 hours per night; others regularly rack up 9 hours or more. Such sleep patterns are genetically influenced (Hor & Tafti, 2009).

In studies of fraternal and identical twins, only the identical twins had strikingly similar sleep patterns and durations (Webb & Campbell, 1983). Today's researchers are discovering the genes that regulate sleep in humans and animals (Donlea et al., 2009; He et al., 2009).

In the United States and Canada, adults average 7 to 8 hours of sleep per night (Hurst, 2008; National Sleep Foundation, 2010; Robinson & Martin, 2009). North Americans are nevertheless sleeping less than their counterparts a century ago. Thanks to modern light bulbs, shift work, and social diversions, those who would have gone to bed at 9:00 p.m. are now up until 11:00 p.m. or later.

With sleep, as with waking behavior, biology and environment interact.

Being bathed in light disrupts our 24-hour biological clock (Czeisler et al., 1999; Dement, 1999). Bright light affects our sleepiness by activating light-sensitive retinal proteins. T

his signals the brain's **suprachiasmatic nucleus** to decrease production of *melatonin*, a sleep-inducing hormone. Our ancestors' body clocks were attuned to the rising and setting Sun of the 24-hour day.

Many of today's young adults adopt something closer to a 25-hour day, by staying up too late to get 8 hours of sleep.

Most animals, too, when placed under unnatural constant illumination will exceed a 24-hour day.

Suprachiasmatic nucleus   A pair of cell clusters in the hypothalamus that responds to light-sensitive retinal proteins; causes pineal gland to increase or decrease production of melatonin, thus modifying our feelings of sleepiness.

Light striking the retina signals the suprachiasmatic nucleus (SCN) to suppress the pineal gland's production of the sleep hormone melatonin.

At night, the SCN quiets down, allowing the pineal gland to release melatonin into the bloodstream.

A *circadian disadvantage*: One study of a decade's 24,121 Major League Baseball games found that teams who had crossed three time zones before playing a multiday series had nearly a 60 percent chance of losing their first game (Winter et al., 2009).

Sleep often eludes those who stay up late and sleep in on weekends, and then go to bed earlier on Sunday to prepare for the new week ahead (Oren & Terman, 1998).

For North Americans who fly to Europe and need to be up when their circadian rhythm

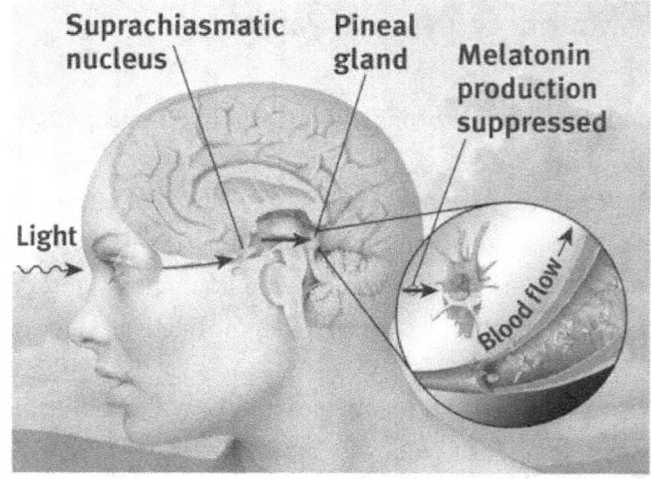

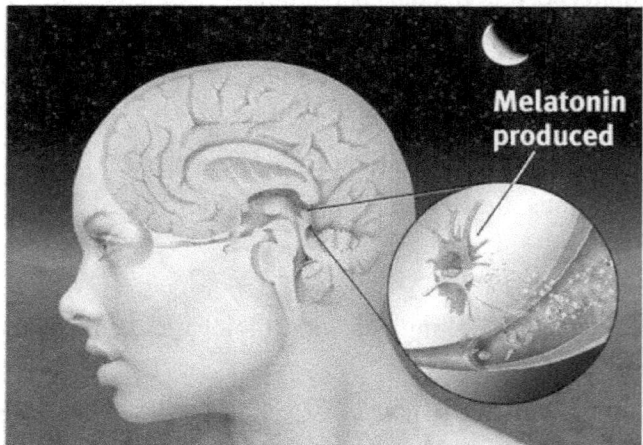

cries *"SLEEP,"* bright light (spending the next day outdoors) helps reset the biological clock (Czeisler et al., 1986, 1989; Eastman et al., 1995).

Sleep Theories

What are sleep's functions?

So, our sleep patterns differ from person to person and from culture to culture. But why do we have this need for sleep? Psychologists offer five possible reasons why sleep evolved.

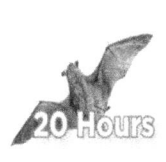 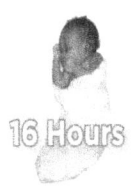 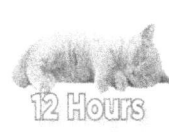 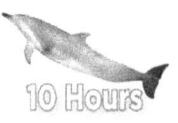 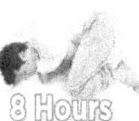 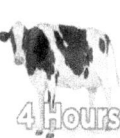 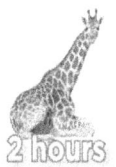

1.   ***Sleep helps us recuperate.*** It helps restore and repair brain tissue. Bats and other animals with high waking metabolism burn a lot of calories, producing a lot of *free radicals*, molecules that are toxic to neurons. Sleeping a lot gives resting neurons time to repair themselves, while pruning or weakening unused connections (Gilestro et al., 2009; Siegel, 2003; Vyazovskiy et al., 2008). Think of it this way: When consciousness leaves your house, brain construction workers come in for a makeover.

"Corduroy pillows make headlines." *Anonymous*

2.   ***Sleep helps restore and rebuild our fading memories of the day's experiences.*** Sleep consolidates our memories—it strengthens and stabilizes neural memory traces (Racsmány et al., 2010; Rasch & Born, 2008). People trained to perform tasks therefore recall them better after a night's sleep, or even after a short nap, than after several hours awake (Stickgold & Ellenbogen, 2008).

After sleeping well, older people remember more.

And in both humans and rats, neural activity during slow-wave sleep re-enacts and promotes recall of prior novel experiences (Peigneux et al., 2004; Ribeiro et al., 2004).

Sleep, it seems, strengthens memories in a way that being awake does not.

3.   ***Sleep feeds creative thinking.*** On occasion, dreams have inspired noteworthy literary, artistic, and scientific achievements, such as the dream that clued chemist August Kekulé to the structure of benzene (Ross, 2006). More commonplace is the boost that a complete night's sleep gives to our thinking and learning.

After working on a task, then sleeping on it, people solve problems more insightfully than do those who stay awake (Wagner et al., 2004). They also are better at spotting connections among novel pieces of information (Ellenbogen et al., 2007).

To think smart and see connections, it often pays to sleep on it.

4.   ***Sleep supports growth.*** During deep sleep, the pituitary gland releases a growth hormone necessary for muscle development. A regular full night's sleep can also "*dramatically improve your athletic ability*," report James Maas and Rebecca Robbins (2010).

Well-rested athletes have faster reaction times, more energy, and greater endurance. Teams that build 8 to 10 hours of daily sleep into their training show improved performance.

As we age, we release less of this hormone and spend less time in deep sleep (Pekkanen, 1982).

Given all the benefits of sleep, it's no wonder that sleep loss hits us so hard.

Sleep Deprivation and Sleep Disorders

How does sleep loss affect us, and what are the major sleep disorders?

When our body yearns for sleep but does not get it, we begin to feel terrible. Trying to stay awake, we will eventually lose. In the tiredness battle, sleep always wins.

In 1989, Michael Doucette was named America's Safest Driving Teen. In 1990, while driving home from college, he fell asleep at the wheel and collided with an oncoming car, killing both himself and the other driver. Michael's driving instructor later acknowledged never having mentioned sleep deprivation and drowsy driving (Dement, 1999).

Effects of Sleep Loss

Today, more than ever, our sleep patterns leave us not only sleepy but drained of energy and feelings of well-being. After a succession of 5-hour nights, we accumulate a sleep debt that need not be entirely repaid but cannot be satisfied by one long sleep. "The brain keeps an accurate count of sleep debt for at least two weeks," reported sleep researcher William Dement (1999, p. 64).

Obviously, then, we need sleep. Sleep commands roughly one-third of our lives—some 25 years, on average. Allowed to sleep unhindered, most adults will sleep at least 9 hours a night (Coren, 1996). With that much sleep, we awake refreshed, sustain better moods, and perform more efficient and accurate work.

The U.S. Navy and the National Institutes of Health have demonstrated the benefits of unrestricted sleep in experiments in which volunteers spent 14 hours daily in bed for at least a week. For the first few days, the volunteers averaged 12 hours of sleep a day or more, apparently paying off a sleep debt that averaged 25 to 30 hours. That accomplished, they then settled back to 7.5 to 9 hours nightly and felt energized and happier (Dement, 1999).

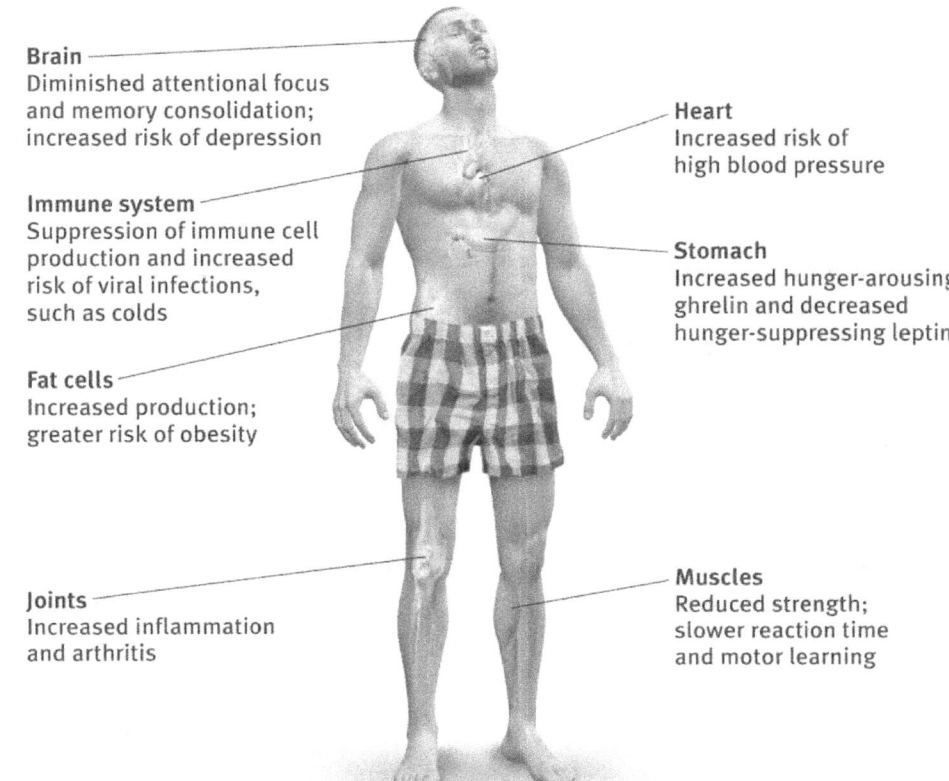

Brain
Diminished attentional focus and memory consolidation; increased risk of depression

Immune system
Suppression of immune cell production and increased risk of viral infections, such as colds

Fat cells
Increased production; greater risk of obesity

Joints
Increased inflammation and arthritis

Heart
Increased risk of high blood pressure

Stomach
Increased hunger-arousing ghrelin and decreased hunger-suppressing leptin

Muscles
Reduced strength; slower reaction time and motor learning

In one Gallup survey (Mason, 2005), 63 percent of adults who reported getting the sleep they needed also reported being "very satisfied" with their personal life (as did only 36 percent of those needing more sleep).

College and university students are especially sleep deprived; 69 percent in one national survey reported "feeling tired" or "having little energy" on several or more days in the last two weeks (AP, 2009). In another survey, 28 percent of high school students acknowledged falling asleep in class at least once a week (Sleep Foundation, 2006).

Sleep loss is a predictor of depression. Researchers who studied 15,500 young people, 12 to 18 years old, found that those who slept 5 or fewer hours a night had a 71 percent higher risk of depression than their peers who slept 8 hours or more (Gangwisch et al., 2010). This link does not appear to reflect sleep difficulties *caused* by depression.

When children and youth are followed through time, sleep loss predicts depression rather than vice versa (Gregory et al., 2009).

Moreover, REM sleep's processing of emotional experiences helps protect against depression (Walker & van der Helm, 2009). After a good night's sleep, we often do feel better the next day.

And that may help to explain why parentally enforced bedtimes predict less depression, and why pushing back school start time leads to improved adolescent sleep, alertness, and mood (Gregory et al., 2009; Owens et al., 2010).

Sleep-deprived students often function below their peak. And they know it: Four in five teens and three in five 18- to 29-year-olds wish they could get more sleep on week-days (Mason, 2003, 2005). Yet that teen who staggers glumly out of bed in response to an unwelcome alarm, yawns through morning classes, and feels half-depressed much of the day may be energized at 11:00 p.m. and mindless of the next day's looming sleepiness (Carskadon, 2002).

"Sleep deprivation has consequences—difficulty studying, diminished productivity, tendency to make mistakes, irritability, fatigue," noted Dement (1999, p. 231). A large sleep debt "makes you stupid."

"Remember to sleep because you have to sleep to remember." *James B. Maas and Rebecca S. Robbins*, Sleep for Success, *2010*

It can also make you gain weight. Sleep deprivation increases *ghrelin*, a hunger-arousing hormone, and decreases its hunger-suppressing partner, *leptin* (more on these in Chapter 10). It also increases *cortisol*, a stress hormone that stimulates the body to make fat. Sure enough, children and adults who sleep less than normal are fatter than those who sleep more (Chen et al., 2008; Knutson et al., 2007; Schoenborn & Adams, 2008). And experimental sleep deprivation of adults increases appetite and eating (Nixon et al., 2008; Patel et al., 2006; Spiegel et al., 2004; Van Cauter et al., 2007). This may help explain the common weight gain among sleep-deprived students (although a review of 11 studies reveals that the mythical "freshman 15" is, on average, closer to a "first-year 4" [Hull et al., 2007]).

Sleep affects our immune system. When infections set in, we typically sleep more, boosting our immune cells.

Sleep deprivation can suppress the immune cells that battle viral infections and cancer (Motivala & Irwin, 2007).

In one experiment, when researchers exposed volunteers to a cold virus, those who had been averaging less than 7 hours sleep a night were three times more likely to develop the cold than were those sleeping 8 or more hours a night (Cohen et al., 2009).

Sleep's protective effect may help explain why people who sleep 7 to 8 hours a night tend to outlive those who are chronically sleep deprived, and why older adults who have no difficulty falling or staying asleep tend to live longer than their sleep-deprived agemates (Dement, 1999; Dew et al., 2003).

Sleep deprivation slows reactions and increases errors on visual attention tasks similar to those involved in screening airport baggage, performing surgery, and reading X-rays (Lim & Dinges, 2010).

When sleepy frontal lobes confront an unexpected situation, misfortune often results. Consider the timing of the 1989 *Exxon Valdez* oil spill; Union Carbide's 1984 Bhopal, India, disaster; and the 1979 Three Mile Island and 1986 Chernobyl nuclear accidents: All occurred after midnight, when operators in charge were likely to be drowsiest and unresponsive to signals requiring an alert response.

Slow responses can also spell disaster for those operating equipment, piloting, or driving. Driver fatigue has contributed to an estimated 20 percent of American traffic accidents (Brody, 2002) and to some 30 percent of Australian highway deaths (Maas, 1999).

Stanley Coren capitalized on what is, for many North Americans, a semi-annual sleep-manipulation experiment—the "spring forward" to "daylight savings" time and "fall backward" to "standard" time. Searching millions of records, Coren found that in both Canada and the United States, accidents increased immediately after the time change that shortens sleep

There is good news! Psychologists have discovered a treatment that strengthens memory, increases concentration, boosts mood, moderates hunger and obesity, fortifies the disease-fighting immune system, and lessens the risk of fatal accidents.

Even better news: The treatment feels good, it can be self-administered, the supplies are limitless, and it's free! If you are a typical university-age student, often going to bed near 2:00 a.m. and dragged out of bed 6 hours later by the dreaded alarm, the treatment is simple: Each night just add an hour to your sleep.

- Exercise regularly but not in the late evening. (Late afternoon is best.)

- Avoid caffeine after early afternoon, and avoid food and drink near bedtime. The exception would be a glass of milk, which provides raw materials for the manufacture of serotonin, a neurotransmitter that facilitates sleep.

- Relax before bedtime, using dimmer light.

- Sleep on a regular schedule (rise at the same time even after a restless night) and avoid naps.

- Hide the clock face so you aren't tempted to check it repeatedly.

- Reassure yourself that temporary sleep loss causes no great harm.

- Realize that for any stressed organism, being vigilant is natural and adaptive. A personal conflict during the day often means a fitful sleep that night (Åkerstedt et al., 2007; Brissette & Cohen, 2002). Managing your stress levels will enable more restful sleeping. (See Chapter 11 for more on stress.)

- If all else fails, settle for less sleep, either going to bed later or getting up earlier

PAGE 219

Supreme Health & Fitness!   Health & Wellness Series Volume 1

*****

Conclusion

*****

Your lifestyle can affect how well your immune system can protect you from germs, viruses, and chronic illness. This in-turn determines the Quality of your Life as well as the amount of time you get to Enjoy it!

Replacing bad health habits with good ones can help keep your immune system healthy. This is how EASY it is to Start Creating Your Own Health and Wellness.

We are Created with the Natural ability to Heal Self … it is through the mis-handling of Ourselves that we lose that Natural Gift.

There are many external influences that contribute to this problem. Many of these are "emotional stress, physical stressors such as inadequate sleep or athletic overtraining, environmental and occupational chemical exposure, UV and other types of radiation, common viral or bacterial infections, certain drug therapies, blood transfusions and surgery."

The way we eat also has an impact on our immune responses. Nutrient deficiencies also cause problems within an immune system. Consuming excessive amounts of fat, alcohol or refined sugars also cause problems.

Another huge cause are certain diseases, such as AIDS. Others, due particularly to genetic abnormalities, also have an impact. In relation to the nutrient deficiency, your weak immune system could be your mother's fault. If she had low nutrients while pregnant with you, it could have transferred to you and given you a lowered immune system.

There are many possibilities that could cause such a thing.

PAGE 220

Supreme Health & Fitness!   Health & Wellness Series Volume 1

If you are suffering from a Deficient Immune system, there are ways to enhance your immune system, such as consuming vitamins and supplements, exercising regularly, and stress management. Drinking plenty of water and getting a good night's rest are also recommended.

This book and its purpose is to help You understand Your Immune System so that You can know how to STOP damaging Self and Increase Your Healing abilities. We Must Be Careful, though, because a weakened immune system can often lead to tumor growth and autoimmune diseases.

Summary

- Leaky gut = Leaky brain
- Inflamed gut = Inflamed brain
- Need healthy foods, but also nutritional supplements to really achieve sufficient good gut bacteria. Avoid inflammatory foods.
- Stress increases bad bacteria/decreases good gut bacteria.
- Probiotics change gut bacteria and treat GI disorders.
- Restore gut function and balance immune system to promote self-healing and wellness.
- Balanced immune system facilitates treatment of mental and emotional health issues.

The correction and means to regain our Healing Gift is In Our HANDS ... As soon as we Start the process ... Healing STARTS!!!!!

The following brief checklist covers the 3 main areas that create a Healthy environment within Self ... they are also one of (if not all) the 3 categories that we are failing in that causes the imbalance and prevents achievement of Homeostasis.

Check this list to see where you could use some improvement. Recognize it and Resolve it!!!

PAGE 221

Supreme Health & Fitness!   Health & Wellness Series Volume 1

1. You're short on sleep.

You may have noticed you're more likely to catch a cold or other infection when you're not getting enough sleep. Studies help bear out that well-rested people who received the flu vaccine developed stronger protection against the illness.

> ## Sleep Patterns Are Determined by the Immune System
>
> IL-1 induces Stage 4 sleep and stimulates the HPA axis.
> In health, IL-1 production is cyclic.
> It is stimulated by muramyl peptides derived from normal gut microflora.
> It is inhibited by glucocorticoids.

Sleep and the circadian system exert a strong regulatory influence on immune functions. Investigations of the normal sleep–wake cycle showed that immune parameters like numbers of undifferentiated naïve T cells and the production of pro-inflammatory cytokines exhibit peaks during early nocturnal sleep whereas circulating numbers of immune cells with immediate effector functions, like cytotoxic natural killer cells, as well as anti-inflammatory cytokine activity peak during daytime wakefulness.

Although it is difficult to entirely dissect the influence of sleep from that of the circadian rhythm, comparisons of the effects of nocturnal sleep with those of 24-h periods of wakefulness suggest that sleep facilitates the extravasation of T cells and their possible redistribution to lymph nodes. Not getting enough sleep can lead to higher levels of a stress hormone. It may also lead to more inflammation in your body.

Although researchers aren't exactly sure how sleep boosts the immune system, it's clear that getting enough - usually 7 to 9 hours for an adult - is key for good health.

"A lot of studies show our T-cells go down if we are sleep deprived," Balachandran says. "And inflammatory cytokines go up. ... This could potentially lead to the greater risk of developing a cold or flu."

Sleep loss not only plays a role in whether we come down with a cold or flu. It also influences how we fight illnesses once we come down with them.

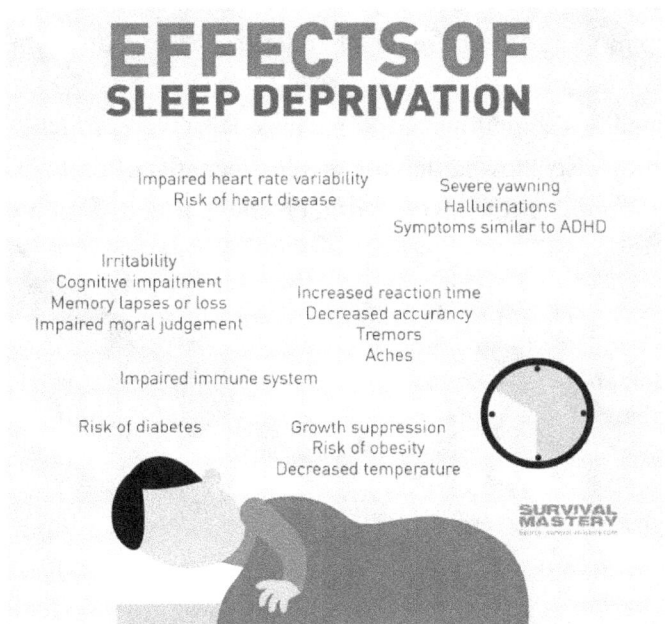

EFFECTS OF SLEEP DEPRIVATION

Impaired heart rate variability
Risk of heart disease

Severe yawning
Hallucinations
Symptoms similar to ADHD

Irritability
Cognitive impairment
Memory lapses or loss
Impaired moral judgement

Increased reaction time
Decreased accurancy
Tremors
Aches

Impaired immune system

Risk of diabetes

Growth suppression
Risk of obesity
Decreased temperature

SURVIVAL MASTERY

For example, our bodies fight infection with fevers. "One of the things that happens when we sleep is that we can get a better fever response," Balachandran says. "This is why fevers tend to rise at night. But if we are not sleeping, our fever reaction is not primed, so we may not be waging war on infection as best we can."

In simple terms, sleep deprivation suppresses immune system function. Or, as Balachandran puts it, "The more all-nighters you pull, the more likely you are to decrease your body's ability to respond to colds or bacterial infections."

2. You don't exercise.

Try to get regular, moderate exercise, like a daily 30-minute walk. It can help your immune system fight infection.

If you don't exercise regularly, you're more likely to get colds, for example, than someone who does. Exercise can also boost your body's feel-good chemicals and help you sleep better. Both of those are good for your immune system.

Exercise is a key factor to boosting your immune system naturally and increasing your overall health, but contrary to popular belief, you don't have to become a gym rat to reap the benefits. Research from the University of South Carolina and the University of Massachusetts shows that light to moderate exercise on a regular basis can reduce your risk of getting a cold by a third.

This includes something as simple as a daily walk, which is even easier to do if you have a dog. The study also showed that the greatest benefits of daily exercise were seen during the fall and winter months. So, grab the leash, or grab a friend, put on your running shoes and get moving!

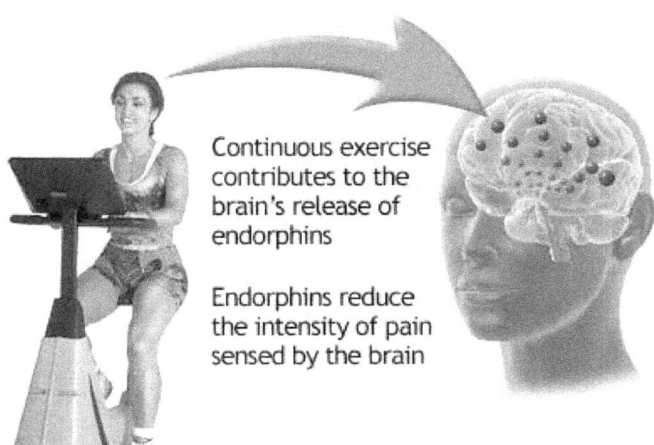

Continuous exercise
contributes to the
brain's release of
endorphins

Endorphins reduce
the intensity of pain
sensed by the brain

Regular Moderate Exercise Boosts Immunity

There are some things that seem to protect us from catching colds and the flu. One of those things appears to be moderate, consistent exercise. Research continues to support a link between moderate, regular exercise and a healthy immune system.

Early studies found that recreational exercisers reported fewer colds once they began running regularly. Moderate exercise has been linked to a positive immune system response and a temporary boost in the production of macrophages, the cells that attack bacteria.

It is believed that regular, consistent exercise can lead to substantial benefits in immune system health over the long-term.

More recent studies have shown that there are physiological changes in the immune system as a response to exercise. During moderate exercise, immune cells circulate through the body more quickly and are better able to kill bacteria and viruses. After exercise ends, the immune system generally returns to normal within a few hours, but consistent, regular exercise seems to make these changes a bit more long-lasting.

PAGE 224

Supreme Health & Fitness!   Health & Wellness Series Volume 1

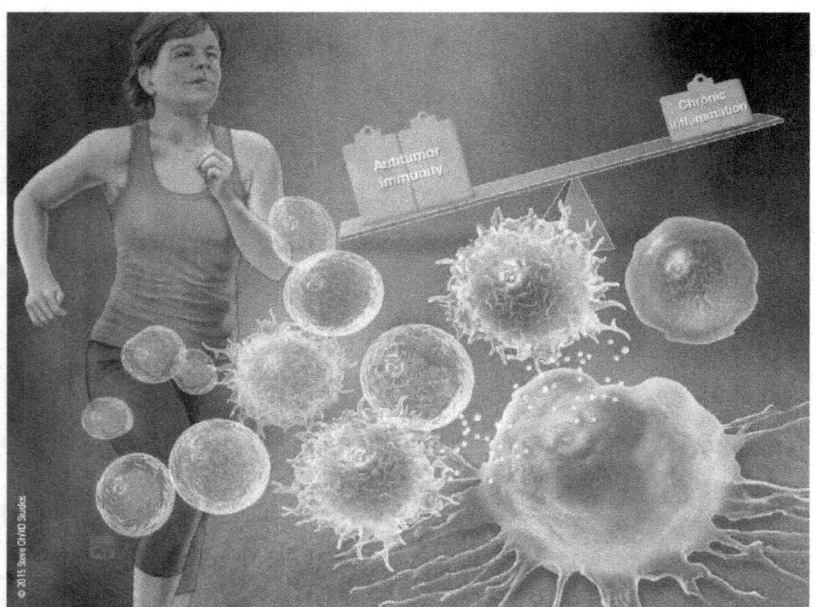

Figure 1. Schematic representation of the postulated role of exercise in shifting the inflammation-immune axis balance in cancer through (1) decreasing chronic inflammation and (2) increasing antitumor immunity, altering the initiation and progression of disease.

According to professor David Nieman, Dr. PH., of Appalachian State University, when moderate exercise is repeated on a near-daily basis there is a cumulative effect that leads to a long-term immune response.

His research showed that those who walk at 70-75 percent of their VO2 Max for 40 minutes per day had half as many sick days due to colds or sore throats as those who

Research is uncovering a link between moderate, regular exercise and a strong immune system.

However, there is also evidence that too much intense exercise can reduce immunity and may even make you sick.

The average adult has two to three upper respiratory infections each year. We are exposed to viruses all day long, but some people seem more susceptible to catching colds or the flu.

The following factors have all been associated with impaired immune function and increased risk of catching colds:

- Stress
- Poor nutrition
- Fatigue and lack of sleep
- Cigarette smoking
- Older age

Supreme Health & Fitness!　　　　　　Health & Wellness Series Volume 1

PAGE 225

Overtraining syndrome – Too Much Exercise Decreases Immunity

There is evidence that too much intense exercise can reduce immunity. Research is showing that more than 90 minutes of high-intensity endurance exercise can make athletes susceptible to illness for up to 72 hours after the exercise session. This is important information for those who compete in longer events such as marathons or triathlons.

Intense exercise seems to cause a temporary decrease in immune system function. Research has found that during intense physical exertion, the body produces certain hormones that temporarily lower immunity.

Cortisol and adrenaline, known as the stress hormones, raise blood pressure and cholesterol levels and suppress the immune system. This effect has been linked to the increased susceptibility to infection in endurance athletes after extreme exercise (such as marathon running or Ironman-distance triathlon training).

If you are training for ultra-endurance events, a key component of your training should be including enough rest and recovery days to allow your body (immune system) to recover. If you are feeling run-down or have other symptoms of overtraining syndrome—such as increased resting heart rate, slower recovery heart rate, irritability or general heaviness and fatigue—you may need to tone down your workouts as well.

If you are already ill, you should be careful about exercising too intensely. Your immune system is already taxed by fighting your infection, and additional stress could undermine your recovery.

In general, if you have mild cold symptoms and no fever, light or moderate exercise may help you feel a bit better and actually boost your immune system. Intense exercise will only make things worse and likely extend your illness.

If you're not exercising intensely but notice yourself sneezing or or battling a runny nose after your workout, your body might be reacting to pollen, allergies, or other environmental factors. Talk to your doctor to get to the root of the cause.

What affects your Immune System?

Stress - *physical and mental and emotional.*
Worries, not enough rest or sleep.

Environmental Stress - *toxins, chemicals,*
medication, radiation, pollution, smoking etc.

Poor Nutrition – *fast foods; overload of sugar &*
carbohydrates, chemicals flavourings &
additives.

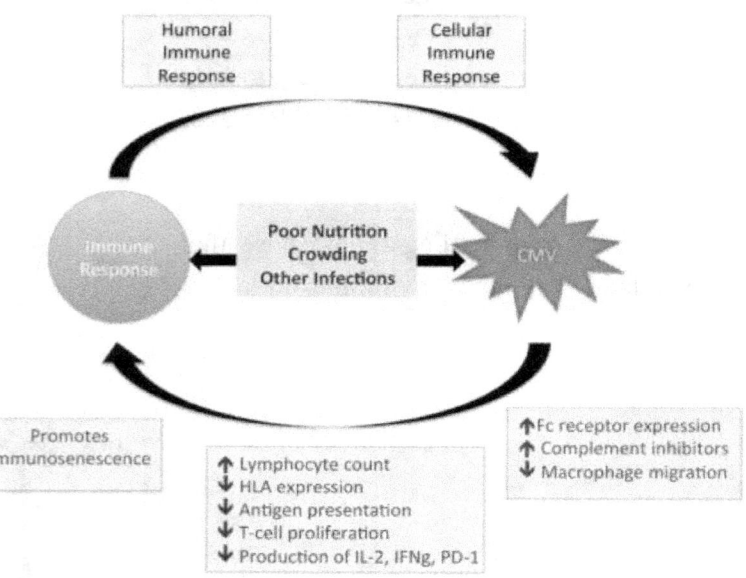

3. Poor dietary choices.

Eating or drinking too much sugar curbs immune system cells that attack bacteria. This effect lasts for at least a few hours after downing a couple of sugary drinks.

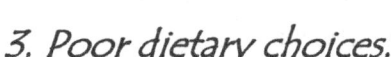

Many experts have argued that vitamin D may be one of the most important nutrients for a healthy immune system.

Thankfully, our bodies produce vitamin D naturally, but we need a little help from the sun for this to happen.

Perhaps this is why we tend to get sick more often in the Fall and Winter when we're not exposed to as much sun as in the Spring and Summer.

Studies have shown that taking a vitamin D supplement could help reduce your chances of getting the flu by as much as 40 per cent. As always, we recommend talking with your doctor before starting any supplement routine. You can even ask your doctor to check your vitamin levels to ensure your immune system is operating efficiently.

Many herbs and spices have great immune-boosting benefits, but Turmeric has been called one of the most powerful anti-inflammatory spices of all.

Eat more fruits and vegetables, which are rich in nutrients like vitamins C and E, plus beta-carotene and zinc. Go for a wide variety of brightly colored fruits and vegetables, including berries, citrus fruits, kiwi, apples, red grapes, kale, onions, spinach, sweet potatoes, and carrots.

Other foods particularly good for your immune system include fresh garlic, which may help fight viruses and bacteria.

Melaleuca oil, or more commonly known as Tea Tree Oil, comes from the leaves of the Melaleuca alternifolia tree and is produced throughout Australia. Tea tree oil is known to have strong antimicrobial properties, meaning it helps kill off harmful germs and bacteria.

A scientific study published in the journal Letters in Applied Microbiology, showed this essential oil to be an effective antiviral against the influenza virus. Tea tree oil is toxic if ingested but it can be used in small amounts as a natural hand sanitizer and some experts recommend carrying a small bottle with you and inhaling the aroma before entering a crowded space where germs are likely to be circulating.

Oregano Oil is an essential oil derived from the leaves and flowers of the oregano plant, that's right, the same herb you probably have in your pantry. Oregano oil has multiple superpowers in the fight against colds and flu as it's a powerful antimicrobial, antibacterial, antiviral, and antifungal.

It also cleanses your gut of harmful bacteria which helps keep you healthy and virus free. It can be taken orally to prevent parasites and infections. Mix with a carrier oil like coconut oil and place under your tongue. Hold it for a few minutes then rinse it out. It can also be used to fight colds and sinus infections by putting a few drops in hot water and inhaling the steam.

Like Turmeric and Garlic, Ginger is also a great natural immune booster.

PAGE 228

Supreme Health & Fitness!   Health & Wellness Series Volume 1

Ginger helps warm the body and break down the accumulation of toxins in your organs, especially the sinuses, lungs and lymphatic system. Keeping these vital organs free of toxins may help prevent against illness and infection.

Ginger is also a very powerful anti-inflammatory and promotes healthy sweating which can help fight the symptoms of cold and flu.

Our Immune System is the Gift from The CREATOR, that is the Solution to the Fountain of Youth and the Foundation for successful Enjoyment of Abundant LIFE!!!

It is designed to keep this Awesome vehicle called the Human Body, which is the God-Body, Alive to continue to House the Force and Power of God and for the Presence of God to manifest through.

When our Immunity compromised it opens the door for our Dis-Ease, Sickness and the lose of the ability to Heal Self.

If we don't know how to CLOSE this door and re-start our Healing process, then we will suffer our Pre-Mature DEATH!

You are not created to get Sick ….. You are not created to DIE!

It's all up to YOU!!!!

Take Charge of Your Healing, Health and Life … Eat To Live and Increase Your Physical Activities and You can create the environment IN Self that facilitates Your Healing, Improves Your Health, Increases Your Power – allowing You to Successfully Enjoy Your Abundant Life!

PEACE!

Sean Ali,

Supreme Health and Fitness by Sean Ali!

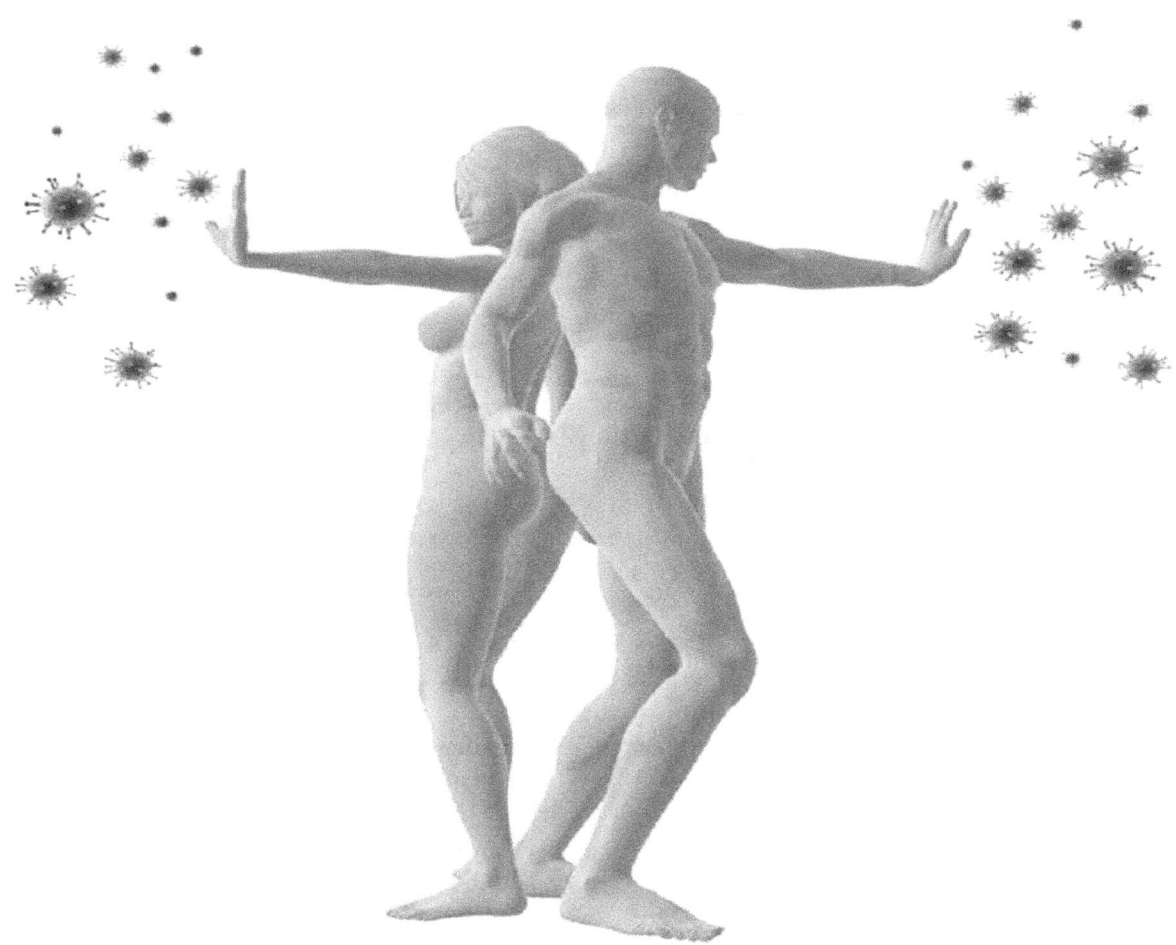

References

*****

- American Dietetic Association. Position of the American Dietetic Association: Nutrient supplementation. *J Am Diet Assoc 109*:2073–2085, 2009.

- Schroder, B.G., Griffin, I., Specker, B.L., and Abrams, S.A. Absorption of calcium from the carbonated dairy soft drink is greater than that from fat-free milk and calcium fortified orange juice in women. *Nutritional Research 25*:737–742, 2005.

- He, K. Fish, long-chain omega-3 polyunsaturated fatty acids and prevention of cardiovascular disease—Eat fish or take fish oil supplement? *Prog Cardiovasc Dis 52*:95–114, 2009.

- Antony, M.L., and Singh, S.V. Molecular mechanisms and targets of cancer chemoprevention by garlic-derived bioactive compound diallyl trisulfide. *Indian J Exp Biol 49*:805–816, 2011.

- Andres, S., Abraham, K., Appel, K.E., and Lampen, A. Risks and benefits of dietary isoflavones for cancer. *Crit Rev Toxicol 41*:463–506, 2011.

- Böhm, F., Edge, R., and Truscott, T.G. Interactions of dietary carotenoids with singlet oxygen (1O2) and free radicals: Potential effects for human health. *Acta Biochim Pol 59*:27–30, 2012.

- Nile, S.H., and Park, S.W. Edible berries: Review on bioactive components and their effect on human health. *Nutrition 30*:134–144, 2014.
- Toh, J.Y., Tan, V.M., Lim, P.C., et al. Flavonoids from fruit and vegetables: A focus on cardiovascular risk factors. *Curr Atheroscler Rep 15*:368, 2013.

- Nogueira Lde, P., Knibel, M.P., Torres, M.R., et al. Consumption of high-polyphenol dark chocolate improves endothelial function in individuals with stage 1 hypertension and excess body weight. *Int J Hypertens 2012*:147321, 2012.

- Khatua, T.N., Adela, R., and Banerjee, S.K. Garlic and cardioprotection: insights into the molecular mechanisms. *Can J Physiol Pharmacol 91*:448–458, 2013.

- Ma, L., Dou, H.L., Wu, Y.Q., et al. Lutein and zeaxanthin intake and the risk of age-related macular degeneration: a systematic review and meta-analysis. *Br J Nutr 107*:350–359, 2012.

- Eussen, S.R., de Jong, N., Rompelberg, C.J., et al. Dose-dependent cholesterol-lowering effects of phytosterol/phytostanol-enriched margarine in statin users and statin non-users under free-living conditions. *Public Health Nutr 14*:1823–1832, 2011.

- Alexiadou, K., and Katsilambros, N. Nuts: anti-atherogenic food? *Eur J Intern Med 22*:141–146, 2011.

- Calder, P.C. The role of marine omega-3 (n-3) fatty acids in inflammatory processes, atherosclerosis and plaque stability. *Mol Nutr Food Res 56*:1073–1080, 2012.

- Yuan, J.M., Sun, C., and Butler, L.M. Tea and cancer prevention: epidemiological studies. *Pharmacol Res 64*:123–135, 2011.

- Borneo, R., and León, A.E. Whole grain cereals: functional components and health benefits. *Food Funct 3*:110–119, 2012.

- Crowe, K.M., and Francis, C. Position of the Academy of Nutrition and Dietetics: Functional Foods. *J Acad Nutr Diet 113*:1096–1103, 2013.

- Ogden, C.L., Carroll, M.D., Kit, B.K., and Flagel, K.M. Prevalence of childhood and adult obesity in the United States, 2011–2012. *JAMA 311*:806–814, 2014.

- U.S. Department of Agriculture and U.S. Department of Health and Human Services. *Dietary Guidelines for Americans, 2010*, 7th Edition. Washington, DC: U.S. Government Printing Office, December, 2010.

- U.S. Burden of Disease Collaborators. The state of US health, 1990–2010: burden of diseases, injuries, and risk factors. *JAMA 310*:591–608, 2013.

- Murphy, S.L., Xu, J., and Kochanek, K.D. Deaths: Final data for 2010. *National Vital Statistics Reports* 61(4), May 2013. Available online at http://www.cdc.gov/nchs/data/nvsr/nvsr61/nvsr61_04.pdf. Accessed May 3, 2014.

- Kaput, J. Nutrigenomics—2006 update. *Clin Chem Lab Med 45*:279–287, 2007.

- Division of Nutrition and Physical Activity. *Research to practice series No. 2: Portion size*. Atlanta: Centers for Disease Control and Prevention, 2006. Available online at http://www.cdc.gov/nccdphp/dnpa/nutrition/pdf/portion_size_research.pdf. Accessed May 3, 2014.

- Institute of Medicine, Food and Nutrition Board. *Dietary Reference Intakes for Energy, Carbohydrate, Fiber, Fat, Protein and Amino Acids*. Washington, DC: National Academies Press, 2002.

- Berryman, D.E., and Hulver, M.W. Cellular and whole-animal energetics. In M.H. Stipanuk and M.A. Caudill (ed.), *Biochemical, Physiological, and Molecular Aspects of Human Nutrition*, 3rd ed. St. Louis: Saunders Elsevier, 2013, pp. 481–500.

- Dinas, P.C., Koutedakis, Y., and Flouris, A.D. Effects of exercise and physical activity on depression. *Ir J Med Sci 180*:319–325, 2011.

- Institute of Medicine, Food and Nutrition Board. *Dietary Reference Intakes for Energy, Carbohydrates, Fiber, Fat, Protein and Amino Acids*. Washington, DC: National Academies Press, 2002.

- Strasser, B. Physical activity in obesity and metabolic syndrome. *Ann N Y Acad Sci 1281*:141–159, 2013.

- Behm, D.G., and Chaouachi, A. A review of the acute effects of static and dynamic stretching on performance. *Eur J Appl Physiol 111*:2633–2651, 2011.

- Garber, C.E., Blissmer, B., Deschenes, M. R., et al.; American College of Sports Medicine. American College of Sports Medicine position stand: Quantity and quality of exercise for developing and maintaining cardiorespiratory, musculoskeletal, and neuromotor fitness in apparently healthy adults: Guidance for prescribing exercise. *Med Sci Sports Exerc 43*:1334–1359, 2011.

- Gallagher, D., Heymsfield, S., Heo, M., et al. Healthy percentage body fat ranges: An approach for developing guidelines based on body mass index. *Am J Clin Nutr 72*:694–701, 2000.

- U.S. Department of Agriculture and U.S. Department of Health and Human Services. *Dietary Guidelines for Americans, 2010*, 7th ed, Washington, DC: U.S. Government Printing Office, December 2010.

- U.S. Department of Health and Human Services. 2008 Physical Activity Guidelines for Americans. Available online at http://www.health.gov/paguidelines/guidelines/. Accessed August 31, 2014.

- National Center for Health Statistics. Health, United States, 2012: With Special Feature on Emergency Care. Hyattsville, MD, 2013.

- Haskell, W.L., Lee, I-M., Pate, R.R., et al. Physical activity and public health: Updated recommendations for adults from the American College of Sports Medicine and the American Heart Association. *Circulation 116*:1081–1093, 2007.

*****

Publications by Supreme Health & Fitness!

*****

Sean Ali

Understanding Carbohydrates: LIFE Energy, Fiber, Sugar and Starch! (Science Of LIFE Series)

ISBN-13: 978-1520559988, **ISBN-10:** 1520559984

#1 New Release in Fiber

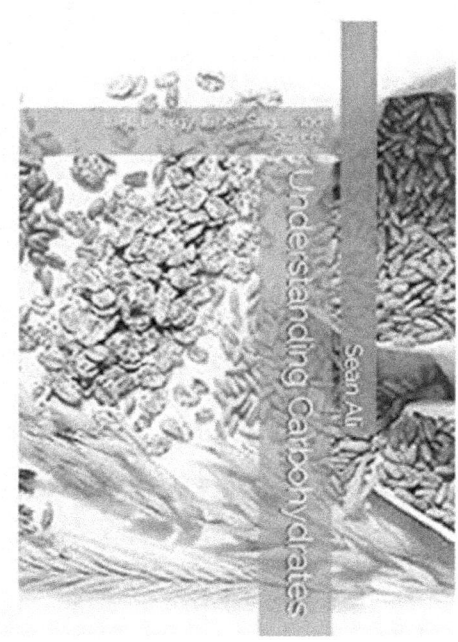

Project Summary
OxyGen!: The Breath Of LIFE In Atomic Form!
Authored by Sean Ali, Authored by Kareem Tyree, Authored by Gabriella Monique, Authored by Khlail Malik

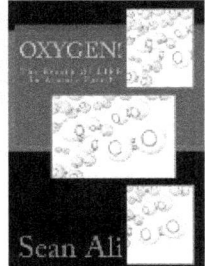

List Price: **$35.00**

7" x 10" (17.78 x 25.4 cm)
Full Color on White paper
182 pages

ISBN-13: **978-1548589561** (CreateSpace-Assigned)
ISBN-10: 154858956X
BISAC: Medical / Healing

Peace and Blessings of Health!

*Do YOU have health issues that YOU want to over-come?
*Do YOU want to Improve the Quality of YOUR Life?
*Do YOU want to achieve ABUNDANT LIFE?
*** THEN THIS BOOK IS FOR YOU!! ***

Oxygen IS the Breath Of LIFE in Atomic form!
This short work is a composition of Scientific, Medical and Spiritually based research , compiled into a comprehensive, easily read and understood format, designed to Help the reader achieve and maintain their own Supreme Health and Fitness!
We have 3 major functions - Eating, Drinking and Breathing, that must be performed in order for us to be considered Alive......... Of these 3 functions, Breathing is the least explored, taught or performed properly - BUT THE MOST IMPORTANT.
We can go 7-10 days without Food before signs of Nutritional deficiency. We can go 3-7 days without Water before we present symptoms .... But, 1 Minute of Oxygen deprivation/deficiency causes Cellular Damage!
Our Cells need 2 elements for Growth and Reproduction = OXYGEN & GLUCOSE !
Let's explore and discover the Amazing Power of Oxygen and the Natural Abilty to Heal Self!
OXYGEN IS THE BREATH OF LIFE IN ATOMIC FORM !
OPEN THIS BOOK - and take the steps to Successfully Build Your own Supreme Health & Fitness!
PEACE!

CreateSpace eStore: https://www.createspace.com/7316042

Project Summary

LIFE Energy!: *The Sun, Gluceose & WHY Humans Are Herbivores!
Authored by Sean Ali, Authored by Kareem Tyree, Authored by Gabriella Monique, Authored by Khalil Malik

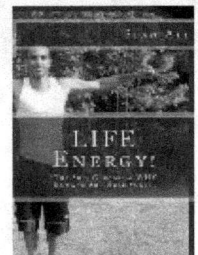

List Price: **$32.00**

7" x 10" (17.78 x 25.4 cm)
Full Color on White paper
166 pages

ISBN-13: 978-1548545017 (CreateSpace-Assigned)
ISBN-10: 1548545015
BISAC: Health & Fitness / Healthy Living

Peace and Blessings of Health!

*Do YOU have a health issue that YOU would like to over-come?

*Do YOU want to Improve the Quality of YOUR Life?

*Do YOU want to experience ABUNDANT LIFE?

*** OPEN THIS BOOK - NOW!!! ***

This small book is written with the purpose of re-examining the role of Nutrition in health care and everyday Life......LIFE IS
ENERGY.....Nutrition is a descriptive term to describe how we replenish our Life Energy.

Understanding Nutrition is the equivalent of understanding Energy and Knowledge of Nutrition enables us to make precise
Energy adjustments through Nutrients to provide the proper Energy needed for all our body functions/tasks – from
achieving Homeostasis, facilitating our Growth, Development and Self- Healing.

We come from the Earth and all our Solutions are manifested from the Earth...... All we have to do is return back to the
Earth and extract what we need.

Food is our naturally occurring vehicle, perfectly designed for administering the Life Energy in the form of Nutrition.

Our Food choices and the Energy released from it, presents as either the root cause of our dis-ease or the base for our
Solution.

From our Cells to our Immune system, we are Created to Heal and Regenerate Self with the aide of proper
Nutrition/Energy.

Our Food is our Medicine ONLY with proper application...... There is no in-between, which means that we are either eating
to die – OR – Eating To LIVE !!!!

Energy is the Key to LIFE and we Know that the Sun is the Source of all Energy, so if we focus on how to obtain as much
Sun in the form of food as possible = the Key to Nutritional Health and Therapy.

Let us explore and examine Life Energy and how to obtain the best Quality and Value so that we may successfully
manifest the Best out of Life and Enjoy a long, active and fruitful Life span!

Achieving and Maintaining Supreme Health and Fitness by increasing the level of Knowledge and Science of Life!

Peace
Sean Ali

CreateSpace eStore: https://www.createspace.com/7310862

PAGE 237

Supreme Health & Fitness! Health & Wellness Series Volume 1

Project Summary

Understanding Carb-O-Hydrates!: *Life Energy, Fiber, Glucose & Starch!

Authored by Sean Ali, Authored by Kareem Tyree, Authored by Gabriella Monique, Authored by Khalil Malik

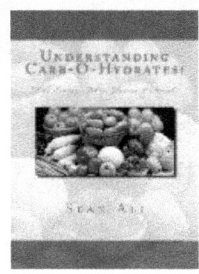

List Price: **$30.00**

7" x 10" (17.78 x 25.4 cm)
Full Color on White paper
158 pages

ISBN-13: **978-1548543143** (CreateSpace-Assigned)
ISBN-10: **1548543144**
BISAC: Health & Fitness / Healthy Living

Peace and Blessings of Health!

*Do YOU have health issues that YOU want to over-come?
*Do YOU want to Improve the Quality of YOUR Life?
*Do YOU want to experience ABUNDANT LIFE?

*** THEN THIS BOOK IS FOR YOU!! ***

There is a disproportionate amount of fad diets and food-like TOXIC items that are available and which we are bombarded with that promote a detrimentally 'low' or 'no' Carb meal plan that goes TOTALLY against ALL Nutritional science and evidence of the function of Carbohydrates.

There is little to no serious governmental regulation of these types of claims or food-like items and most are cases of clever advertisement vs actual claims of quality and value.

This small book has been produced to provide understanding of the Nutritional and Life value of Carbohydrates - from a Scientific analogy, while simultaneously shedding light on these false claims and food-like products so that YOU can make the Best Life choices for YOUR successful Growth & Development!

Let us explore and learn about our Primary Energy source and become able to make the best Nutritional choices.

OPEN THIS BOOK - and Begin the steps to Successfully Build and Maintain Your own Supreme Health and Fitness!

Peace !
Sean Ali

CreateSpace eStore: https://www.createspace.com/7310656

Project Summary

Enjoying Abundant LIFE!: Scientific Concepts to Successfully Build YOUR Supreme Health!
Authored by Sean Ali

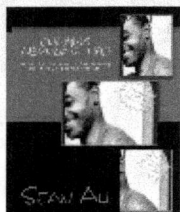

List Price: **$35.00**

8" x 10" (20.32 x 25.4 cm)
Full Color on White paper
170 pages

ISBN-13: **978-1546732075** (CreateSpace-Assigned)
ISBN-10: 1546732071
BISAC: Medical / Healing

Peace and Blessings of Health!

*Do YOU have a health issue that YOU would like to over-come?
*Do YOU want to improve the Quality of YOUR Life?
*Do YOU want to experience ABUNDANT LIFE?

*** OPEN THIS BOOK - NOW!!! ***

This small book is written with the purpose of re-examining the role of Nutrition in health care and everyday Life......LIFE IS ENERGY.....Nutrition is a descriptive term to describe how we replenish our Life Energy.
Understanding Nutrition is the equivalent of understanding Energy
Knowledge of Nutrition enables us to make precise Energy adjustments through Nutrients to provide the proper Energy needed for all our body functions/tasks – from achieving Homeostasis, facilitating our Growth, Development and Self-Healing.
We come from the Earth and all our Solutions are manifested from the Earth...... All we have to do is return back to the Earth and extract what we need.
Food is our naturally occurring vehicle, perfectly designed for administering the Life Energy in the form of Nutrition.
Our Food choices and the Energy released from it, presents as either the root cause of our dis-ease or the base for our Solution.
From our Cells to our Immune system, we are Created to Heal and Regenerate Self with the aide of proper Nutrition/Energy.
Our Food is our Medicine ONLY with proper application...... There is no in-between, which means that we are either eating to die – OR – Eating To LIVE !!!!
Energy is the Key to LIFE and we Know that the Sun is the Source of all Energy, so if we focus on how to obtain as much Sun in the form of food as possible = the Key to Nutritional Health and Therapy.
Let us explore and examine Life Energy and how to obtain the best Quality and Value so that we may successfully manifest the Best out of Life and Enjoy a long, active and fruitful Life-span!

Achieving and Maintaining Supreme Health and Fitness by increasing the level of Knowledge and Science of Life!

Peace
Sean Ali

CreateSpace eStore: https://www.createspace.com/7174743

PAGE 239

Supreme Health & Fitness!   Health & Wellness Series Volume 1

Project Summary

Understanding Our Human Energy!: Energy Cycle & Transformation to Achieve Abundant LIFE!
Authored by Sean Ali

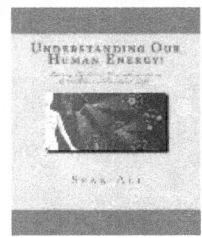

List Price: **$45.00**

8" x 10" (20.32 x 25.4 cm)
Full Color on White paper
224 pages

ISBN-13: 978-1546343462 (CreateSpace-Assigned)
ISBN-10: 1546343466
BISAC: Medical / Alternative Medicine

Peace and Blessings of Life!

•Do YOU Have health ailments/issues that YOU would like to over-come??
•Do YOU want to Improve the Quality of YOUR Life??
•Do YOU want to Experience and Enjoy ABUNDANT LIFE??
** Then this book is for YOU!

This small book is written so that we can explore and gain an Understanding of what our Human Energy System is, with a particular focus on What our Energy is, the Best sources and What to avoid to successfully Grow and LIVE so that we can Enjoy to the fullest, our GOD-Given potential of a Long and Abundant LIFE !!!!!!!
Understanding our Human Energy is synonymous with Understanding our LIFE...it's what keeps us Alive and the main difference between Us and a body in the grave - Human Energy !!!!
Human Energy is manifested in the form of FOOD....Growing Our Own Food is the ONLY way that ensures we recieve the Highest Quality Life Energy - Straight from the Source!

OPEN THIS BOOK and Begin the neccessary steps to Improve the Quality of YOUR LIFE!

Building and Maintaining Supreme Health & Fitness by increasing the level of Knowledge and Science of Life!

Peace!
Sean Ali, BS Health & Wellness

CreateSpace eStore: https://www.createspace.com/7126564

PAGE 240

Supreme Health & Fitness!   Health & Wellness Series Volume 1

Project Summary
The Manual Of Healing Herbal Elements!: *Earth-based Solutions for Healing, Health & Life!
Authored by Sean Ali, Authored by Kareem Tyree, Authored by Gabriella Monique, Authored by Khalil Malik

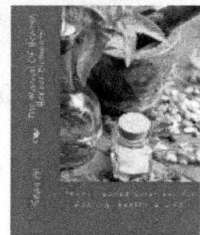

List Price: **$65.00**

8" x 10" (20.32 x 25.4 cm)
Full Color on White paper
336 pages

ISBN-13: **978-1547137985** (CreateSpace-Assigned)
ISBN-10: 1547137983
BISAC: Medical / Holistic Medicine

Peace and Blessings of Health!
This small work is being presented as a Manual of Healing, Health and Life. A comprehensive and scientific Handbook of Analysis and Research on over 80 Clinically & Commonly accessible Life & Healing Energy Herbal Elements. Each Herbal Element is categorized to include the latest research on the Uses, Actions, Dosages, Client Considerations, Contraindications & Interactions.
As many of Us are witnessing the RISE in Life-threatening dis-eases, especially in childhood Obesity and Diabetes, we are looking for more Natural ways to Heal.
This Manual Of Healing is a Professional Grade handbook to Help YOU choose and use the BEST Naturally occurring Life Elements to Successfully Heal YourSelf!
We come from the Earth and ALL our Solutions come from the Earth!

PEACE!
Sean Ali

CreateSpace eStore: https://www.createspace.com/7225520

PAGE 241

Supreme Health & Fitness!   Health & Wellness Series Volume 1

Project Summary

Understanding & Creating Herbal Healing!: Teas, Decoctions & Tinctures!
Authored by Sean Ali, Authored by Khalil Malik, Authored by Kareem Tyree, Authored by Gabriella Monique

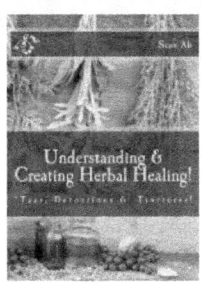

List Price: **$22.00**

7" x 10" (17.78 x 25.4 cm)
Full Color on White paper
108 pages

ISBN-13: **978-1548105457** (CreateSpace-Assigned)
ISBN-10: **1548105457**
BISAC: **Medical / Healing**

Peace and Blessings of Health!

This small work represents Volume 2 of my Science Of Healing Series and is being presented as a Handbook of Healing through the vehicles of Teas, Decoctions and Tinctures.

This is a comprehensive and scientific Handbook of Analysis and Research on over 30 Clinically used & easily accessible Life & Healing Energy Herbal Elements.

This Handbook Of Healing is Professional Grade and designed specifically to Help YOU choose and use the BEST Naturally occurring Life Elements to Successfully Heal YourSelf!
We come from the Earth and ALL our Solutions come from the Earth!

PEACE!
Sean Ali

CreateSpace eStore: https://www.createspace.com/7257513

PAGE 242

Supreme Health & Fitness!   Health & Wellness Series Volume 1

Supreme Health & Fitness by Sean Ali!

Achieving and Maintaining Supreme Health by increasing the level of Knowledge and Science of Life!